MIND AND MEDICINE

Pittsburgh Series in Philosophy and History of Science

Series Editors:

Adolf Grünbaum
Larry Laudan
Nicholas Rescher

MIND AND MEDICINE

Problems of Explanation and Evaluation in Psychiatry and the Biomedical Sciences

Larry Laudan, Editor

UNIVERSITY OF CALIFORNIA PRESS
Berkeley   Los Angeles   London

University of California Press
Berkeley and Los Angeles, California

University of California Press, Ltd.
London, England

Copyright © 1983 by The Regents of the University of California

Library of Congress Cataloging in Publication Data
Main entry under title:

Mind and medicine.

    (Pittsburgh series in philosophy and history
of science ; v. 8)
    Includes index.
    1. Psychoanalysis—Philosophy.   2. Psychiatry—
Philosophy.   3. Medicine—Philosophy.   4. Knowledge,
Theory of.   5. Causation.   I. Laudan, Larry.   II. Series.
[DNLM: 1. Concept formation.   2. Philosophy, Medical.
3. Logic.   W 61 M633]
RC506.M53   150.19'5   82-40094
ISBN 0-520-04623-4   AACR2

Printed in the United States of America

1 2 3 4 5 6 7 8 9

Contents

Preface

Since 1962, the Center for Philosophy of Science at the University of Pittsburgh has been issuing volumes devoted to an exploration of the conceptual foundations of science. Volumes one through seven were issued under the title of "Pittsburgh Series in the Philosophy of Science." In 1980, as the publication of the series was moved to the University of California Press, the title was changed to "Pittsburgh Series in Philosophy and History of Science." The present volume is the eighth in the series published under the Center's auspices.

Adolf Grünbaum
Larry Laudan
Nicholas Rescher,
Series Editors

Editor's Introduction

Ever since Aristotle, the problem of explanation, especially scientific explanation, has loomed large among the puzzles of philosophy. Linked as it is to such issues as understanding, coherence, causation, and intelligibility, the problem of explanation brings us face to face with the central question of epistemology: what is the relationship between our theoretical knowledge and that externality which is its object? During the 1940s and 1950s, several discussions of the nature of scientific explanation appeared that have since become minor classics. Particularly noteworthy were the studies by Hempel, Popper, and Nagel. In each case, these authors took certain fairly simple patterns of inference in the natural sciences as archetypes around which to construct models of explanation that purported to be perfectly general in scope. Very quickly, these "covering-law" or "deductive-nomological" models became the benchmark against which all putative explanations were to be judged. The logical, epistemic, and pragmatic features of these models came to be widely acknowledged, at least within the tradition of analytic philosophy, as capturing something essential about explanation.

But for all the progress and clarification these models represented, two central issues have remained unresolved: (1) how is one to characterize that crucial species of explanation called "causal explanation"? and (2) how far can the covering-law model go toward capturing the structure of explanation in the highly complex sciences of human

1

behavior? On the first point, it was clear from the outset that the covering-law model did not "capture" the causal relationship. All sorts of interrelationships satisfy the covering-law model without being causal. Thus, one can use Boyle's law to predict that certain changes in the volume of a gas will be accompanied by certain changes in its pressure. One can even cast this reasoning into the form of a covering-law explanation. But few would say that we had thereby identified the causes of gaseous behavior. Contrariwise, there *seem* to be many cases where we give a causal account of some process without citing or presupposing any nomic regularities of the kind required by the covering-law model. Minimally, it has become clear that in order to characterize the structure of *causal* explanations, further refinements are called for in the received model. More radically, it has been suggested that the modeling of causal explanations requires a wholesale repudiation of the covering-law account.

Concurrent with these criticisms was a growing set of concerns about the capacity of prevalent models of explanation to do justice to patterns of explanation in the sciences of man. Efforts to apply the covering-law model to cases of teleological explanation, motivational explanation, rational explanation, intentional explanation, and functional explanation met with decidedly mixed success. A plethora of rival models emerged in the 1960s and 1970s, each designed to bring philosophical accounts of explanation into closer correspondence with existing scientific practice. This was particularly true for history and biology.

But many of the sciences of man remained largely outside this framework, especially medicine and psychiatry. It was simply unclear whether those scientific disciplines utilized patterns of explanation unique to themselves or whether their modes of inference and explanation could be assimilated to existing philosophical models. This concern was more than purely academic. After all, one of the best-known proponents of the covering-law model, Karl Popper, has singled out psychoanalysis as a pseudoscientific discipline that offers only bogus explanations. On the medical side, it seemed that many forms of explanation and diagnosis were counterinstances to the received view of explanation (recall Scriven's discussion of the syphilis-paresis case).

Even with the explosion of rivals to the covering-law picture in the 1970s, the explanatory structure of medicine and psychiatry remained largely unstudied and unanalyzed. Particularly untouched was the notion of causal explanation in these disciplines. Can unconscious motives causally explain human actions? Is there a clear distinction between the symptoms and the causes of a disease? Are there laws of human behavior, and do they play the same role in explanation as physical laws do?

These specific questions, urgent and timely as they are, harken back to an older and larger question to which several of the essays in this volume are indirectly addressed. Concurrent with the rise of classical positivism and its commitment to a univocal sense of "explanation" for all the sciences, one can trace a dissenting and rival view. Associated chiefly with Dilthey and Rickert in the nineteenth century and with hermeneutics in our own, this point of view insisted that human actions were susceptible to a distinctive kind of understanding, and hence a distinctive form of explanation. It was suggested that being humans ourselves (rather than, say, octopi or falling stones), we are suited—when dealing specifically with human behavior—to go beneath the descriptive externalities that characterize our efforts to explain nonhuman objects and processes. We can, it was said, "get inside another man's head," "rethink his thoughts" (Collingwood), intuitively "empathize" or "identify" with his situation, thus coming to see it from the "inside." More generally, it was argued that we have a form of "privileged access" to the mental life of our fellow human beings, and this makes possible a form of explanation in the sciences of man that is quite different from other forms of explanation. Numerous subtle variations of this theme have been a commonplace in the literature of psychoanalysis, and the appraisal of this position is one of the central concerns in the essays by Morris Eagle and Michael Moore.

Questions arise not only about the logical form or structure of explanations in the human sciences but also about their evidential status. As we have already noted, models of explanation address themselves simultaneously to the logical form of an explanation and also to the epistemic status of its premises. An explanation, many want to say, is an explanation only if its premises have successfully survived exacting tests. Without well-tested theories, it is said, the task of explanation cannot even begin. But what makes for "well-testedness"? It may be reasonably clear how to test *macroscopic* hypotheses such as Boyle's law or the law of gravitation, but how do we test much more complex theories, particularly if they involve unobservable entities? At an even more complex level, how do we test etiological and therapeutic theories in psychiatry and medicine, where subjective judgments of therapeutic efficacy seem open to all manner of distortions? Adolf Grünbaum explores a variety of claims about the widely touted methods for testing the psychodynamics of Freudian theory and shows them to be, at best, highly problematic. Even if one leaves aside the intricate complexities presented by psychiatry, it is clear that the assessment of causal hypotheses, particularly if they are probabilistic in character, poses challenges more demanding than standard discussions of the logic of theory testing generally acknowledge. Some of these challenges are directly addressed by Kenneth Schaffner in his discussion of causal explanation in medicine.

These three themes—explanation, causation, and evaluation—form the central foci of the essays in this volume. More specifically, all the essays, except that by Joseph Margolis, address these issues within the context of psychoanalytic and biomedical concerns. It is our hope that this volume will demonstrate by example how much can be learned from the conceptual analysis of explanation and validation in sciences frequently ignored by philosophers.

The Nature of Psychoanalytic Explanation

Michael S. Moore*

INTRODUCTION

It has become something of an orthodoxy in the "philosophy of psychoanalysis" of the past three decades to assert that typical psychoanalytic explanations are motivational in character.[1] This is sometimes put by saying that psychoanalytic explanations give *reasons* for *actions*, rather than *causes* of mechanical *movements* or processes; that the specific explanations of particular actions in terms of their motives are fruitful, but that the broader, theoretical overviews attempted in psychoanalysis are useless; that such typical explanations are framed in terms of ordinary, mentalistic language rather than in the technical

*This article was initially presented as part of the Eighteenth Annual Philosophy of Science Lecture Series at the Center for the Philosophy and the History of Science, University of Pittsburgh, March 1978, and later at a seminar in philosophy and psychoanalysis, philosophy department, University of California, Los Angeles. My thanks go to the participants at these discussions for their many helpful comments, to Robert Audi, Michael Green, and Adolf Grünbaum for their detailed commentaries, and to Dan Dennett, Alan Garfinkel, Herbert Morris, Stephen Morse, and Alan Stone, with whom I have discussed these topics for years and from whom I have learned much. My thanks also go to my research assistant, [now Professor] Carol Tsuchida, for her painstaking work on the references for the final draft.

5

language of a theoretical science; or, that psychoanalytic explanations deal with phenomena that themselves have meaning, as opposed to the colorless phenomena with which natural science deals.

Although my title might suggest it, it is not my purpose to defend or attack this thesis (not frontally, at least, although I do believe this article has some bearing on it). Rather, I wish to examine the purportedly motivational explanations offered by psychoanalytic theory and to ask, first, whether such explanations *could* make good sense since the motives are said to be unconscious, and second, whether such typical psychoanalytic explanations in fact square with the prima facie sense of the phrase 'unconscious motive'. My conclusions, simply put, are that the idea of there being unconscious motives for our actions makes perfectly good sense, but that psychoanalysts rarely make use of motivational language in that sense. As often as not, a deceptively uniform motivational language masks a variety of different kinds of explanations.

I have not attempted a comprehensive survey of motivational language in all of psychoanalysis. Sufficient to demonstrate my theses, I think, is the set of explanations given in one aspect of the discipline, the theory of dreams. The psychoanalytic theory of dreams is an apt example for a number of reasons. To begin with, it is sufficiently rich in different levels of purportedly motivational explanations to illustrate the variety of types of explanations being offered. Because of this richness, it is sometimes pointed to as the best example of motivational explanation in psychoanalysis. Also, it is one of the most accessible bodies of theory in psychoanalysis, because of its comparative lack of revision after Freud's original theorizing.[2] Thus, one may, with some appropriateness, focus on *Freud's* theory of dreams and ignore more recent developments (which I, in any event, intend to do). Finally, the psychoanalytic theory of dreams may have some intrinsic interest of its own. It is, for example, sometimes well regarded even by critics otherwise quite hostile to psychoanalysis generally.[3] Freud wrote of his own dream theory that "insight such as this falls to one's lot but once in a lifetime."[4] The editors of a recent edition of *Daedalus* apparently agreed, including *The Interpretation of Dreams* as one of the classics of the twentieth century.[5] Hence, this often well-regarded and, in any event, historically important example of scientific theorizing in the raw may *ceteris paribus* be preferred to other examples of motivational explanation in psychoanalysis.

I shall proceed by sketching briefly an overview of the psychoanalytic theory of dreams. I shall then analyze the sense of the notion of unconscious motive and compare that sense with other types of explanations. Finally, I shall conclude with an interpretation of the theory of dreams that construes its purportedly motivational explanations as more aptly framed in the language of functions and mental causes.

A SKETCH OF THE PSYCHOANALYTIC THEORY OF DREAMS

Freud's explanation of dreams presents one of the most strikingly complex explanations in terms of 'motive' and its related terms that one may find in psychoanalysis. The levels of *meanings*, the degree to which motives are given for everything in the content, form, or process of formation of dreams, is matched only by his explanation of neurotic symptoms in the most complex of case histories.

This is to some extent a result of the task Freud set for himself in explaining dreams: he stated that he was going to *interpret* dreams, to find their meaning,[6] the task of the ancient soothsayers. His search was, from the start, for the meaning of dreams, and it should be no surprise that the explanations he found are couched in the language of meaning, i.e., in terms of motives, wishes, intentions, and the like.

Freud accused those who dismiss dreams as having no meaning, or who explain dreams solely by reference to physiological or external causes, as abandoning strict, scientific determinism.[7] With such explanations, he thought, one could not explain the content of dreams (why a hen rather than a rabbit, for example).[8] Freud here confused determinism in the sense of "every event has a cause" with his rather animistic version: "every (mental) event has a meaning." There is nothing unscientific about assuming that dreams are perfectly meaningless and yet are strictly determined by (as yet unknown) causes.[9]

In any event, for good reasons or ill, Freud was committed to finding meanings for dreams. It is not a task unsuggested by the phenomena, inasmuch as dreams do seem to be expressed in some kind of hidden language. What is surprising is the extent to which all aspects of dream phenomena are found to have meaning by Freud.

The rockbed of Freud's dream interpretations, as everywhere in psychoanalysis, rested on the technique of free association. Freud interpreted each element of the dream as described by the patient, and constructed the meaning of the dream from those associations and the elements of the remembered dream. Thus the Freudian attempt to explain dreams rests at least initially on the consciousness of the individual whose behavior (dreaming) is to be explained.

Basic to Freud's explanation of dreams is his distinction between the manifest content of a dream and the latent dream thoughts. The manifest content was defined as what the dreamer could remember of a dream and relate to others: "whatever the dreamer tells us must count as his dream."[10] In fact, Freud paid very close attention to the precise wording, hesitations, and order of presentation of his patients' remembrances. He recognized that the dreamer's memory of dreams, as of anything else, could be faulty, and that remembering the dream at different times could produce different descriptions of it. Freud acknowledged that, since there is no independent check on the patient's memory of what he dreamt, any and all such descriptions should be treated with equal respect and called the manifest content of the dream. The dream as variously described was explicable by reference to the same set of latent dream thoughts, but how the dream was related at different times was itself the subject of motivational analysis. For example, where descriptions of the same dream given at different times differed, Freud believed he had a clue to the sensitive area of the dream. Similarly, for the forgetting of parts of a dream: what we forget, we have a reason for forgetting.[11]

Since dreams as remembered simply do not fit explicitly the pattern of meaning (wish fulfillments) Freud believed they had, or any single pattern for that matter, he felt compelled to invent the notion of the latent dream thoughts. Only by reference to thoughts other than those that we could remember did Freud believe he could justify his discovery of the meaning of dreams without appearing to be obviously wrong.

The latent dream thoughts are "entirely rational" and "have their place among thought processes that have not become conscious— processes from which, after some modification, our conscious thoughts, too, arise."[12] They are not to be conceived of as the forgotten thoughts occurring during a dream—whether remembered or not, those thoughts are all part of the manifest content. If I read Freud correctly, all of the thoughts or images occurring during dreaming that are potentially the subject of recall are the manifest content of the dream. What that leaves one wondering is what is left over to be referred to as *latent* dream thoughts, for Freud's distinction between manifest and latent places all recallable contents in the 'manifest' basket, and there doesn't seem to be anything left to put in the one labeled 'latent'.

One possibility that recurs in Freud's writing is to regard the latent dream thoughts as a set of processes or states that *cause* the manifest dream thoughts to occur. This raises a very general problem about the status of such processes or states that I will discuss later in connection with the dream work. Briefly: to escape the charge of Molière — defining the cause of the manifest dream as "the dream-causing state" — Freud would have to give some independent definition of the latent dream thoughts and of the processes of the dream work that distort them. Since we still know little of the brain physiology involved, "latent dream thoughts" might be regarded as the name of those functional states (whose physical structure is unknown) that must exist if dreams indeed have the form Freud said they have, *viz.*, wish-fulfillments.

An alternative (but equally problematical) possibility is to relate the latent dream thoughts to the manifest content of dreams in some logical way, rather than in a causal way. That is, one might regard the latent dream "thoughts" not as experiential or physiological carriers of the meaning of the dream (and certainly not as Ryle's ghostly nonphysiological carriers) but as that meaning itself. Freud on occasion made this equation himself.[13] So conceived, the latent dream "thoughts" then become whatever we can infer of the meaning of the dream from its manifest content and from the trains of association produced in psychoanalysis. Assigning them this logical status does not commit one to assuming that there exist processes known as latent dream thoughts measurable in ways independent of the meanings to be inferred in dreams. On the other hand, as we shall see, such a "hermeneutic" interpretation of what the latent dream thoughts are, is in danger of trivializing completely Freud's theory of dreams. I shall put aside for now this ambiguity in the status of the latent dream thoughts, since it is resolvable only by considerations raised later in this article.

The overall hypothesis in Freud's explanation of dreams is that dreaming is a means of staying asleep. The problems we have during the night in remaining asleep are, for Freud, the result of the activities of three potential sleep disturbers: (1) the accidental stimuli occurring during the night, such as a fallen bedcover or a bout of indigestion; (2) continued thoughts from the perceptions or activities of the preceding day; and (3) a repressed, unconscious wish from childhood seeking expression during the night. The latter item is the crucial one in Freud's explanation. Such wishes arise during the night because our normal censorship of them is weakened during sleep, presumably in line with the lessened mental activity generally characteristic of the sleeping state.

In any event, in whatever way they arise, such wishful impulses would awaken us if they were directly expressed in thought, since, being repressed, they are "unthinkable" for the subject. Hence, such wishes are potential disturbers of sleep. The problem for the subject who wishes to remain asleep is how to defuse them. Our normal form of dealing with such wishes—some form of behavior indirectly expressing the wish—is not available because we are asleep. The only other alternative is fantasy. Hence, the content of the dream represents the repressed wish as satisfied. Freud hypothesized that fantasy relieves the cravings (unconscious wishes) that give rise to it to some extent, a fact somewhat supported perhaps by the phenomenology of daydreams.

Since the unconscious wish is repressed, on Freud's account it cannot even be given expression in a dream that fantasizes its fulfillment. Thus, what we dream (the manifest content) is distorted from what, in one sense, we would really like to dream (the latent dream thoughts), namely, that our repressed wish is fulfilled. The processes of the dream work are introduced by Freud as mechanisms by which the dreamer gets the best of both worlds: he is allowed to remain asleep by the fantasized fulfillment of his otherwise disturbing wish, and yet he does not pay the usual cost of recognizing such a wish, because it is so distorted in its fantasized fulfillment that he cannot perceive (except in psychoanalysis) the actual meaning of his dream.

The use of motivational language in this explanation of dreams may be grouped into three levels: (1) Freud explains dreaming as such (as opposed to the particular content of a given dream) as being the result of the overriding wish to sleep; (2) Freud explains the particular (manifest) content of a dream as being motivated by the fulfillment of a repressed wish; and (3) Freud further explains certain peculiar aspects of the content of the dream by reference to the processes of the dream work, themselves explicable by reference to motives the dreamer had for distorting his dream. These three levels of explanation together constitute the heart of Freud's theory of dreams.[14] Each of them, it is worth emphasizing, is couched in terms of motives or related terms. Just what the actual meaning of such purportedly motivational terms is in each of these three contexts is the topic of this article.

A TYPOLOGY OF EXPLANATIONS: MOTIVE AND ITS COUSINS

One of the reasons for the lack of influence of the philosophy of psychoanalysis on the discipline itself is the failure in the philosophical literature to make explicit the distinctions being relied on. One of the most typical offending approaches is to rely on some version of the distinction between motivational and causal explanations, without it ever being made clear what the differences are supposed to be. I shall accordingly set forth, with no particular claims to originality, what I mean by motivational explanation, and then contrast that form of explanation (whether the motives are conscious or unconscious) with causal and functional explanations. Only then will I return to the dream theory sketched earlier to review its purportedly motivational accounts.

THE PRIMA FACIE SENSE OF PSYCHOANALYTIC MOTIVE EXPLANATIONS

THE BASIC PATTERN OF EXPLANATION IN TERMS OF MOTIVES

There are a host of things one may say in response to the question of *why* one performed a certain action. One may have opened a window, for example, "because one was too hot"; or "in order to chill the wine"; or "because one believed that the Englishmen present preferred the room cooler," etc. All such explanations fit a relatively straightforward pattern of explanation modeled on what Aristotle called "practical syllogisms."[15] Although in ordinary speech we often cite only one of the premises (and sometimes give only an elliptical expression of one premise), the full explanation requires two premises: the major premise, specifying the agent's desire (goals, objectives, moral beliefs, purposes, aims, wants, etc.); and the minor premise, specifying the agent's factual beliefs about the situation he is in and his ability to achieve through some particular action the object of his desires. The conclusion of the syllogism was, for Aristotle, the action itself.

Thus, if X opens the window in order to chill the wine (alternatively "because he believes the wine is warm," or "because he wants to chill the wine"), we will have explained his action by citing explicitly or implicitly (1) his desire that the wine be chilled, and (2) his belief that opening the window will chill the wine. Knowing this desire and belief set of X, we can understand his action in the fundamental way in which we understand all human action, in terms of the agent's reasons or motives for acting.

There are two quite distinct components to the understanding generated by this mode of explanation, which has given rise to much confusion in contemporary philosophy. Reasons for action both *rationalize* an action and *causally* explain it.[16]

Taking these aspects in order: a belief/desire set rationalizes an action in the sense that it exhibits the action as the rational thing to do, given the agent's beliefs and given his desires. We understand the action in this sense because we can understand that a rational agent would so act—that *we*, had we a similar belief/desire set, would so act. We can see the action as a means to something the agent wants. As long as the object of the agent's desire is intelligible to us as something a person in our culture could reasonably want, and so long as the factual beliefs are not themselves irrational, we can empathize with the action even if we disagree with it morally or aesthetically; empathize, because knowing the belief/desire set we perceive the activity to be the rational thing to do for an agent with such desires and beliefs.

This aspect of reasons for acting, or motives, is sometimes expressed by saying that there is a logical connection between the sentences describing the belief/desire set and that describing the action. There is not any straightforward logical connection, as examination of the example above will show. Practical "syllogisms" do not fit any of the rules of inference of our standard logic. It was perhaps this that led Aristotle to separate practical reasoning from theoretical reasoning, practical syllogisms from true logical syllogisms. Still, there is some logical connection between the *content* of the belief/desire set and the action. The content of X's belief about means (constituting the minor premise) will necessarily include the same description of the action to be explained (opening the window) as was given in the conclusion, and the content of such belief will also necessarily include the same description of the object of the desire (chilling the wine) as was given in the major premise. One may schematize this as a practical syllogism as follows:

$$D(q)$$
$$\underline{B(p \supset q)}$$
$$p$$

Where "$D(q)$" in the example means "I desire that the wine be chilled," "$B(p \supset q)$" means "I believe that if I open the window, then the wine will be chilled," and "p" means "I open the window." The logical relationships are simply those of identity, $p = p$ and $q = q$. That the logical relationships hold for practical syllogisms is but to say that we presuppose the rationality of the agent who will see them in acting for a reason.[17] To say there is a logical relationship in such patterns of explanation is to say that an action is *rationalized* in such fashion.

The second sense in which we understand an action when we understand its reason is that we understand which of an agent's many beliefs and desires actually caused this action.[18] When we say that A opened the window *because* of his beliefs and desires, the 'because' is necessarily causal. For *A* might have had any number of belief/desire sets that would equally well rationalize his actions. He might have desired, for example, to offend his guests, and believed that an intentional opening of the window would accomplish that; yet even if he has such a desire, and even if he intentionally opens the window, it need not be for the latter reason at all. He may be much too polite for that. His reasons may be simply as stated earlier: to chill the wine. Which reason is *his* reason for opening the window is a straightforwardly causal hypothesis: whichever belief/desire set caused him to act as he did explains his action.[19] Thus, the etymology of 'motive': something that moves us to action.

A true motivational explanation requires that both of these features be present. A belief/desire set will be a reason for action, a practical syllogism, if and only if it both rationalizes and causes the action it is given to explain. For clarity it may be useful here to distinguish preliminarily the incomplete modes of explanation/justification. (I shall take each of these up in the later section.) There are two cases: rationalization without causation, and causation without rationalization.

'Rationalization' was a word coined by Ernest Jones, Freud's biographer and a member of Freud's inner circle, to describe the citing of belief/desire sets for actions when the sets cited were not the true reasons for action.[20] Belief/desire sets cited in this way are often given to *justify* an action by showing it to be the rational thing to do relative to the (presumably good) end cited. Such sets do not *explain* an action, however, because they did not cause it. Rationalization in Jones's sense is an attempt to parade belief/desire sets that would justify an action if they were the reasons for which it was performed, as the reasons that do explain it. It is justification, or an attempt at it, not explanation at all. Motives must *explain* as well as justify in Jones's sense of *rationalization*, or else they are not the motives of an action.

Two examples of causation by beliefs and desires without rationalization are:

1. His desire to beat Bobby Fischer caused his heart attack.
2. His belief that a murderer was prowling down the hall caused his heart to palpitate.

In such cases, a desire or a belief causes an event, but such beliefs or desires do not rationalize that event. We do not, in such examples, come to see the heart attack or palpitation as the action of a rational agent pursuing an end that is intelligible to us. The desires and beliefs, accordingly, do not operate in such explanations as parts of a practical syllogism, as a reason for action. (Nor for that matter are the events usually explained in such ways actions at all.) The desires or beliefs simply *cause* the event that they explain.

To summarize the results of this discussion: a desire that a state of affairs q take place is the motive for an action p by actor X if and only if:

1. X desired q
2. X believed that doing p would produce q
3. X's doing of p was caused by his desire for q and his belief that doing p would produce q
4. X's doing of p was an intentional action by X[21]

The event to be explained, p, is both exhibited as the rational thing to do (because of its relationship to the content of the beliefs and desires in the first two criteria) and explained (because of the causal hypothesis in the third criterion). There is admittedly some stipulation involved in giving such a definition of 'motive' (although I also believe it to conform to a substantial body of ordinary usage of the term). The justification for this "regimentation of ordinary usage," in Quine's phrase, is to sharpen and to systematize those distinctions that are important to us in our explanations and evaluations of the intentional actions of persons.

CAN MOTIVES BE UNCONSCIOUS?

Most of the motives suggested in psychoanalysis, for dreams and other phenomena, are *unconscious* motives. It has often been suggested that unconscious motives are a conceptual impossibility. For quite divergent reasons, many philosophical critics of psychoanalysis share Ernst Nagel's sentiment that "the notions of unconscious, causally operative motives and wishes...are just nonsense..."[22] If this were correct, then this article could be considerably shorter. Since the mental states cited by Freud to explain dreams are unconscious mental states, it would follow very quickly that the various explanations of dreams propounded by Freud could not be motivational in character.

There are some notoriously bad arguments leading to the conclusion that the idea of unconscious mental states makes no sense. These should be put aside at the start. One of these stems from Freud's own analogy of unconscious mental states as Kantian kinds of "ding-an-sich," objects that can never be known directly.[23] Such comparisons, if accepted, easily lead to skepticism about the existence of things (unconscious mental states) that are unknowable, in principle, to anyone. Yet such skepticism is unwarranted because the analogy is a poor one to begin with.[24] Although necessarily the holder of an unconscious mental state will not know that he has it, other people (such as his analyst) may well possess such knowledge. Indeed, if therapy is successful, he himself may come to know that fact as well. There is nothing "unknowable in principle" about unconscious mental states.

Also to be ignored here are both radical Behaviourist and phenomenological rejections of unconscious mental states. With regard to the first, Skinnerians deny the causal efficacy of unconscious mental states in producing behavior, even if they do not deny the existence of such states themselves. To quote Skinner:

> Freud's contribution [with regard to the unconscious] has been widely misunderstood. The important point was not that the individual was often unable to describe important aspects of his own behavior or identify important causal relationships, but that his ability to describe them was irrelevant to the occurrence of the behavior or to the effectiveness of the causes. . . . We may say that he is conscious of the parts he can describe and unconscious of the rest. But the act of self-description, as of self-observation, plays no part in the determination of action.[25]

Such denials are no more than part of what Michael Scriven once called Skinner's "allergic" reaction to explaining behavior by *any* kind of mental states, conscious or unconscious.[26]

Some phenomenologists, following Merleau-Ponty, have also urged that "unconscious mental states" are not the terms in which human behavior is to be explained. David Levin urges that "what Freud tries to explain by means of the notion of an unconscious idea or motive, we can now explain solely by reference to the bodily constituted field of phenomena."[27] What Levin means by the latter phrase is no easy matter to specify. The replacement for Freud that Levin has in mind, he tells us, "is a theory which integrates mind and body by interpreting both in terms of the phenomenological notion of an intentional field of behavior."[28]

In any case, these latter two attacks on there being causally operative (and thus explanatory) unconscious mental states can be put to the side here. For each is hostage to the very general programs in psychology that each represents. These theory-based attacks are *not* the basis for the popular suspicion about the sense of the idea of unconscious mental states. Such suspicions are better captured by those forms of skepticism themselves rooted in the common understanding of mind.

There are two levels at which such popular suspicions are to be captured: at the level of *things*, where the suspicion is that mind is consciousness; and at the level of *words*, where the suspicion is that "mind" means "conscious of." I shall discuss each of these, and then close this section with a less general skepticism about unconscious mental states presented by Ernst Nagel.

An Old Debate: Mind Is Consciousness

The "conceptual impossibility" argument is an argument with a history. The philosophical critics contemporary with Freud often took the view that the nature of what mental states are required that one be aware of his own mental states. Moreover, this requirement that one be conscious of his mental states was not thought to be some incidental feature of mental states but rather, their essence, so that in *no* sense could one properly be said to have a motive if he were not conscious of it. That being so, statements such as Freud's, to the effect that the only point in which unconscious motives differ from conscious ones "is just in the lack of consciousness in them," were thought to be "preposterous": "It is just like Mr. Churchill's cannibals in all respects except the act of devouring the flesh of victims."[29] As another contemporary critic more fully spelled out:

When I reflect on what I mean by a wish or an emotion or a feeling, I can only find that I know and think of them simply as different forms of consciousness. I cannot find any distinguishable element in these experiences which can be called consciousness and separated from the other elements even in thought so as to leave anything determinate behind. And to ask us to think of something which has all the characteristics of a wish or a feeling except that it is not conscious seems to me like asking us to think of something which has all the attributes of red or green except that it is not a colour.[30]

Freud was aware that "philosophers find difficulty in accepting the existence of unconscious processes," and that their line of attack was "based on [his] alleged abuse of the word 'conscious.'"[31] His reply to this line of criticism raises an interesting methodological question. Freud's reply was that such criticism "sounds like an empty dispute about words";[32] that "it is a matter of convention of nomenclature," and being such, is "of course, like any other convention, not open to refutation";[33] and that the identification of 'mind' and all its concepts with conscious processes was simply an old prejudice embedded in our language.[34] Freud opposed his critics' logical analysis of language sometimes with the brute facts of his empirical discovery that there are unconscious motives,[35] and sometimes with his right as a scientist to create a new concept, the only test for which is "whether the convention is so expedient that we are bound to adopt it."[36]

Such replies misconceived the thrust of an analysis into the reference of terms such as 'wish' and 'motive'. If the reference of mental state terms were conscious processor states, then it does make no sense to speak of 'unconscious motives', etc. And it is no reply to assert as a matter of fact that one has discovered their existence — for Freud would already have stipulated that the only criterion for their existence (consciousness) is not met. If there are no other criteria, there is nothing one could discover factually that would entitle one to speak of a motive.

Nor would Freud have been free to postulate a new theoretical concept and call it 'unconscious motive'. As a scientist, one may be free to invent any terms one likes, in which event we defer judgment on the utility of their creation until we are in a position to judge the entire scientific system in which they appear. But if one chooses a household word like 'motive' for such a theoretical term, one can only mislead others as well as oneself about the nature of the claims being made when the concept is used. Nor on such a view can Freud's claim that he discovered motives and wishes strictly analogous to those of everyday life be made out;[37] and without the latter claim, what could one make of the imputations of wishes and motives in therapy, which are supposed to make the patient accept responsibility either for the character such wishes are a part of, or for the actions such motives explain? Such responsibility may follow if one was *motivated* to act, or at least if his acts express his wishes, but only if 'motive' and 'wish' here mean what they ordinarily mean. For no one accepts responsibility for his "psychogens" or other inventions of psychological theory.[38]

While Freud's replies claimed a freedom from the ordinary meaning of 'motive' and 'wish' that he himself did not really want to claim, the philosophical criticisms themselves were not founded on an adequate analysis of mental concepts. Particularly since the work of Ryle and later Wittgenstein, few philosophers would agree that motive and its related mental states are to be thought of "simply as different forms of consciousness." For one could adopt any nondualistic position in the philosophy of mind and *not* assume that there is "nothing left behind" if consciousness is subtracted. If 'desire', for example, names a set of dispositions to behave, or a set of dispositions to further mental states, or a physical state with as yet unknown features, or a functional state, consciousness or the lack of it would simply be an incidental feature. Only if one were a follower of Descartes would one hold that nothing else is meant by mental words such as 'desire' but conscious mental experience.

A Contemporary Debate: 'Mind' Means 'Conscious of'

There is a contemporary version of this "conceptual impossibility" objection. This version follows the "linguistic turn" of contemporary philosophy by focusing not on what mental states might be but on certain aspects of the use of mental words. In modern guise, the philosophical objection to Freud's "discovery of the unconscious" would be that the distinctive feature of mental words lies precisely in the agent's ability to avow (that is, his consciousness of) what it is that he intends, hopes, fears, desires, etc. First-person, present-tense statements are often said to be mental statements only insofar as they possess this distinctive epistemic feature.

Consider, as an example of this kind of argument, F. A. Siegler's argument about the concept of an intention. Siegler has concluded that:

[I]t is a mistake to speak of a person's finding out, discovering, detecting or in any way identifying his own intentions. It makes no sense to talk in this way, and so it makes no sense to speak of a person's *failing* to find out, detect, or identify his own intentions. Consequently, it makes no sense to speak of a person's being mistaken in saying 'I intend to do X.' But this is exactly what Freud requires . . . [39]

Careful analysis of this conclusion will reveal that Siegler has conflated three distinct epistemic claims. The first is that mental words are asymmetrical with respect to the modes of their verification in their first- and third-person usages. This may be called the claim of *privileged access*.[40] If I have knowledge of my desires, intentions, pains, etc., that knowledge is acquired in a way distinct from the way in which others come to have the same knowledge of my mental states. I do not observe my own behavior in order to conclude that I am in pain, that I intend to go downtown tomorrow, or that I believe that it is raining. Others may use behavioral evidence to make third-person statements about my mental states, but I do not perform any acts of observation, inner or outer, to learn my own mental states. If I know them, I know them in a nonobservational way.

Second, some first-person, present-tense mental statements are *incorrigible*. Distinct from the mode-of-verification claim of privileged access is the claim of infallibility in one's judgments about one's own states of mind. The claim of incorrigibility is that, if I say I am in pain, or desire a yacht, and I am sincere about it, then it must be true that I am in pain or desire a yacht at the time I say so.[41] Predictions of my future states of mind, or memories of past states of mind, are fallible; the claim of incorrigibility is that *present*-tense statements in the first person are infallible if sincere.

Third, mental states are often said to be *self-intimating*.[42] This is the converse of the incorrigibility claim, which was that if I think I am in pain, I am in pain. Here, what is asserted is: if I am in pain, I think I am in pain (*mutatis mutandis* for other mental states). There can be, in this view, no unfelt pains, no unperceived afterimages, no unknown desires.

Siegler in the passage quoted begins with a claim of privileged access: we do not "discover" or "detect" our own intentions as we do the intentions of others. As Siegler elsewhere elaborates:

[I]t is absurd to suggest that I find out what my intentions are by observing my behavior, still less by hearing myself say 'I intend to...'. Do I then find out on the basis of some 'internal' evidence, do I observe what is going on in my mind and infer from that what my intentions are? This sounds equally absurd.[43]

From here Siegler moves to the claim of self-intimation, when he concludes that a person cannot *fail* to find out his own intentions. As he puts it elsewhere: "Normally I can come right out and state what my intentions are..."[44] The next move is to incorrigibility, Siegler's conclusion that a person cannot be mistaken in his beliefs about his own intentions.

If one is to have any chance of understanding the conceptual impossibility argument, one has to do a better job than this of keeping these three distinct claims separate. For the truth of each of these claims is *not* dependent upon the truth of the others. In particular with regard to Siegler, it will not do to assume that because we have privileged access to our own mental states then we must also be incorrigible about them and such states must be self-intimating to us. As John Wisdom once pointed out:

It is a common mistake to identify the fact that a person has, necessarily has, a way of knowing what's in his own mind which no one else has, with the claim that he can't be mistaken about his own mind. That's a very different matter indeed.[45]

It is an equally common mistake to confuse privileged access to one's own mind with the kind of "perfect" access to one's own mind that self-intimation would give one if it were true.

Keeping these epistemic claims separate allows one to state more precisely the alleged conceptual problem with unconscious mental states; for a mental state to be unconscious is to lack just that knowledge held by the claim of self-intimation to be a necessary prerequisite to being in the state in question. Further, such an unconscious mental state would be unaccompanied by the *noninferential* knowledge held by the claim of privileged access to be a necessary prerequisite to being in the state in question. In addition, if one were conscious of some particular mental state, and the incorrigibility thesis were right, that would not seem to leave any room for contradiction by the psychoanalytic suggestion of other, unconscious mental states. Thus, from each of these epistemic claims seemingly arises a version of the "conceptual impossibility" objection. I shall examine each version and each epistemic claim separately.

The Claim of Privileged Access

First, consider the least problematic of the three claims, that of privileged access. On these occasions when we do know what we desire, what we believe, or that we are in pain, do we come to such knowledge in a nonobservational or noninferential way? Rather plainly, it is usually true that we do. Except to a well-conditioned behaviorist, it is surprising to be asked how one knows, for example, that he wants an ice-cream cone, or believes that going downtown will get him one, or that his left foot hurts. Yet this feature of privileged access to such states in no way renders nonsensical the idea that one may be unconscious of his desires, his beliefs, or other mental states.

To begin with, one might urge that the lack of privileged access to beliefs, desires, and other mental states in no way changes the *meaning* of the words referring to those states. The sense or criteria of 'motive' (and of 'belief' and 'desire') is not to be confused with the modes of verifying whether those criteria are satisfied. Unless one is a verificationist about meaning (meaning *is* the mode of verification), then the fact that one mode of verification is lacking (because the actor is unaware of it) in no way changes the meaning of the mental terms used.

Hence, a tempting construction of 'unconscious motive' would be to assume that the same criteria are meant as for 'motive' generally, with the proviso that the modes of verification of these criteria are no longer different in first- and third-person usages. This construction is so straightforward that numerous philosophers have given all unconscious mental states such an (inevitably behaviorist) interpretation.[46] Freud himself gave support to such a view by analogizing our knowledge of our own unconscious to our knowledge of other minds.[47]

There are problems with this point of view that I will not address here, for I do not believe that even this small innovation was meant when Freud spoke of unconscious motives. Freud seemed to think that one had what might be called "deferred privileged access" to one's unconscious mental states, namely, that if one became conscious of such states, he did so noninferentially (through memory). Freud throughout his writings emphasized that in psychoanalysis one does not become conscious of an unconscious mental state just by looking at the evidence, namely, his own behavior patterns and the authoritative interpretation of his analyst. He has to *remember* it as his motive, to know that it was his motive in such a way that he is surprised he did not know it before.

What, then, must we do in order to replace what is unconscious in our patients by what is conscious? There was a time when we thought this was a very simple matter: all that was necessary was for us to discover this unconscious material and communicate it to the patient. But we know already that this was a short-sighted error. Our knowledge about the unconscious material is not equivalent to his knowledge. . . . We must look for it in his memory.[48]

One has such memory because, the theory asserts, in successful therapy one comes to *re* –experience the (formerly unconscious) mental states.

Psychoanalytic therapy requires, in short, the same kind of nonobservational knowledge to confirm its interpretations as one has of one's conscious mental states outside of analysis. The modes of verification for ascribing a mental state to a person are thus still asymmetrical with respect to first- and third-person usages. The only difference a mental state being unconscious makes is that at the time at which it is unconscious, one cannot verify that one has the mental state in the accustomed manner. It may require a good bit of jogging of memory, either by free association, by re–experiencing the emotion via transference, or otherwise, before the subject recognizes the mental state as his. Indeed, for various reasons he may in some cases never recognize such unconscious mental states. But in principle, the way in which he comes to know his own mental states is the same irrespective of whether they were conscious or unconscious.[49]

For two reasons, then, the claim of privileged access to anything that can truly be called a *mental* state can be admitted to be true; yet the implication sought to be drawn from it—that there can be no unconscious mental states—should be denied as false. To summarize these two reasons: either privileged access is applicable to unconscious mental states, albeit it is deferred privileged access; or, even if it is not applicable to unconscious mental states, there is no reason to think that a mode of verification such as privileged access is even a *part* of the meaning of mental state terms such as "wish," "belief" and the like (let alone so central a feature of the meaning of such words that its absence renders usage of such words "nonsense").

The Claim of Self-Intimation

Unlike the claim of privileged access, the claim of self-intimation, if true, would preclude there being any things properly called unconscious mental states. If mental states must be transparent to their holders (self-intimating) in order to be mental states at all, unconscious mental states would be (in Siegler's words) "incoherent and self-contradictory." We can have unconscious mental states only if the claim of self-intimation is false.

With respect to the causal connections between mental states and behavior there is little or no plausibility to a claim of self-intimation. Many causal connections which we readily admit to exist between mental states and behavior are not known to the actor. A pain in my foot may be the cause of my gruffness to a colleague, yet even if the pain itself were a self-intimating state, the causal connection between that state and my behavior is not. I may know I am in pain and I may know that I am being gruff to a colleague; there is not even a hint from ordinary usage that the proper use of the word "pain" requires that I know the causal connection between the two. For belief/desire states the same arguments may be made as were just made for pain states, that is, even if beliefs and desires were self-intimating states, there is nothing to suggest that their causal connection to behavior (as a reason for action or otherwise) need be self-intimating.

Saying this does not, unfortunately, dispose of that part of the "conceptual impossibility" objection stemming from the claim of self-intimation. Even if the causal connection between belief/desire states and behavior is not self-intimating, if the states themselves are self-intimating, then *unconscious* beliefs or desires would make no sense. One could talk of "unconscious reasons," but only in a very limited sense, namely, one where conscious beliefs and desires cause behavior without the actor being aware of their doing so.

Are beliefs, desires and other mental states themselves self-intimating states? One historically important reason for thinking that they are has been rejected earlier. This was the idea that such states were defined solely by the ability of their possessor to avow that he was in such a state. One would, in other words, be in state S if and only if one had the ability to avow, "I am in state S." This ontologically very spare account (which reduces mind to linguistic competence) does not seem very appealing in light of more substantial theories about what minds are. (Even in a "functionalist" view of mind, mental states are characterized by functions other than that the subject has certain linguistic abilities.)

Another historically important argument with the conclusion that mental states are self-intimating has only partial applicability to mental states. With experiential states, such as pain, one might think that the following two entailments hold: if one is in pain, one *feels* the pain; if one feels the pain, one knows (and can avow) that one is in pain. By virtue of such entailments, unconscious pains (or other experiential states of sensation, emotion, or imagination) would make no sense. Desires and beliefs, however, are not experiential states. Although one can experience a strong craving or a passionate desire, or one can recite to oneself one's beliefs, such occurrences are incidental to being in the states named by "belief" and "desire." Beliefs and desires are not plausibly interpreted to be occurrences, as philosophy at least since Ryle seems to have recognized. The argument to self-intimation from the immediacy of mental experience is accordingly nonexistent for those mental states connected to reasons for action.

Even for experiential terms such as those like 'pain' that name sensations, the alleged entailments are very problematic, to say the least. Being in pain can entail feeling in pain, and feeling in pain can entail awareness of the pain, only according to a very questionable view about meaning. This theory of meaning freezes our present guides to correct usage as *criteria* in the logical positivists' sense of necessary and sufficient conditions. Since 'pain' as we presently use the word always, when correctly used, is accompanied by painful feelings (and the latter, accompanied by awareness), this view of meaning freezes painful feelings as the meaning of 'pain'. On such a view an unfelt pain is quite literally "nonsense" (i.e., not in accordance with the *sense*, the criteria, of the word).

The general problem with this theory of meaning is that it cuts off our ordinary understanding from the progressive insights of science. It limits our insights into what pain might be, by a kind of conventional fiat: whatever aspect of pain we have stumbled across first is all there is to pain. This leaves those psychologists who discover, say, the functions pain may serve in learning, as talking about something else the moment they treat pain as a state more importantly characterized by those learning functions than by the feelings of its subject. Similarly, physiologists who wish to characterize pain as a certain form of C-fiber stimulation (even if there are occasionally no painful feelings) would be talking about something else on such an insular view of meaning.

As a last example, consider pain-thresholds. Talk of people having different pain-thresholds must be nonsense if 'pain' entails feeling and knowing. For what sense could be made of saying that someone had a "high pain-threshold," i.e., that he didn't notice and didn't feel pains that others would notice and feel? If he didn't notice it and didn't feel it, then on the theory of meaning here considered he shouldn't be said to be in pain at all. Nor can such a person be said to "stand more pain" than others — because he has pains only in proportion to what he feels, and if he doesn't feel much pain then he doesn't have much pain. His threshold, in such a case, is mislabelled a *pain*-threshold.

Psychologists cannot be shut out of talking about pain in these ways. It may turn out that persons have pains only when they feel them. If this is the case, however, it will only be the case because the best scientific theory we are able to muster about what pain really is, tells us it is the case. It cannot be shown to be the case by freezing one present guide to usage as a meaning-connection, an analytic truth, violation of which is "self-contradictory." The short of it is that the entailments that could justify self-intimation as a characteristic of mental states, do not exist even for experiential mental terms.[50]

A different argument for self-intimation focuses on mental terms such as "belief" and "desire," terms which take objects. For such words the most serious argument for self-intimation I take to stem from the nature of Intentional[51] (or intensional)[52] objects. Desires and beliefs, like all mental states taking intensional objects, are individuated in part by those objects. What counts as one desire as opposed to another desire in part depends on what the object of that desire is. One of the striking facts about mentalistic language is that it is nonextensional, that is, that the substitutivity of identicals does not hold for referring terms when parts of the objects of mental states. Even if the room referred to by the description "the dirtiest room in the inn" is the very same room as that referred to by the designation "Room 10," that identity does not allow one to conclude that Ralph desired the dirtiest room in the inn just because Ralph desired Room 10. A desire for the dirtiest room in the inn is different from a desire for Room 10 — even though the things seemingly referred to in the propositional objects of the two desires is in reality one thing.

The upshot of this Intentionality for present purposes is this: whatever account one gives for what sorts of things mental states are, one must make room for this essentially linguistic mode of their individuation. This may seem to require self-intimation, because the most obvious source for fixing the descriptions of the objects of belief and desire are the descriptions uttered by the person whose beliefs and desires they are. The subject can give such descriptions, the argument concludes, only if he is conscious of what his beliefs and desires are.

The crucial step in this argument for the self-intimation of states of desire and belief is that which requires a connection to exist between the subject's having a certain belief or desire, and his possession of the speech dispositions sufficient to identify it. Requiring such a connection is motivated by the fact that our present abilities to fix the objects of beliefs and desires do depend heavily upon the linguistic abilities of the subject. This is true of our conscious mental states, but is also perhaps true of unconscious ones for which one can invoke extended memory as the means of fixing the relevant objects. Behavior, the most obvious alternative source of evidence here, can only take us so far in pinpointing the object of a belief or a desire. For even if behavior seemingly "pointed to" some object in the world as the goal of the actor, it would not differentiate that object under one description as opposed to another. Yet as the *goal* of the actor, it is so differentiated. This is what the nonsubstitutivity of descriptions of identicals in Intentional contexts means. Without some verbal behavior, one could not, for example, distinguish a desire to occupy Room 10 from a desire to occupy the dirtiest room in the inn, on the basis of behavior of someone tending to place himself in that room; for there is only one room, and the behavioral tendency is to occupy *that room* (without regard to how it is described).

The essential problem for this step of the argument is the same problem that confronts the claim that *experiential* words are self-intimating: one cannot prevent better and better scientific theories about what sort of states beliefs and desires really are by this kind of freezing of present indicators into unassailable entailments (meaning-connections, analytic truths, etc.). A theory about what desires are, it is true, must include features not needed to be included in a theory about pain; it must, that is, include features that account for the linguistic way in which such desire states are individuated. To account for such features, a theory about desires might well include the controversial brain-writing thesis. Alternatively, perhaps some more complicated relation will be found between the content of mental states, language, and brain physiology. However such theorizing comes out, one cannot rule it irrelevant—as not being about *desires*—simply because it may go counter to our present indicators of the content of such desires; any more than one can rule irrelevant theorizing about pain that does not utilize our present indicator of pain, *viz.*, painful feelings. In short, neither "pain" nor "desire" can name self-intimating states because such words are open to revisable scientific theory, not hostage to a fixed linguistic convention.

Self-intimation cannot thus be made out as a necessary condition of any state being a *mental* state. Our minds are not transparent to us, and nothing in ordinary usage binds us to such a view.

The Claim of Incorrigibility

If the incorrigibility claim were true, it would not rule out the possibility of unconscious mental states. For the incorrigibility thesis only concerns the correctness of any beliefs the subject has about his mental states. It does not preclude him from having other mental states, even contradictory ones, that are unconscious. Suppose someone, X, thinks he desires to help a friend. The incorrigibility thesis only claims that X must have the desire he thinks he has. It is silent about whether he has other mental states of which he is unaware, including perhaps a desire to hurt (rather than to help) his friend.[53]

The claimed incorrigibility of first person awareness only becomes a problem for the unconscious with regard to unconscious motives (reasons for action). For with regard to motives, psychoanalysts do need to be able to contradict the actor's beliefs about his motives if they are to have the ability they claim, to divine the "real reasons," the unconscious ones, that motivated an actor to do what he did. The claim of incorrigibility, if true, does seem to stand in the way of there being unconscious motives, and I shall accordingly examine the correctness of this claim with regard to motives specifically.

Richard Peters once advanced a version of this incorrigibility claim against there being unconscious motives. According to Peters, it makes no sense to ascribe unconscious motives to those actions for which we have a perfectly intelligible, conscious motive: "some actions have such obvious and acceptable reasons that reference to unconscious wishes seems grotesquely out of place."[54] It is only when there is no conscious motive, or when the alleged conscious motive was suspect in some way, that Peters thought that unconscious motives could appropriately be ascribed.

Such a claimed incorrigibility of the subject does not rule out there being unconscious motives. For sometimes the actions explained by Freud are actions whose motives puzzle the actor. He may even think that he had no motives.[55] (People who are not Freudians probably think this is so about most of their dreams.) If the actor is in such a state of puzzlement, then he has no incorrigible knowledge of his motives to be contradicted by a psychoanalyst's discovery of his unconscious motives.

Still, unconscious motive ascriptions, both in psychoanalysis and in everyday life, often do contradict the beliefs of the actor about his motives. If the claim of incorrigibility were right with respect to our use of 'motive', then the latter subclass of unconscious motive ascriptions could make no sense. As it turns out, the incorrigibility claim is simply wrong with respect to even this subclass of unconscious motives.

There are a number of avenues to be pursued here. One might start with the observation that most of the motives that psychoanalysts and laymen talk about are motives cited to explain *past* behavior. The temptation might be to say that by 'unconscious motive' one means only that the actor cannot now recall what the motive was, even though at the time the action was performed he did know what it was with certainty. On such a construction one could well think he recalls what his motive was, and yet be mistaken in his recollection. The apparent incorrigibility of one's expressions of his own motive would then be no barrier to speaking of unconscious motives, even in situations where one believes he knows his motive to be different from the unconscious motive suggested by the psychoanalyst. Such an interpretation might have particular force in the case of unconscious motives for dreams, since the motives will *always* be attributed in the past tense (psychoanalysis not taking place when one is asleep).

If 'unconscious' as used by Freud meant only that one lacks a *present* ability to recall one's motive, some such construction could be made out. But plainly, psychoanalytic explanations are not limited to situations where one was conscious of his motive when he performed the action, but now has no memory of what he earlier knew. In fact, it is hard even to find an example in psychoanalysis where 'unconscious motive' is so used.[56] Rather, Freud's striking claim is that we perform actions, think with certainty that we know why, yet in fact do not know our true motive even as we are acting because of it. Freud challenges, in other words, the incorrigibility of our first-person statements, not just in the past tense, where they are clearly open to challenge, but in the present tense as well. The claim is that we do not know what we *are* about, even if we think we do; not just that we cannot correctly recall what we *were* about at some time in the past, even though we think we do recall what it was.

Another avenue that may appear tempting is to grant that present-tense expressions about one's own motives are not subject to contradiction, but to deny that psychoanalysts really contradict them when they cite one's unconscious motives. One may have both a conscious motive and an unconscious motive in performing a given action; one can be certain that the former was his motive, and be correct, and still the latter may also have been one's motive.

On this construction an unconscious motive, when cited as the explanation of an action for which the actor appears to know his motive, never means *the* (single) motive; it only means one of the *mixed* motives. The conscious and unconscious motive together cause the performance of the action. Citing the unconscious motive as one of the set of the mixed motives does not contradict the actor's knowledge that he had conscious reasons as well for doing what he did. Both were his motives for doing it.

There is nothing implausible about this account. We do act for mixed motives, and there is no reason some of them may not be unconscious. Yet neither in psychoanalysis nor in ordinary speech is our use of 'unconscious motive' limited to such situations. The very language that we often employ to describe an unconscious motive as "the real motive" belies our assumption that sometimes we do contradict the actor's apparent certainty about his motives.

The good sense with which we may question the testimony of the agent as to his own motives stems directly from the meaning of 'motive' elucidated earlier. Unlike pains, future intentions, imaginings, etc., one does not "have a motive" except in the sense that some action is explicable by reference to it. One may feel pains, imagine things, intend to do various things, and yet perform no action for which these items may serve as an explanation. By contrast, I cannot have a motive as I "have" a pain or a future intention in the absence of an action; a motive is always given as an explanation of an action.[57]

It is always in point to ask whether an explanation, of an action or of anything else, is a good one or not. If one is citing his motive in the first person, he is explaining his action no less than is a third-person observer who cites his motive in the third person. In both cases, to be an explanation at all it must have the possibility of being false. It must be possible that the conscious motive is not the cause of the action being performed, even if the actor believes that it is.

The moment one uses 'pain' or 'intention' in an explanation of an action, our expressions using these terms also become clearly subject to contradiction. If I tell a colleague that my gruffness is the result of a pain in my foot, I could easily be said to be mistaken. If I say that I am speaking rapidly because I intend to catch the next bus, I can be mistaken. 'Intention' and the like could be incorrigible only insofar as we do not use them to explain an action. The difference with 'motive' is that motive can be used only to explain one's actions. Hence, all uses of 'motive' in the first person allow one to be mistaken about his motives, because all such uses purport to be contingently true explanations.

This last argument, of course, shows only that one is not incorrigible about the causation element in motivational ascriptions (the third criterion of 'motive'); one might still be incorrigible with respect to the mental states of desire and belief (the first and second criteria of 'motive'). Yet to make perfectly good sense of there being unconscious motives that contradict the actor's own view as to his motivation, it is not necessary to address the question of the incorrigibility of our usages of 'desire' and 'belief'. For even if one is incorrigible about his own present desires and beliefs, that knowledge is not contradicted at all by an ascription of unconscious motives to an action. For if the incorrigibly known desires and beliefs are not causally relevant to the action, then the field is open to the analyst to suggest other (unconscious) desires and beliefs as the true motives of the action. Such suggestions in no way contradict the agent's assertions that he does desire X or believe Y; they contradict only the causal influence of such beliefs and desires, as to which the agent has no special authority. Only if there is something illegitimate about saying there are beliefs and desires of the agent of which he is not conscious, is there a problem here. This would be a problem stemming from the supposedly self-intimating nature of such states, a problem that I have argued does not exist.

The upshot of this analysis is that there is nothing suspect about attributing unconscious motives even when the subject believes his motives to be something entirely different. Our ordinary usage reflects this unproblematic character of unconscious motive ascriptions by the idioms of "real reasons" and "deeper reasons."

It might be thought that our present use of 'motive' in this way is only the result of the "pollution" of the language brought on by the immense popular currency of Freud's ideas about unconscious motives. To some extent, our use of "real motives" probably has expanded since Freud began writing. Yet well before Freud, our language allowed the use of 'motive' such that the person whose motive it was, was not conscious of it. (Indeed, Freud himself rather charmingly admitted, in reminiscing about his discovery of unconscious processes, that his only claim to discovery was by being ill-read.) George Eliot's novels, for example, are replete with discernment of the hidden motives that activate her characters. Yet no one to my knowledge criticized books such as *Middlemarch* because its characters acted for motives of which they were not aware. We all seem to understand without difficulty that one such as Bulstrode could well act for a reason of which he was not aware, and moreover, could even believe with apparent certainty that his motive was something entirely different. Eliot's readers also seemed to understand that well enough, based on their ordinary concept of 'motive'.

Although not strictly necessary to make sense of unconscious motives, it is perhaps worth noting in closing this section how very suspect the incorrigibility claim is with regard to desires and beliefs themselves (not just, that is, with regard to their causal connection to behavior). Such suspicions are particularly justified about "desire." "Desire" as ordinarily used is a theoretical word tied to satisfaction states, behavioral tendencies, tendencies with regard to other desires and beliefs, perhaps to physiology as well. One can no more freeze the conscious belief of the subject about what he desires into a sufficient condition of desire (which is what the incorrigibility thesis does) than one could make such belief into a necessary condition (which is what the self-intimation thesis would do); and for the same reason: there are no analytic truths about "desire," only scientific theories about desire. Such fallibility about "desire" is easily observed in everyday speech, when we say, "he thinks he wants...(a new car, a new wife, etc.)." Such locutions make sense only because things may not be as they seem to the subject, that is, because he is *not* incorrigible about his own desires.[58]

On Unconsciously Wishing for the Impossible

Separate from any of the epistemic claims about mental states is Ernst Nagel's conceptual argument toward his earlier quoted conclusion that unconscious wishes and the like are "just nonsense." Nagel reasoned that "there is an important failure of analogy between conscious motives and unconscious mental processes";[59] that because of this failure, "it is only by a radical shift in the customary meanings of such words as 'motive' and 'wish' that Freudian theory can be said to offer an explanation of human conduct in terms of motivations and wish-fulfillments."[60] Nagel's charge here is that Freudians can explain behavior by unconscious mental states only if they gerrymander the idea of mental states enough to allow for unconscious mental states.

The crux for any such charge is to see whether there *is* any failure of analogy between ordinary wishes and motives, and unconscious wishes and motives. For Nagel the failure of analogy is to be found in the enduring nature of Freudian wishes:

[T]hese unconscious motives have an enduring character and tenacious attachment to specific objectives that conscious wishes do not exhibit. Indeed, in Freudian theory a thwarted wish of early childhood, directed toward some person, may not completely vanish, but may enjoy a repressed existence in the unconscious, and continue to operate in identical form into the present even though that person has long since died.[61]

It is important at the outset to see that Nagel's kind of argument, even if it is succeeded, can only be directed against certain kinds of unconscious mental states; these are the unconscious wishes of childhood so much a part of Freud's developmental metapsychology. *Not* at stake here is the conceptual possibility of there being unconscious wishes or unconscious motives at all.

In any case, even restricted to the unconscious wishes of childhood of Freud's developmental metapsychology, Nagel's alleged failure of analogy does not have much to do with the kind of states such wishes are. Rather, Nagel's point has to do, first, with the degree of attachment Freud says we have to the *objects* of our childhood wishes, and second, with the nature of those *objects* themselves — Freud allows that we may wish for the obviously impossible, as in an Oedipal wish toward a dead parent. Yet neither of these points should convince us that Freud abused the ordinary meaning of "wish" or "motive." Even if these differences in *what* people wished for were large ones, the kind of state that wishing *is* would not differ. And, in any event, these are not really departures from our ordinary pre-Freudian ideas about wishes and their objects. People sometimes at least do orient their lives around some early formed wishes. And they do this even after the original objects of such passions have become impossible of attainment. Perhaps this is not very rational of people (in the sense of "rational" having to do with mastery of the passions); but it is very human.[62]

For my own part I find one of the most attractive features of Freudian theory to be its emphasis on this tragic aspect of man. In any case, even if Freud's thesis that our deepest longings are to be found in the enduring wishes from childhood is only a tragic picture, aesthetically attractive but literally false, it is *not* a conceptual howler. Freud's developmental metapsychology conceptualized in terms of unconscious wishes enduring from childhood, is not suspect on these conceptual grounds.

My conclusion is that there are no conceptual grounds on which one can write off talk of unconscious motives as "nonsense." Such an expression, *prima facie*, makes very good sense; that is not to say, however, that psychoanalysts, in fact, always use it in that sense. Three other alternatives must be considered before we return to psychoanalytic usage in the theory of dreams.

INCOMPLETE PRACTICAL SYLLOGISMS: MEANING AND CAUSATION

As earlier pointed out, a practical syllogism generates two kinds of understanding of an action: it exhibits an action as rational and intelligible, and it causally explains it. There are, accordingly, two sorts of cases where a purportedly motivational explanation may go wrong: it may rationalize an action but not explain it; or it may causally explain the action without rationalizing it. Since each such case of a "partial practical syllogism" is a plausible interpretation of part of Freud's theory of dreams, I shall address each briefly.

RATIONALIZATION WITHOUT CAUSATION

Freud's discoveries, for dreams particularly but elsewhere as well, are often said to be a discovery of the *meaning* of such phenomena, or that such phenomena *had meaning*. What one wants to see here is the variety of things that can be meant by this claim *short of saying* that Freud discovered unconscious motives for dreams, slips, symptoms, etc. The most natural way to order this variety is by starting with a likely consequence of an action and seeing what else has to be said before that consequence would be eligible to rationalize fully that action, in the way that motives do.

Suppose an actor X strikes another (Y), and that the likely consequence of this (R) is that there will be violent retaliation. One sense in which we may say that X's action "has meaning" is the sense of 'meaning' in which we might say, "This means trouble," or more specifically, "This means that Y will retaliate."[63] An action has meaning in this sense only because we, the observers, perceive that R is a likely consequence of the action. There is no implication about the actor's state of mind at all, no implication that he in any sense perceived this meaning or acted because of that perception.

This "observer meaning" can be what one discovers when one "finds the meaning" of a painting or other work of art. Often the motives with which the painter painted the painting are judged totally irrelevant to what the painting means. The (observer) meaning of the painting is what we, the observers, think to be a plausible interpretation of its elements, and our interpretive judgments are guided by what we think to be the likely impressions produced by various elements of the painting.

There is undoubtedly more to art interpretation than this, but the example, even when supplemented by a more adequate analysis, is illustrative of the basic distinction proposed: between the meaning the painting may have for us as we observe the effects its elements produce within us, and the meaning it had for the actor. Much of our "finding meaning" in phenomena consists only of our perceiving likely consequences of those phenomena.

If we are to move beyond the minimal sense of (observer) meaning to begin to rationalize the action, we must come to see some likely consequences as a "possible motive" for an action.[64] This involves two steps: first, we must judge that it would not be irrational for an actor in X's position to have believed that striking Y would lead to retaliation; second, we must judge that it would be intelligible for Y to want to retaliate. If the belief is wildly irrational—e.g., saying that "storks" rather than "stocks" will make one a mother—then we cannot fully understand the action as that of a rational agent.[65] Similarly, if the desire is so bizarre as to be unintelligible to us—say, a desire to keep one's elbow in the mud all afternoon for no further reason—we again cannot understand the action as that of a fully rational agent.[66] Only if there is a set of rational beliefs promoting intelligible desires can we exhibit an action as fully rational.

It is true that any set of beliefs and desires that fits the general form, X desires O, X believes A will produce O, will exhibit an action A as rational in some sense.[67] Let us say of such cases that an action is exhibited as being *minimally rational* if we can hypothesize a set of beliefs and desires whose content exhibits the required logical relationships, no matter how bizarre or irrational those beliefs and desires themselves may be. Let us say that an action is *fully rational* only if the beliefs are themselves rational and the desires are themselves intelligible.

Notice that to say any of these things about an action is still not to say anything about the actor. To say that an action may be seen as either minimally or fully rational is only to say that we, the observers, can hypothesize a set of beliefs and desires that, if the actor had them and acted on them, would render his action rational. Hence, to say that an action "has meaning" in this second sense still says nothing at all about the actor.

To exhibit some particular action as rational is to do more than perceive that it has some likely consequence about which an intelligible desire and a rational belief might be formed. To exhibit an action as rational is to say that the actor had the requisite set of beliefs and desires, and that in light of *his* beliefs and desires, the action was the rational thing to do. It was minimally rational if he had the beliefs and desires with the requisite logical connection between their content and the action described; it was fully rational if, in addition, his desires and beliefs are themselves intelligible and rational. To exhibit an action in such light is still not to explain it motivationally (or at all), because no causal connection is asserted between the belief/desire set and the action. Yet it is to do more than discover possible motives.

To summarize this discussion, one may find an action to have meaning in any of three senses: (1) it has an observer's meaning; (2) the action "would make sense," i.e., the actor was in a situation such that he had a possible motive for doing what he did; or (3) the action was a rational thing to do, in light of the actor's beliefs and desires. Only the last of these is to exhibit an action as rational, but the first two must also be mentioned, because they are plausible reconstructions of what the psychoanalytic discovery of meaning is about, in dream theory as elsewhere.

CAUSATION WITHOUT RATIONALIZATION

A belief or a desire may cause an event without constituting part of a motivational explanation. The examples given earlier were of two kinds: (1) a desire alone caused an event ("His desire to beat Bobby Fischer caused his heart attack"), and (2) a belief alone did so ("His belief that a murderer was prowling down the hall caused his heart to palpitate"). Because it turns out to be more pertinent to Freud's explanations of dreams (and probably also generally), I will focus on the first kind of partial practical syllogism alone, i.e., where *desires* cause events.

From the examples of such explanations that most readily come to mind, there seems to be a lack of two characteristics of a truly motivational explanation: first, the minor premise is missing entirely. Our ambitious chess player did not *believe* that having a heart attack would get him what he wanted: beating Bobby Fischer in chess. Second, the chess player did not perform an *action* in having a heart attack; it was something that happened to him, not something *he did*.

Lack of each of these features is sufficient to disqualify such explanations as motivational in character. With respect to the first: without the belief that A leads to O, the desire will not *rationalize A* in any sense, nor need the desire even be a possible motive for acting. It is the content of the belief that makes the action the rational thing to do in order to obtain the object of the desire. Without such a belief, a desire with any object may be cited as the cause of any event. A desire to be an artist may cause one to live a long time, to kill one's mother, to cut off an ear, etc. Without the belief, the intensional object of the desire need have no rational connection to the action; the desire with such an object need only be contingently connected to the action.

With respect to the second deficiency, the lack of an *action* to be explained: there is a long-noticed conceptual connection between the concept of a motive and that of an action. Often, indeed, in contemporary accounts of action the one is used as a sufficient criterion for the other.[68] If an event is motivated, then that event is an action, on this account. This of course means that if some event is not an action, then whatever is cited to explain it cannot be a motive. The range of items that motives explain is limited to actions. Accordingly, to cite a desire as an explanation of a heart attack, which is not an action, cannot be a motivational explanation.

There is nothing wrong with thinking that there is *some* connection of action and motive. Motives are reasons *for acting*. If we acted for a reason, necessarily we acted. What is overlooked by those who use motives as their criterion of action is the Freudian possibility: the discovery of hidden motives *ipso facto* transforms the events explained by them into full-fledged human actions. If one has as his only criterion of action that the action be explicable by reasons, then there is nothing to prevent a Freudian from expanding the extension of 'action' by discovering hidden motives. What one needs is some criterion of action other than motives, in order to make the objection here interposed—no action—a significant objection. I shall defer discussion of this until I return to dream theory, where it is obviously of great importance.

Assuming we have some criterion of action independent of motivation, then the earlier chess player example remains distinguishable on both grounds, no belief and no action. It turns out that the first is the more crucial of the distinctions in any event, for there are explanations of events that are admittedly actions, and that nonetheless are not motivational explanations. Suppose X is a prisoner who wants very much to get out of prison. He rattles the bars of his cell "because he wants out." His rattling the cage is an action he performs, and his desire causes it; yet he does not rattle the bars *in order to* get out, because he does not believe for an instant that he can shake loose the bars. His desire, in other words, is not his motive for action. He must adopt his action as a means to attain the object of his desire, which he does not do because he does not have the requisite belief in the causal efficacy of his action. He expresses his desire, if you like, but he does not act on it as a motive.

There is a large literature, mainly in the "philosophical psychology" of the 1950s and '60s, which argued that causal explanations of action by desires is not logically possible. Most of that literature is directed at a point different from that made here; namely, that desires, *as used in motivational explanations*, cannot function as causes.[69] I, of course, disagree with that point, too, in light of the earlier explication of motivational explanation; but irrespective of that controversy, most of the arguments of that literature having nothing to do with whether nonmotivational usages of 'desire' may not function as the names of causes of actions.[70]

NONEXISTENT PRACTICAL SYLLOGISMS: FUNCTIONS

The word *purpose* has two quite distinct usages: one usage as a member of the family of concepts that are the subject matter of this article ('motive', 'intention', 'desire', etc.); the other as specifying the function some process, object, or action may serve. If I distribute leaflets protesting the continuation of nuclear testing in the atmosphere, my purpose (motive) in doing so can be to end the tests; a social scientist, however, might explain my action as serving the purpose (function) of alienating local law-enforcement officials, if in fact that is what occurs as a result of my activity. The apparent discrepancy between my statement of purpose and the social scientist's is not like the disagreement an actor sometimes has with an observer as to the actor's motives. Rather, two different forms of explanation have been given; both of them could be correct, and yet I still may not have acted from mixed motives.

Functional explanations share a common vocabulary with motivational explanations. 'Purpose' can indicate either, as the leaflet example illustrates; the phraseologies "in order to" or "for the sake of" are equally appropriate to either type of explanation. Both types of explanation are often classified as "teleological." Both concepts share a common historical origin in primitive animism. Because of these superficial grammatical similarities and historical background, it is common to find one form of explanation being confused with the other. This is particularly true of both popular and psychoanalytic discussions of unconscious purpose. Because of this potential for confusion, and actual confusion in fact, a brief examination of the logic of function statements, and of the ways in which functional explanations differ from motivational ones, is pursued in this section.

THE LOGIC OF FUNCTIONAL EXPLANATIONS

A familiar use of 'function' is one such as: "The function of the heartbeat is to circulate the blood."[71] This could be paraphrased without change of meaning to: "The heartbeat serves the purpose of circulating the blood" or, "The heart beats in order to circulate the blood." Four elements are most commonly found in the unpacking of such statements: a system (S) is tacitly assumed; an end state of the system (ES) is also tacitly assumed; an identifiable part of the system or a process (P) occurring within the system (which is the item for which an explanation is sought) is expressly mentioned; and an effect (E) of the process of part (which is also a state of the system) is expressly mentioned.

In such an explanation the information content is that the existence or activity of the part or process P is a contingently *necessary condition* to the occurrence of the effect E; the tacit assumption further asserts that E is itself a contingently necessary condition to the maintenance of the system as a whole in some general end state ES. Thus, "the function of the heartbeat is to circulate the blood," implies the existence of a system (the human body), labels an identifiable part (the heart) or process (the heart's beating), and specifies an immediate effect of that process, namely, a state of the system in which the blood circulates. The function assigned to the heart is the effect named in the statement (the circulation of blood), and the information content is that in certain living systems with which we are familiar (namely, vertebrates), the heart's beating is a necessary condition for the circulation of blood. This effect (the circulation of blood) is of interest to us only because it is, in turn, a necessary condition for the survival of such organisms. Hence, the ultimate empirical content of such a functional statement will be that the beating of the heart is a necessary condition for the survival of the organism.

It is important to stress that P is a necessary condition to E (and to ES) only relative to some system S. Hearts are not *logically* necessary for blood to circulate in all living systems; some other mode of circulation is certainly logically possible. Hearts are necessary for the survival only of those living systems we classify as vertebrates. Since the class of vertebrates is not defined as "creatures with a heart," the asserted connection between having a heart and being a live vertebrate is a genuinely empirical claim.

It is equally important to stress that it is only relative to some end state ES in system S that a function may be assigned. Absent the end state of health of the human body, one would be free to pick any consequence E of the heart's beating (Hempel's example is the noise it makes in the chest cavity) as its function; for freed of the requirement that E itself causally contributes to the maintenance of some general end state ES, one consequence of the heartbeat is as good as another to be emphasized as *the* function of the heart.

Thus, although the statement with which we began did not expressly mention either a system or an end state, both must be tacitly assumed if sense is to be made of such statements. In fact, of course, the contexts in which such statements are made will often expressly provide definitions of S and of ES.

What such explanations tell us is that there is a causal connection between the part or process to which a function is attributed and the existence of the end state. In vertebrates, the heart must beat in order for blood to circulate. This is a genuinely empirical claim that may be expressed equivalently in nonfunctional language as, "The blood circulates (in vertebrates) *only if* the heart beats."

Thus, functional explanations involve causal laws, but "in reverse": rather than explaining the heart's beating by reference to its *causes*, a functional explanation explains it by reference to one of its *effects* (the circulation of blood). The relationship of cause and effect is asserted in such explanations, but we are told what has been *caused by* the part or process about which we are curious, not what *causes it* to be or do what it does.

It has struck many people as decidedly peculiar that an *effect* of an event should be cited to explain it; it sounds much like the Aristotelian notion of a Final Cause, where some end causally determines the events that are its means. Yet nothing of the sort need be asserted in one's use of 'purpose' in the sense of function. In the first place, much of the use of functional statements such as that about heartbeats is not explanatory of the heartbeat at all; the attribution of functions in such statements is often merely a description of the heart or heartbeat that emphasizes certain of its features. Secondly, where function is used in an explanation, the effect *E* (e.g., the circulation of blood) that is called the function does not play the role of a cause of the item to be explained, the heartbeat. Each of these two legitimate uses of 'function' merits some discussion.

1. Where scientists share a common concern for a particular system and the maintenance of some particular end state in the system, the attribution of functions is a useful descriptive task. Thus, in medicine one is concerned with the human body, and there is widespread agreement among doctors on the desirability of maintaining that system in the particular end state we call health (a state seemingly characterized by the absence of pain, survival, and by the ability to engage in the normal activities of daily life). In such circumstances it is useful for medical texts to attribute functions to organs and other physical structures, or to their activities. Formulating medical information in this way serves to emphasize the causal contribution each organ or process makes to the maintenance of an end state that doctors seek to preserve. By classifying a great deal of information in such a way, one knows immediately the contribution of each part of the system to the end state desired for that system.

To be sure, the classifying of a good deal of causal information in this way, so as to emphasize just those features relevant to a particular undertaking, does not lead to *explanations* of why, for example, a heart beats. Functional statements in such situations are simply a mode of organizing information about parts of a system and their relationship of one another around a central concern. One can see this by schematizing functional statements such as the one quoted, as: for all S, ES only if P. From such a premise nothing can be deduced about any particular individual's heart beating or not. Yet such a premise does tell us that, *if* in general we are interested in maintaining system S in state ES, we must make certain P occurs. If we wish to keep patients alive, we must keep their hearts beating.

2. Beyond the organizational benefits of attributing functions, one may use such attributions as part of a genuine explanation of the event in question. To do this one must add the premise that the system in question will tend (within certain boundary conditions here ignored) to return to some particular end state. The structure of the argument is then: (1) the heart's beating (P) is a necessary condition for health (ES) in vertebrates (S) [ES only if P for all S]; *and* (2) the body will maintain itself in a state of health [for all S, ES]. From these premises, the conclusion P, follows by the rules of elementary logic. Thus, for systems that do in fact tend to return to some end state despite varying conditions in the environment, it is a legitimate form of explanation of a part or process to cite its function in the maintenance of some larger system. It is a matter for empirical discovery to what extent such self-regulating systems are to be found in nature or in human artifacts, such as homing devices on missiles, thermostats for furnaces, etc.; where there are such regularities, the attribution of functions and explanations in terms of them are appropriate.

Medicine is an obvious example that fits both of these requirements. It is concerned with a well-defined system in which numerous homeostatic balances are maintained (e.g., body temperature), and the maintenance of a particular state of that system is one about which doctors are much concerned. The latter is a sufficient ground for *attributing* functions to parts and processes in the body; the former allows one, in addition, to use that attribution of function as part of a genuinely empirical explanation of why we should expect to find that part or process occurring in some particular vertebrate's body.

The suspicions that functional explanations engender outside of medicine or biology largely result from the fact that functions are assigned in situations that do not meet either of the two criteria just discussed. Rather, some effect of a social practice or habit is singled out as *the* function of the practice in question, and treated as an explanation of such practice, without (1) any reason being given as to why we should be concerned about the particular end state of the system relative to which the function is assigned; or (2) any reason being given to believe that the system in fact tends to achieve the end state relative to which the function is assigned. We may be told, for example, that the function of a ceremonial rain dance among certain tribes is to reinforce group solidarity. While the reinforcement of group solidarity may be an effect of the practice in question, so are a lot of other things—tired feet, satisfaction at the completion of exercise, relaxation of group anxieties, etc. Absent some stipulation of an end state about which we are most concerned to maintain in such systems (societies), or which is in fact maintained in such systems, there is little to be gained by selecting this one effect of the action in question over a host of others for the emphasis as "the function." It is about as useful as saying that the function of the heart is to produce sounds in the chest cavity. Functions can be assigned only relative to end states, and are usefully assigned only when such end states are a matter of great interest to us to preserve, or are preserved irrespective of our interests in nature.

MOTIVES AND FUNCTIONS

The difference between functional explanations and motivational explanations should be relatively apparent from the foregoing exposition. Functional statements, if they explain an event at all, explain it in neither of the two ways that motives explain human actions: (1) assigning a function to an event is not to render that event intelligible in the same way that a possible motive renders an action intelligible, *viz.*, by exhibiting it as the *rational* thing to do; (2) nor does the function an action may serve in any way involve the mind of the actor—he need not believe his action will have the effect called its function, nor need he desire (in any sense) to bring about this effect. Each of these two fundamental distinctions is amplified below.

   1. Actions are rendered intelligible to us by motivational explanations because the latter presuppose a set of beliefs and desires that are intelligible in a given culture (since they are familiar to the members of that culture), and because such explanations exhibit the action in question as the rational thing to do in light of such intelligible beliefs and desires. Explaining an action by reference to some function it serves, however, is not to show the action as intelligible in this way. This is true, first, because one is not exhibiting the activities of hearts and of individuals in societies as rational when one assigns them a function. One is simply stating in rather peculiar form a causal connection between certain events and the maintenance of certain states in a larger system. Secondly, the effects that are labeled functions are often not the kinds of affairs men intelligibly desire, in any culture. As Peters once noted, "end-states are not goals like hunting a man, marrying a girl, or becoming Prime Minister. They are more mysterious states of quiesence, satisfaction, tension-reduction, and so on."[72]

2. Even more fundamentally, assigning a function to an action does not entail anything about the mind of the actor. To say that the function of my distributing leaflets is to aggravate local law-enforcement officials is to assert that such alienation was in fact a consequence of my action — a causal assertion that says nothing about my state of mind (although it has some other implications for further effects on some larger system, as discussed above). For such a result to have been my motive, I must have *believed* that such a causal connection existed; whether such an event is a consequence of my action is not only not sufficient but it is irrelevant, for I could well act with such a motive on the basis of a mistaken belief about a causal connection that does not exist. It is my beliefs and not the objective facts of the matter that are relevant to motive explanations, but not to functional ones. Similarly, for police baiting to have been my motive I must also have *desired* that the end state come about. Unless we all desire all those consequences of our actions that have some conservative impact on some system, the fact that my action has a function is irrelevant to whether I desired that one effect that the function picks out for emphasis over all the other effects of my action. Moreover, functional explanations do not exhibit the asymmetry in the modes of verification for first and third person usages that is characteristic of mental states. If I should know the functions my actions serve in some large system, I will have no privileged access to such knowledge; rather, I will arrive at it through the same recourse to observation and inference as any third-person observer. I have no such privileged access to what functions my actions serve as I may have over what I believe and what I desire. In short, functions have nothing to do with the actor's mind, and 'function' is not a mental word at all.

To these two differences may be added the highly related point that the scope of functional explanations is considerably different from the scope of motivational explanations. Except for metaphorical extensions to the actions of animals or of complex machines, our motive vocabulary is used to explain the *actions* of human beings. 'Function', however, shares no such restriction. While functions may be assigned to explain human actions (usually as having some contributing role in some larger social system), they are also used to explain purely physiological processes, or the movements of parts in man-made machines, or in fact any natural, unintelligent phenomenon with an end state meeting one of the criteria set forth earlier.

For each of these three reasons, then, functional explanations differ markedly in character from explanations in terms of motives. None of this is to say that in certain cases the function an action serves may not also be the actor's motive, in fact. Thus, for example, a historian writing about John Stuart Mill might assert that the writing by Mill of his autobiography served the function of placing before numerous readers the story of an unusual education. By implicit reference to a system (nineteenth-century English society), and to an end state for that system (a better-educated society, itself thought of as a possible necessary condition for successful democracy), a functional attribution could perhaps be made out here. Yet even if it can, the function served by Mill's action could also turn out to be Mill's motive for having written the book. If Mill adopted an outlook whereby he thought it desirable for society to be educated, and if he believed that publishing the tale of his own education would serve that purpose, and if in fact his beliefs and desires in this respect were the cause of his action, then the end was also his motive. All that is necessary for such a coincidence of function and motive is that the actor adopt the end state of the system as a goal for himself. The most obvious type of motive where such overlap may be most expected is in the moral sphere, where goals may be adopted as a social duty, that is, for social (i.e., systemic) reasons. For well-socialized individuals, the functions served by their actions in society (relative to certain end states, such as public order) will often be their motive, in fact, for those actions.

Such coincidences, of course, do not affect the differences in the logic of each of the two types of explanation. They do make more comprehensible the confusion between them.

Although there is a clear enough distinction between 'purpose' used as 'motive' and its use as 'function', functional explanations are often misunderstood as being motivational in nature. The upshot of this is not just that authors and audiences misapprehend the type of explanation that is being given (although this can be serious enough, because one then mistakes the proper methods of confirmation); this confusion also often leads to the framing of explanations that pass muster neither as functional explanations, nor as motivational explanations, but which *sound* explanatory because they are framed in the familiar idiom of motives. As Carl Hempel has observed:

This psychological association of the concept of function with that of purpose, though systematically unwarranted, accounts to a large extent for the appeal and the apparent plausibility of functional analysis as a mode of explanation; for it seems to enable us to 'understand' self-regulatory phenomena of all kinds in terms of purposes or motives, in much the same way that we 'understand' our own purposive behavior and that of others. . . . It tends to encourage the illusion that a profound understanding is achieved, that we gain insight into the nature of these processes by likening them to a type of behavior with which we are thoroughly familiar through daily experience.[73]

MOTIVES FOR DREAMING

With this typology in mind, I shall now return to the psychoanalytic explanation of dreams. It is most fruitful to proceed by giving a separate analysis of each of the three levels of purportedly motivational explanations earlier distinguished.

THE WISH TO SLEEP

Freud often spoke of the "double wish fulfillment brought about by dreams."[74] The two wishes to which he was referring are the preconscious wish to sleep, on the one hand, and the unconscious wish that is fantasized as fulfilled in the dream, on the other. The second is dealt with in the next subsection. The first, Freud thought, is "universal, invariably present, an unchanging wish to sleep." This wish to sleep *"must in every case be reckoned as one of the motives of formation of dreams, and every successful dream is a fulfillment of that wish* [emphasis in original]."[75]

The notion is that we dream in order to remain asleep. Freud thought that "all dreams are in a sense dreams of convenience: they serve the purpose of prolonging sleep instead of waking up."[76] Dreams serve this purpose by fantasizing the satisfaction of some disturbing impulse, usually a wish in its own right, and by so doing, lessening the demands of such impulses. If we dream of drinking a glass of water when we are thirsty, Freud's thesis is that this helps to relieve the feelings of demand for the water. If we dream of riding a horse when we, in real life, have a painful boil in a position that would make such an action difficult, this potentially sleep-disturbing sensation is diminished by a dream that denies it. "The currently active sensation is woven into a dream *in order to rob it of reality* [emphasis in original]."[77]

It should first be noted that this explanation does not, and was not intended to, explain the particular content of individual dreams. It is an explanation of dreaming as an activity in general. It is given in answer to the question, "Why do we dream?" not to the question, "Why did *he* dream *that*?" The content of the dream is explained by the wish or otherwise disturbing impulse (dealt with in the following section);

showing why the dreamer lessens the awakening tendency of such impulses by creating a dream at all is the burden of the wish-to-sleep hypothesis. "You dream to avoid having to wake up, because you want to stay asleep."[78]

The nature of the question posed gives a clue to the kind of answer we should expect. To seek an explanation, in *general*, of dreaming should not produce a motivational explanation at all. For our common experience renders highly unlikely that any one motive is always operative for a universal activity such as dreaming. People do not operate from just one motive on all occasions of working or joking or running. One usually has a variety of motives, some operative on some occasions, and some on others.

One might think that the same should be true of dreaming. On some occasions, we may wish to sleep as a means of getting away from a foreseeably unpleasant morning. Yet this is rare, and there is no reason to think that we *always* dream because we have some such want. Motives are usually assigned only for individual acts of individual persons, not across the board for human processes continually engaged in by us all.

A second clue to the nature of the explanation being given here may be found in the total lack, in all of Freud's work, of a single example where Freud got the patient to acknowledge the presence of a wish to sleep. In the case studies, and in the theoretical work on dreams, Freud simply postulated the presence of this supposedly preconscious wish.[79] Nowhere did he make the same kind of interpretive effort at recapturing the content of this preconscious wish as he made at recapturing the unconscious wishes of his patients. There is simply no evidence of a wish to sleep, nor did Freud even bother looking for any.

It is perhaps true that we do remain asleep when we dream, and there is thus some "behavioral evidence" of a wish to sleep. But it is also true that we move our eyes when we dream. Do we therefore wish to engage in rapid-eye-movement behavior, and is this a motive for dreaming?

There is, similarly, no evidence of a belief by the dreamer that dreaming will tend to keep him asleep. Freud again simply postulates the existence of the minor premise of the dreamer's supposed practical syllogism: "I am driven to conclude that throughout our whole sleeping state we know just as certainly that we are dreaming as we know that we are sleeping."[80] Freud was driven to such a strange conclusion only because he thought he had to complete a practical syllogism for the dreamer.

What he failed to perceive was that his central insight about dreams could be presented without any talk of a wish, motive, or intention to sleep (Freud used all such terms),[81] nor need he be "driven" to unnecessarily animistic conclusions because of the requirements of a practical syllogism. Freud's explanation of dreaming as an activity simply need not be motivational in character. In this instance, I think it rather clear that what Freud had in mind was an explanation of dreaming in terms of the *function* it served, not the motive dreamers invariably have for dreaming. Indeed, to speak of dreams as serving "the purpose of prolonging sleep" is the language of function, not of motive. Freud occasionally noticed the true nature of his explanation, as in his analogy to dreams of convenience:

The thirst gives rise to a wish to drink and the dream shows me that wish fulfilled. In doing so it is performing a function.... If I can succeed in appeasing my thirst by dreaming that I am drinking, then I need not wake up in order to quench it. This, then, is a dream of convenience.[82]

The language of wish and motive in such a case is wholly unnecessary to convey the insight Freud wished to convey. One of the *effects* of dreaming is that we are allowed to continue sleeping. Dreaming is (in those circumstances in which we are subject to disturbing stimuli) a necessary condition of sleeping.

In his transformation of this causal connection between dreaming and sleeping into a functional attribution (the purpose of dreaming is to sleep), Freud is consistent with the requirements examined earlier for significant functional accounts. A general end state (health) is assumed, inasmuch as one may at least plausibly think that sleeping is a contingently necessary condition of our health.[83] One thus has all the elements of a typical functional attribution: a system (the human organism), a process (dreaming) in the system to be explained, an effect of that process (sleep), and an end state, itself the effect of sleeping (health). One effect (the prolongation of sleep) is emphasized by labeling it as the function of the process, dreaming. Since sleep is necessary to health, that mode of emphasis is perhaps as justifiable here as elsewhere in medicine, *viz.*, if one is greatly interested in maintaining that particular end state, it is useful to index information by the causal contribution each part or process makes to the maintenance of it.

Beyond the advantages of classification by function, Freud also seems to hypothesize that the system is a self-adjusting one, so that the emphasis on the one effect of the process labeled its function is justified. Despite varying disturbances, dreaming tends to produce the same effect, namely, sleep. This, I think, is all that Freud is attempting to say when he states, in characteristically animistic fashion, that "all through the night the preconscious is concentrated upon the wish to sleep."[84] That is, like other teleological mechanisms, this one tends to produce one effect despite the intervention of varying conditions. Car governors, hearts, and guidance mechanisms in missiles do the same thing.

To translate Freud here as giving a functional account rather than a motivational one eliminates the problems earlier mentioned. There is no peculiarity in assigning *one* function to all occurrences of dreaming as there is in assigning one motive universally present. A "universal, invariably present, unchanging" biological function served by dreaming (namely, the preservation of sleep) is not nearly as implausible as is a psychological wish to sleep with the same characteristics. A functional interpretation also eliminates the difficulty of the lack of evidence of the existence of a wish to sleep. It also eliminates the need to posit beliefs of dreamers about the connection of dreaming and sleeping. One also avoids, with a functional interpretation, the thorny issue of whether a dream is an *action* that can be explained by motives. For as noted before, the range of explanations is broader for function than for motives; any sort of event or process may have a function, whereas only actions are explained by motives.

Construing the theory functionally also eliminates some of the confusions and puzzles of contemporary psychoanalytic dream theory. One need not wonder whether, to be consistent with the wish-to-sleep hypothesis, we should also hypothesize that "every person who is awake wishes to remain awake";[85] in neither case do we *wish* for such states. Nor need one puzzle over the lack of the "dynamic" character of the wish to sleep;[86] construing sleep as a function of dreaming eliminates any necessity of thinking of some dynamic state that *causes* dreaming. The dual nature of the wish to sleep—as a psychological wish and as a biological need—is also eliminated in the functional interpretation, for all the theory need postulate is a biological need to sleep, and thus to dream.[87] In addition, one would hardly debate "the obvious theoretical importance [of the] discovery of the omnipresence in dreams of the wish to sleep,"[88] if one understood that it is omnipresent only because it is the function assigned to all dreaming. Freud did not discover one of man's universal wishes, but only an unnoticed but perhaps important characteristic of dreams, namely, that one of their effects is that they tend to preserve sleep.

Whether in fact Freud's hypothesis here is correct is another matter. Does dreaming preserve sleep? The contemporary evidence suggests that it does not.[89] But in any case, translated functionally, the question can be resolved empirically, for one knows how to test an alleged causal connection of dreaming and sleeping. Cast a wish, however, disconfirmation of the causal connection of dreams to sleep would not disconfirm the "guardian-of-sleep" hypothesis. (For one's wishes may cause one to act, though the action fails to realize the object of the wishes. Indeed, in another context Freud regularly availed himself of this sort of escape hatch from disconfirmation; if the object of a wish is not fulfilled by a dream, "you can say nevertheless that a dream is an *attempt* at the fulfillment of a wish.")[90] Given the total lack of criteria for the "wish" to sleep, those who would test the hypothesis under its wish construction must simply wonder what else they are to test once they have disconfirmed the causal connection.[91]

WISH FULFILLMENT IN DREAMS

Unlike the preceding explanation, Freud's second "motive" in the formation of dreams is not universal, has no one content, and indeed, varies with each action. Freud cannot here be assigning a function to dreams, but must be attempting some more legitimate use of motivational terms in his explanation of why it is we dream of certain things. The claim of Freud to explain dreams as being fulfillments of wishes rests solely and squarely with this use of 'wish', 'motive', etc.

A convenient example with which to begin is Freud's explanation of his dream of a patient's injection. Freud dreamed that he had met his patient, Irma, in a hall with numerous guests. After admonishing her that any pain she still felt was her fault, Freud examined her throat. In doing so he attracted the attention of two other physicians who were Freud's real-life acquaintances. Freud in his dream placed nonsensical diagnoses in the mouths of one of these friends, and accused the other (Otto) of having given the patient an improper injection.

Analyzing the dream phrase by phrase, Freud believed he discovered the motives for such a dream in his desire for revenge against Otto for the latter's real-life reproaches against Freud, and in his desire to be exonerated from any responsibility for the failure of Irma's cure:

The meaning of the dream was borne in upon me. I became aware of an intention which was carried into effect by the dream and which must have been my motive for dreaming it. The dream fulfilled certain wishes which were started in me by the events of the previous evening (the news given me by Otto and my writing out of the case history). The conclusion of the dream, that is to say, was that I was not responsible for the persistence of Irma's pains, but that Otto was. Otto had in fact annoyed me by his remarks about Irma's incomplete cure, and the dream gave me revenge by throwing the reproach back on to him.

The dream acquitted me of the responsibility for Irma's condition by showing that it was due to other factors—it produced a whole series of reasons. The dream represented a particular state of affairs as I should have wished it to be. *Thus its content was the fulfillment of a wish and its motive was a wish* [emphasis in original].[92]

The evidence by virtue of which Freud inferred these wishes on his part was by and large limited to his waking thoughts, specifically, the preconscious thoughts produced by free association with each element of the manifest content of the dream. Thus, in deciding that one of his motives for the production of a dream of Irma's injection was revenge on Otto, Freud recalled: "I seemed to remember thinking something of the same kind that afternoon when his words and looks had appeared to show that he was siding against me."[93] As evidence of his "wish to be innocent of Irma's illness," Freud further noted: "I called to mind the obscure disagreeable impression I had when Otto brought me the news of Irma's condition."[94]

It is important to note that Freud did not remember having dreamed that he wished for these things—what he dreamed is just what he remembered and served only as the starting point for his free association. Rather, the phenomenological evidence on which Freud here relies is his memory of consciously thinking of such wishes in his waking life at some time prior to the dream. Neither did Freud have any memory of having dreamed what he dreamed because of such desires. The causal relevance of such wishes to the dream as dreamed is inferred by Freud in the same way Hume says we generally infer causation: we notice a regular concurrence between the two classes of events.

It is also interesting that many of the dreams reported in *The Interpretation of Dreams* are said to be wish fulfillments on precisely the same kind of evidence, that is, rather direct recall of consciously known wishes when the dreamer's memory is prompted by free association. None of them is explained by reference to the repressed unconscious wishes from childhood that Freud consistently throughout his career claimed were necessary to produce a dream.[95] Elsewhere, however, Freud did produce specimens of dreams (not his own) that were explained by a repressed, unconscious wish. It might seem that in such cases the evidence for the existence of such a wish must be different, but in fact it is not: in all cases the primary evidence for the existence of the wish responsible for the particular content of a particular dream is the dreamer's own subjective recall of what he has wished for in waking life. If the wish is repressed, then presumably the trains of association are less clear in their direction, or cannot be produced at all;

but in principle it is the same procedure that ultimately leads to the "motivating wish" of the dream, no matter how deeply such a wish may be repressed.

There is thus in none of Freud's examples or procedures any contradiction of the epistemic peculiarities of mental words, as long as one accepts the notion of "deferred privileged access" introduced earlier. Unlike the wish to sleep, there is evidence of the required sort for the existence of the unconscious wish, which Freud proposes as the explanation of the content of dreams. Problematic, however, is Freud's claim that this wish is the *motive* the dreamer has for dreaming the dream he dreams.

It strikes me that there are three main candidates for the kind of explanation possible here. First, we could take Freud at his word and try to make out a motivational explanation of an action. Freud's wish to be freed of responsibility for the failure of Irma's cure was his motive for dreaming the particular dream he dreamed. Secondly, one might claim that Freud was not really explaining how the particular dream occurred; rather, he was *interpreting* the dream, finding its *meaning*, not discovering its (motivational or nonmotivational) causes. On this account, the rationalizing but noncausal wishes discovered after the dream by free association have nothing to do with producing the dream; they are after-the-fact discoveries made by juxtaposing the manifest content of the dreams with the material produced by free association—an interpretive technique that may tell you something about yourself, but nothing at all of what caused your dreams. Finally, one might construe Freud's account as a nonmotivational, causal account of why this dream was produced; its (nonrationalizing) cause was the wish experienced previous to the dream's production. Each of these possibilities deserves separate consideration.

WISH FULFILLMENTS AS MOTIVES

There are two related reasons why Freud cannot be giving a motivational explanation with the wish-fulfillment hypothesis in dreams, despite all of the language of 'motive', 'intention', etc. First, there is no action to be explained by a motive here. Freud did not actively bring about the dream of Irma's injection, not for the motive he claims nor for any motive. His dream happened to him in the same way that the death of his father happened to him—in neither case did he bring about the occurrence (which is not to deny, in either case, that he might have had some wishes related to each event). Dreaming is like non-directional thinking—sudden inspirations, revelations, or images and the like—in that it just happens without the will or agency of the subject. And this does not mean that dreams and nondirectional thinking are chaotic; it means only that *we*, our acting selves, did not give such thoughts the order that they possess. We are not causally responsible for such thoughts or their order. Since motives make sense only when given to explain actions, 'motive' cannot here be intended by Freud.

In making such an objection one must, as earlier pointed out, have some criterion for action other than the "existence of a motive" criterion used by some contemporary action-theorists. Otherwise, Freudians could simply reply to the foregoing objection that the discovery of unconscious wishes is also the discovery that the seemingly unwilled *events* such wishes cause are really *actions* persons perform. This reply seems to be one of the major points of Roy Schafer's influential, recent book, *A New Language for Psychoanalysis*.[96] Because Schafer believes that "action is human behavior that has a point; it is meaningful human activity; it is intentional or goal-directed performance by people; it is doing things for reasons";[97] and because Schafer believes that psychoanalysis has shown that (almost) all human thinking and behavior is goal directed, he also conceives of all such thinking and behavior as human action: "thoughts come and go only as we think them or stop thinking them, or, in other words, that thinking is a kind of action engaged in by persons. We are responsible for all our thoughts, including as Freud pointed out, our dreams."[98] To assess the force of this Freudian rejoinder requires a brief excursion into contemporary action theory.

What an action is, is still an at best partly answered question in the philosophy of action. Much of the earlier work of the past several decades incorrectly interpreted various attributes incidentally true of certain species of *complex* actions as constituting the essence of human action itself. Much may be said about the various features of complex actions—that in our action descriptions we may incorporate reference to the consequences of the action,[99] the motive or intention with which the action under another description was done,[100] the circumstances under which it was done, or we may presuppose in our description the rules or conventions surrounding the activity in question, e.g., "castling a king."[101] Yet these features of action are not what we seek, for the relevant question about dreaming is not whether it is one or the other of these kinds of *complex* actions. Rather, the question necessary for a Freudian to answer is whether dreaming is a *basic* action.

A basic action is an action I do without there being some other action that I do in order to do it.[102] Usually, for example, when I raise my arm,

I do not do some (even more basic) action in order to raise my arm; I just raise my arm.[103] Hence, usually raising one's arm is a basic act. If, in contrast, I use wires and pulleys and my foot in such a way as to raise my arm, the action of raising my arm is a complex action because more basic actions were done (namely, moving my foot) in order to cause my arm to go up.

There are undoubtedly ways in which one can cause oneself to dream, and thus make a particular instance of "having a dream"[104] into a complex action. By drinking too little water, for example, one might wish to cause, and succeed in causing, a dream of convenience. Such examples hardly answer the relevant question here, however. Being satisfied with such examples would be like ending an investigation into whether most people can wiggle their ears by finding out that most people can wiggle their ears by wiggling them with their hands.

Hence, the relevant question is whether dreaming is a basic act that persons do (or can) perform. And to answer that question requires that we have a criterion of "basic act" that allows us in general to distinguish bodily movements or mental episodes that are our (basic) actions from those that are not. What we seek is an answer to Wittgenstein's famous question, "What is left over if I subtract the fact that my arm goes up from the fact that I raise my arm?"[105]

The answer of some contemporary action-theorists has been to explain, in terms of causation of movements by belief/desire sets, the difference between actions I do perform and movements of my body that I do not perform. Alvin Goldman, for example, defines a movement of a person's body as an action of that person if and only if the movement is intentional, and further specifies that a basic act is intentional if and only if that act is caused "in a certain characteristic way" by the agent's beliefs and desires.[106]

If this were an adequate analysis of action, then the objection interposed here would be no objection, for the discovery of unconscious wishes causing dreams (assuming *arguendo* that all elements of a practical syllogism were made out) would necessarily imply that dreams were actions we performed, not mere events that happened to us. Such analyses, however, are not adequate analyses of action.

The problem such accounts run into stems from counterexamples of the following kind: suppose an actor, Clyde, wishes to kill his pregnant girlfriend, Roberta, and believes that by throwing himself to one side of the rowboat in which they are sitting he will succeed in causing Roberta to drown. (She cannot swim, as Clyde well knows.) Suppose further that Clyde's desire, together with the belief that his desire could easily be fulfilled, causes him to slip and fall on one side of the boat, capsizing it and drowning Roberta. Clyde had a set of desires and beliefs of the requisite form ($p = p$ and $q = q$), and that set of mental states caused the event in question. Yet it is possible that the slip by Clyde was just that—a slip—and not an action on his part. It surely is not nonsense for an omniscient novelist to explain Clyde's motion in the foregoing way, and also to tell his readers that the movement of Clyde's body was *not* an action of his. True, we might be very suspicious that Clyde did perform the action of capsizing the boat (as were the police and the psychoanalyst surrogate in Dreiser's novel); but there is at least a factual question to be debated about whether Clyde's movements were an action. If the Goldman account of action were correct, then there would be nothing to argue about once we knew that Clyde's movements were caused by a rationalizing belief/desire set.

What such thought experiments show is that as a criterion of action, "causation by a belief/desire set that also rationalizes an action" is inadequate. What action theorists of Goldman's persuasion must do is refine their criterion of action to exclude counterexamples of the kind just discussed (usually called "deviant causal chains"). While there is no dearth of such attempts,[107] none thus far seems persuasive. Furthermore, such refinements as are usually offered to exclude these "deviant causal chains" would be of little comfort to Freudians of Schafer's persuasion. For such refinements usually exclude the unwanted counterexamples from the realm of action by supplementing the criterion of "belief/desire set causing a movement" with further mental states of intention or belief;[108] and for dreams, there is no evidence of the existence of such further states, leaving dreaming still on the "nonaction" side of the line. The end result is the same: one cannot show an event to be a human action just because it is caused by the subject's wishes and beliefs.

None of this is intended to suggest that there is no "conceptual connection" between the concepts of action and motivation. The proper domain for motive explanations is limited to actions. What is denied is that one can show an event to be an action by discovering unconscious motives; rather, one can discover unconscious motives only if what they are cited to explain turns out to be an action.

While the foregoing is sufficient to dispose of Schafer's kind of rejoinder, a Freudian might try a different line of attack to reach the desired conclusion that dreaming is an action. In the context of urging that we accept moral responsibility for the content of our dreams, Freud thought that we should not be "artificially limited to the metapsychological ego"; that "obviously one must hold oneself responsible for the evil impulses of one's dreams, because such an impulse not only 'is' in me but sometimes 'acts' from out of me as well"; that while it may be true that in the metapsychological sense this bad repressed content does not belong to my ego, but to the id, still "this ego developed out of the id, it forms with it a single biological unit, it is only a specifically modified, peripheral portion of it, [and] it is subject to the influences and obeys the suggestions that arise from the id."[109]

This comes close to saying that we really do perform an action when we dream, even if that overly proud part of ourself Freud calls 'ego' did not have a hand in it. Freud seems to be urging, first, that our *id* performs an action in sending forth a wish to be fantasized as fulfilled in a dream, and second, that we should identify ourselves as much with our id as with our ego.

Yet these assertions presuppose the structural aspect of psychoanalytic theory, not in its modern sense in which 'ego', 'id', and 'superego' name aggregations of functions—for how can an aggregation of functions perform an action? Rather, the structuralism presupposed is the negative idea that the self cannot be analyzed as a unitary agent, that we have no coherent sense of a person being one self, but only a series of agents, each of which is capable of performing actions for reasons.

Some regard this fragmentation of the self of Freudian metapsychology as a virtue, and anything that leads to it (such as motives for dreaming) thus acceptable. It may turn out that some characteristics of human beings force this fragmented view of the self upon us; self-deception is sometimes proposed as a candidate, but recent philosophical analyses of that phenomenon suggest that it does not necessitate the "little people" hypothesis.[110] Unless some such showing is made, it seems to me that stories about motivated actions of subagencies "within" a person differ not at all from the animism of primitive peoples, who might explain the movement of planets as resulting from their love of one another.[111]

In a unitary concept of self, we do not perform an action when we dream.[112] Our impulses (wishes) "arise" from the id—we do not do anything to call them forth; the censorship does metaphorical battle with such impulses, and a dream results. We—our personal selves—have nothing to do with all of these supposed events. In fact, not too surprisingly, *we* sleep through the whole process!

The second reason that the wishes fantasized as fulfilled in a dream are not the motives for dreaming it is the lack of any minor premise for the dreamer's practical syllogism. There are no *beliefs* by the dreamer that his "action" of dreaming would be a means to achieving the object of his wish. Freud did not believe that if he dreamed of Otto making an improper injection, then this would give him his desired revenge on Otto, nor did he believe that he could in fact be exonerated from responsibility for Irma's incomplete cure if he dreamed of a host of other factors causing her to remain ill. Freud reports no memory of such a belief, either as part of his dream or as part of his waking belief set. Nor is free association said to produce a memory of such a belief. Yet without such a belief, a crucial element of practical reasoning is missing, which leads one to conclude that the "action" is not to be understood on the model of practical reasoning (motives) at all.

There is a very small minority of dreams for which the requisite beliefs might more plausibly be suggested to be present in the dreamer, namely, counterwish dreams. Freud notes two types: those dreams that are created to demonstrate that he and his theories are wrong; and those he characterizes as mental masochism. To a patient who produces a dream that does not express a fulfilled wish, no matter how interpreted, Freud produced the following explanation: "Thus it was her wish that I might be wrong, and her dream showed that wish fulfilled."[113] To those dreams that appear only to frustrate, rather than to fulfill, the dreamer's wishes, Freud stated that they fulfilled the wish of the patient to be frustrated, i.e., to torture himself by refusing to allow the fantasies of dreaming to assuage his desires.

These are rather suspect formulations, to say the least (in light of the otherwise disconfirming nature of such dreams for Freud's wish fulfillment hypothesis). They are, however, used here only to illustrate a point about the more typical character of the dreams Freud talks about. Such counterwish dreams do bear the customary means/end relationship to the wish that is given to explain them. The motive in each case—a desire to prove the doctor wrong, or a desire to frustrate one's self—is fulfilled by the doing of the "action," i.e., the production of a dream with these contents. The patient does not fantasize in her dreams, "Freud is wrong," either verbally or by depicting a situation in which he is wrong. Rather, the having of the dream itself proves him wrong—that is one of its effects. Counterwish dreams are thus more like normal actions for which we can give motives, because Freud ascribes an actual effect they produce in waking life as their motive. In ordinary dreams, however, it is only the *fantasized* effect of the "action" that Freud ascribes as the motive.

For almost all other specimens of dreams that Freud analyzes, no such belief about the dream being a means to the actual attainment of the object of the desire can be made out. The sort of syllogism Freud could plausibly construct for such specimens is at most:

$$\frac{\begin{array}{l} D(q) \\ B(p \supset q) \end{array}}{\text{Dreams that } p}$$

(where "$D(q)$" means "Freud desires that he was not responsible for the failure of Irma's cure"; "$B(p \supset q)$" means "Freud believes that if Otto was responsible for the failure of Irma's cure, then he, Freud, was not responsible for the failure of Irma's cure"; and "Dreams that p" means "Freud dreams that Otto was responsible for the failure of Irma's cure.")

Such a practical syllogism cannot rationalize the "action" it is given to explain, because the logical relationships required do not obtain. More specifically, there is no identity between the antecedent in the content of the belief and the "action," i.e., the dream. "P" is not identical in meaning to "Dreams that p."

To make the above schema a practical syllogism requires a second belief. The kind of belief Freud would have to ascribe to his subjects would be a belief in the causal efficacy of fantasy. In the example used, this would be a belief by Freud that if he had the dream about Otto, then Otto would really be responsible for the failure of Irma's cure [B (Dreams $-$ that $- p \supset p$)]. Now it is at least arguable that the required relationships obtain. For if Freud believes "$p \supset q$," and Freud believes "Dreams $-$ that $- p \supset p$," then he arguably believes also "Dreams $-$ that $- p \supset q$," for the content of the latter belief is implied by the conjunction of the contents of the former two beliefs. It is only arguable because it is very unclear to what extent we are entitled to ascribe beliefs to a person simply because the contents of such beliefs are logically implied by the contents of beliefs that person clearly has. Assuming for purpose of argument that such a movement is legitimate, then Freud would make out a full practical syllogism:

$$\begin{array}{l} D(q) \\ \underline{B \text{ (Dreams} - \text{that} - p \supset q)} \\ \text{Dreams} - \text{that} - p \end{array}$$

The logical relationships required now obtain, namely $q = q$, and Dreams $-$ that $- p =$ Dreams $-$ that $- p$. The crux of the matter is to see whether Freud can justifiably posit a belief (during sleep) that fantasy is just as good as reality for the satisfaction of desire, in order to complete the practical syllogism for himself or his patients.

This is, I think, approximately what Freud attempted to do in his "Metapsychological Supplement to the Theory of Dreams," published sixteen years after the first edition of *The Interpretation of Dreams*.[114] For Freud held that the "dream-wish. . .is hallucinated, and, as an hallucination meets with belief in the reality of its fulfillment."[115] Freud likened the state of dreaming to amentia, or hallucinatory wish-psychosis, and to earliest infancy, when reality testing has not yet deprived us of the tendency to hallucinate the satisfying object when- ever we feel the need of it. In all such states, Freud asserted, hallucina- tion brings belief in reality with it.

The question one wants to raise about such a belief is the question of criteria. By no ordinary criterion can Freud be said to have believed that by dreaming the dream he reports, Otto would be made responsible and Freud exonerated. At no point does Freud acknowledge such a belief, nor does he ever seek an acknowledgment from his patients of such a belief (as he does for the companion wish). Rather, Freud gives an elaborate theoretical account of such belief in terms of his topo- graphical metapsychology. Thus, we are told that there is "topographi- cal regression" in the dream work: the dream-instigating unconscious wish enters the preconscious in the guise of a wish-fulfilling fantasy; while in ordinary waking life such an impulse would enter conscious- ness or be "discharged" by motor activity, in dreams the impulse "pursues a retrogressive course, through the unconscious, to percep- tion, which forces itself upon consciousness." Since perception (itself a "system" in chapters 7-8 of *The Interpretation of Dreams*) is bound up with our beliefs in reality, Freud's thought is that the retrogressive course of this impulse allows it to enter consciousness as real: "when once a thought has followed the path to regression as far back as to the unconscious memory-traces of objects and thence to perception, we accept the perception of it as real."[116]

Whether such speculation by Freud is a good or a bad theory is not a point I need address. The only point important here is that it makes 'belief' a term defined by some such theory, not the name of a familiar mental state that has an assigned place in the scheme of explanation that is the practical syllogism. While one may define theoretical terms as one pleases, and even call them 'belief' if one chooses, one may not substitute such terms in to satisfy the demands of an existing schema and claim that the schema is satisfied just because the word 'belief' was used. To make out a motivational explanation, Freud needed to dis- cover a belief, not postulate a new theoretical entity labeled 'belief'.

For each of these reasons, the wishes that Freud tells us are fanta- sized as fulfilled in dreams cannot explain dreams as motives explain actions performed in waking life. A more difficult question is whether such wishes explain dreams at all.

WISHES AND MEANINGS

One possibility that has gained much favor is to construe Freud's wish- fulfillment hypothesis as nonexplanatory.[117] According to this view,

Freud did not set out to explain the content of dreams by their causal antecedents, but merely wished to build an interpretative "map" that would allow him to see the *meaning* of dreams. Support for this view is garnered by Freud's likening his task to that of one who must interpret a picture puzzle,[118] for the meaning one is to find in picture puzzles need not be motivational. Such meaning need only be the "observer meaning" earlier mentioned. Construing the wish-fulfillment hypothesis in this way would result in it being a maxim of interpretation, restricting the (observer) meanings to be sought to: (1) fantasized fulfillment of wishes, and (2) those wishes that are unconscious wishes of the interpreter who is also the dreamer. Following such a maxim of interpretation would allow one to exhibit the dream as minimally rational, because there is a belief/desire set that could have been a motive for dreaming the dream. It would be only minimally rational, because of the irrational belief required (fantasy is reality) in order to complete the practical syllogism. In addition, it does not exhibit the action as rational for the particular dreamer, because only one element of the practical syllogism is a mental state possessed by the dreamer.

Such an interpretation of Freud's theory of dreams has two startling consequences. First, the theory would not be a theory of dreams. It would be a theory about the laws of association, to the effect that if one free associates to elements of one's own dream, one will eventually uncover one's own unconscious wishes. Yet if all one is doing is after-the-fact interpretation—if, that is, the wishes do not *explain* the dream—this law of association would seem to hold for any subject matter relatively rich in suggestive symbols. Free association to the elements of another person's dream, a picture, a cloud formation, etc., would also probably lead to discovery of one's own wishes, even though the starting points for the trains of association were not authored by the interpreter. Hence, the wish-fulfillment hypothesis would be a hypothesis only about what happens when a person free associates; there would be no hypotheses about dreaming as such at all.

Moreover, the wish-fulfillment hypothesis would be only one interpretive maxim among others equally good. To get around the obvious fact that most dreams do not directly express wish fulfillments, Freud hypothesized the distortion of the dream work; most dreams express *in distorted form* the fulfillment of wishes. Yet once one allows the introduction of such secondary interpretive principles to account for all the obvious counterexamples, then seeing a dream as a fulfillment of wishes is only one of many possible interpretive schemata. It is probably true that as many dreams directly express, say, anxiety as directly express wishes as fulfilled. It is also probably true that free associations also lead to those anxieties of the subject. As long as one allows the considerable leeway for "distortion" that the dream work allows, the "anxiety maxim" at interpreting dreams is just as good as the wish-fulfillment maxim. Both are merely interpretative maxims, heavily qualified by secondary principles of interpretation — the principles of distortion. There might be therapeutic grounds for preferring one to the other, but therapeutic efficacy is hardly to be confused with truth. Telling a patient that his dream is a fantasized fulfillment of his wishes may help him, just as telling a religious patient that God will watch over him may help him; but in both cases the truth of what is told the patient is not affected by the therapeutic efficacy of the statements.

The result of this "hermeneutic" interpretation of Freud's dream theory is to trivialize it completely. Freud himself was careful to eschew any such interpretation of his work.[119] Although he did see his task as *in part* being interpretation, the interpretation of dreams as fantasized fulfillment of wishes was a therapeutic interpretation only because it was also a true explanation of dreams. He sought, in other words, to explain dreams as well as to interpret them. Since the explanations cannot be motivational, Freud must be taken to provide the kind of causal explanation in terms of wishes, to be examined next.

WISHES AS CAUSES

Freud's intent was pretty clearly to explain dreams as caused by unconscious wishes. Although he may have thought his explanation to be motivational, it is not. Rather, it is the kind of partial practical syllogism earlier analyzed as causation without rationalization. Such an explanation depends on two testable hypotheses: do dreams always express unconscious wishes, which free association to the dreams will reveal? And if so, do such wishes cause the dream to have the manifest content it has?

Whatever might have been Freud's intentions, it may of course turn out that the most his theory can amount to is a set of maxims of interpretation, such as just discussed. Whether that is so depends on whether his explanatory account of dreams is true. One of the striking facts about dreams for a Freudian has to be that most dreams do not, in any straightforward way, express wishes. One need not even resort to counterexamples such as punishment dreams, anxiety dreams, counterwish dreams, or other unpleasant or distressing dreams; dreams with no emotional tone at all also do not express wishes in the straightforward way that many of the dreams of children do. Accordingly, if the wish-fulfillment hypothesis is not to be regarded as just obviously false, Freud needed some account of how the unconscious wishes that cause the dream to have the content of a wish fulfillment come to be so unrecognizably distorted. Explaining this was the function of that complicated set of processes Freud called the dream work. This is the last of the three major levels of explanation in the psychoanalytic theory of dreams, to which I now turn.

THE PROCESSES AND THE MOTIVES OF DISTORTION

"Why is it," Freud asked, "that dreams... do not express their meanings undisguised?"[120] Freud's answer came in two parts. First, he purported to discover a series of processes known as the dream work; then he explained why each of the processes occurred by reference to the unconscious motives of the dreamer.

THE DREAM WORK AS A PROCESS

How one conceives of the dream work depends on how one conceives of the wish-fulfillment hypothesis. If the latter is only an interpretive maxim to exhibit the dream as minimally rational, then the former need not be thought of as a process at all but only a second interpretive maxim qualifying the first. But if one construes Freud as intending an explanation with the wish-fulfillment hypothesis, then the dream work must be thought of as a set of processes that occur and cause the latent dream thoughts (unconscious wishes) to be transformed into the manifest content of the dream. Consistent with his intent regarding the explanatory nature of wishes, Freud intended "the dream work" to name a set of processes.

Freud referred to four things by his use of "the dream work": condensation, displacement, considerations of representability, and secondary revision. By condensation, Freud meant that one element in the manifest content of a dream could represent many latent dream thoughts, as, for example, one person in a dream appears to represent several people we have known in waking life. Our latent dream thoughts are "condensed" into one image in our dream.

Displacement is an off-centering of these "psychical intensities" of a dream. What is "off center" is the meaning of the dream: the true meaning is not to be found by implication from the manifest content, but rather it has been "displaced" in various ways, as by displacing our true feeling for one person onto another about whom we are in waking life indifferent. In such a case, one ends up with an emotion inappropriate to the manifest content of a dream, which is good (but not inevitably present) evidence of a displacement.

By "considerations of representability," Freud meant to say that a condition of a dream thought being expressed is that it doff verbal garb for a pictorial representation. Thinking in dreams is done largely in terms of pictorial images, and Freud takes some pains to deny the apparent counterexamples to that hypothesis—solving problems, forming judgments, and making arguments in dreams are not in fact done at the time of dreaming but are lifted wholecloth from memory of having done so before in waking life.

"Secondary revision" is a kind of repiecing of the puzzle. It is, Freud tells us, the first interpretation of the dream performed while we are yet asleep, a performance that gives the dream a nominal order and a semblance of sanity.

While displacement is "nothing less than the essential portion of the dream work," and is "one of the chief methods by which . . . distortion is achieved,"[121] each of the four parts of the dream work distorts the true meaning of a dream. To condense many dream thoughts into a composite is to disguise each of them. The necessity for transforming thoughts into visual images helps to "explain the appearance of the fantastic absurdity in which dreams are disguised."[122] Secondary revision, while allowing dreams to "appear to have a meaning," in fact "creates a meaning for dreams as far removed as possible from their true significance."[123]

The problem for all of this is that there is no direct evidence for the dream work as a *process* (rather than as an interpretive maxim). We have no phenomenological evidence for the dream work considered as a process—while we can remember, sometimes only via analysis, the wish that was the cause of the dream, we cannot remember the condensation of ideas into one, the displacement of them, ordering, etc. We can only observe: (1) that certain words in dreams, particularly those referring to people, seem via their associations to lead to a rather diverse variety of things; (2) that the inappropriateness of affects to the manifest content of a dream does on occasion strike us as peculiar upon remembering a dream; (3) that dreams are largely cast in visual images; and (4) that dreams often exhibit, not chaos, but a certain insane order, as if they were put together hastily by an idiot.

This kind of phenomenological evidence must have been the basis of Freud's insight into the dream work. Freud does not and cannot, however, label these characteristics of dream memories themselves by the names of the four types of dream work. Rather, he infers from these characteristics the existence of processes taking place during the dream and producing memories, with these characteristics as their corresponding effects. (These processes do not follow one another in time, seriatim, but are conceived by Freud as occurring together throughout the dream. Freud nonetheless believes them to be processes.) So considered, Freud's explanation of the distortion in dreams then becomes an attempted causal explanation: that dreams are remembered in distorted form is caused by the occurrence of these processes.

Since the subcategories of the dream work are not experiential terms—and Freud never claimed that anyone experienced or remembered experiencing these things—there is no way of giving definition to the dream work as process. Without some definition independent of that which we would explain—distortion—then the purported explanation is merely tautologous. Perhaps physiology will save the day here, by giving such processes some independent definition. Unless and until it does so, however, the dream work as a process is a specification of the functional steps that would have to be performed if the wish-fulfillment hypothesis is true; but the physical realization of those functional steps can only at this stage be speculated upon.

The dream work as a process thus remains a problematical hypothesis. It is at most a research program not yet begun, not an established proposition in a well-tested theory. Without some adequate account of the dream work as a process, Freud's wish-fulfillment hypothesis is equally problematic, for without an adequate explanation of distortion, Freud's theory that every dream represents a fulfillment of a wish is quite obviously false as a causal theory.

If the dream work is as yet only a specification of the functional steps that would have to exist if the wish-fulfillment hypothesis were true, then any *explanation* of the dream work is equally the hostage of successful future research. Still, it is worth examining briefly Freud's account, for it again purports to be a motivational account of why we distort our dreams.

MOTIVES FOR THE DREAM WORK

Freud gave a variety of specific explanations for each of the processes of the dream work. Condensation, for example, occurs because of the necessity of overdetermination for any latent dream thought to become manifest. What Freud had in mind here was that latent dream thoughts themselves have "psychic intensities." Presumably the most intense find expression in dreams. Yet even the most intense dream thought must "join forces" with others to find its way into the dream; thus they form composite images, and we find condensation. To understand the purportedly motivational character of the dream work, however, one must focus on displacement. Freud considered displacement to be "nothing less than the essential portion of the dream work," and one of the "chief methods by which distortion is achieved."

Freud explains displacement (and thus distortion, too) as the means by which the latent dream thoughts escape the censorship imposed by repression. To be expressed in the manifest content of a dream, a latent dream thought must not only be conjoined with other unconscious thoughts (leading to condensation), pictorially represented, and given a semblance of order (by secondary revision), it must also be distorted so that it may escape undetected the censorship supposedly attached to our repressed desires.

What Freud seems to be saying is that distortion is a form of pain-avoidance behavior. Since certain latent thoughts (namely, those that are repressed) are too abhorrent to be given direct expression, they must be distorted to find their way into the dream at all.

For what is distressing may not be represented in a dream; nothing in our dream thoughts which is distressing can force an entry into a dream unless it at the same time lends a disguise to the fulfillment of a wish.[124]

For example, in the dream of Irma's injection Freud displaced affection onto a colleague for whom it was not appropriate in the context of the dream. "The affection in the dream...was calculated to conceal the true interpretation of the dream....Distortion was shown in this case to be deliberate."[125]

Consider also two examples of distortion that are not displacements (and do not fit neatly into the four categories of dream work): (1) the judgment in dreams that "this is only a dream" "is intended to detract from the importance of what is being dreamt"; and (2) when one dreams that he is dreaming, the wish fulfilled by the dream is one of resistance, to disguise the repressed wish so that it may not be recognized: "the intent is, once again, to detract from the importance of what is being dreamt in the dream, to rob it of its reality."[126]

Despite the considerable language of deliberation, calculation, and intentional action, I do not think Freud could make out a motivational explanation here (the motive for distortion being the avoidance of distressing thoughts), nor need he have tried. The former, because *none* of the elements of practical reasoning analyzed earlier are even asserted by Freud to be present here. First, we plainly do not perform an action when we distort our dreams via displacement. Indeed, in this case the lack of an action is particularly glaring, since there is not even any behavior of a person here at all, voluntary or involuntary; displacement is an internal process Freud postulated to occur within the organism during sleep. It is thus unlike dreaming itself, slips of the tongue, or neurotic symptoms, since each of these is at least an overt behavior (although often not an action). Freud again resorts to his metapsychological thesis of the fragmented person: the motives for distortion are not assigned to the subject as an integrated person, but to some hypothetical subagency, the censor, who performs the "action" to be explained. "The purpose of which the censorship exercises its offices and brings about the distortion of dreams: it does so *in order to prevent the generation of anxiety or other forms of distressing affect* [emphasis in original]."[127] Whatever may be the merits of this early version of Freud's structuralism, in no event is this to say that *we* perform an action, the distortion of our dreams.

Secondly, as might be expected, when *we* do not perform any actions for motives (but our "censors" do), we as persons do not have any first-person knowledge or memory of: (1) a belief that distortion via displacement will conceal from ourselves otherwise distressing thoughts; (2) a desire or wish not to be distressed. Nor (3) is there any evidence that such a belief and such a desire caused the distortion of the latent dream thoughts. In short, none of the elements of practical reasoning essential to a motive explanation (whether of the conscious or unconscious variety) is present for the nonaction that a hypothetical subagency within ourselves performs.

What Freud could have meant is that distortion has as its *function* the avoidance of pain. Like repression itself, the assertion would be that our thoughts, in dreams as elsewhere, through some as yet unknown mechanisms, avoid direct expression of painful ideas. Since avoidance of pain is thought to be both the effect of a distortion and the cause of a more general end state of well-being, we may emphasize its importance by saying that it is *the* function of distortion.

Stating it in this way, I believe, identifies more precisely what is and what is not being claimed about displacement and distortion. If displacement did not occur, so that dreams would be dreamed and remembered in undistorted form, we would wake up from the disturbing wish that causes us to dream; since we need to sleep in order to remain healthy, displacement (ultimately) is a necessary condition for the general end state of health, because it allows sleep to go on while the fantasized wish fulfillment defuses the otherwise disturbing wish. Such, I think, is the core of Freud's claim here, none of which requires talk of "the motives of distortion."[128]

It is worth re-emphasizing, of course, that even so construed, the explanation is hostage to some independent definition of displacement as a process. For as it stands, displacement is simply a hypothesis about the kind of process that would be necessary if the contents of dreams are caused by wishes. Only if there really is some process that answers to this hypothesis can one assign to *it* the function of pain-avoidance.

CONCLUSION

The conclusion of this last part of the article may be simply stated: despite the motivational regalia with which Freud clothed his various explanations of dreams, none of such explanations are truly motivational in character. I suspect that a similar analysis of other phenomena explained by the theory, such as parapraxes or neurotic symptoms, would reveal similar results, although the explanation of *some* slips and some symptoms are probably genuinely motivational in character because one can legitimately make out an action and the required beliefs.

The importance of this conclusion lies in several directions. First, clarity can be a goal in itself. Freud himself was concerned with "introducing the right abstract ideas whose application to the relevant material of observation will produce order and clarity in it."[129] An interpretative effort such as the foregoing can be seen as a continuation of Freud's concern for the clearest exposition of his theory. Secondly, those who would test the theory must know what it is they would test. To look for a function *served by* dreaming is to look for something different from a wish *causing* dreaming; to search for nonrationalizing but causally operative wishes is to search for something other than motives for dreaming.

Thirdly, the implications of psychoanalytic theory for our assessments of responsibility in morals and law depends on the conclusions reached in an enterprise such as this. A psychoanalytic explanation of a dream (or a slip or a symptom) is often thought to show that the person was responsible for the dream, that it was something he did for motives; such an implication seems to hold even if the motives are unconscious.[130] Yet such an implication holds only if psychoanalytic explanations are truly motivational in character. For once we perceive that dreams are not productions we stage for reasons, but are events caused by wishes, then we can be said to be morally responsible for dreams only in the attenuated, Aristotelean sense that we are responsible for the character that includes such wishes.[131] Most of us, the Bible notwithstanding, do not equate responsibility for a wish with that for an action that fulfills it. Hence, to say that our character (which includes our wishes) is revealed by our dreams, is not to say that dreams are motivated actions for which we are responsible.

Fourthly, the interpretation suggested herein may drive a wedge between theory and therapy in psychoanalysis. For if success in therapy depends upon getting the patient to accept a dream, slip, etc., as a motivated action for which he is responsible, whereas in fact the explanation the theory generates is such that no such implication of responsibility holds, then successful therapeutic suggestions will not be successful because they are also true explanations. We would not be cured because we have come to see the truth about ourselves; rather, we are cured because we have come to accept an account that is not true and a responsibility that is not ours.[132] If such a "wedge" is to be avoided, then successful therapy cannot be seen as getting us to accept responsibility for dreams as motivated actions we perform; rather, therapy would be successful when the patient accepts responsibility for being the sort of person he is, that is, a person who has the wishes his dreams express. If that is all successful therapy requires, then there need be no "wedge" between theory and therapy, for the latter would only presuppose a form of explanation that the former can deliver.

Fifthly, and finally, the general thesis with which I began—about the chasm that exists between motivational parts of the theory and its supposedly causal accounts—will have to be redrawn. There are, I think, valid distinctions to be drawn between the particular accounts of particular actions given by psychoanalysts, and the more general accounts attempted by the more abstract parts of the theory. The only point here is that such distinctions may not be so simply drawn as some distinction between motives and causes.

NOTES

1. See A. Flew, "Psychoanalytic Explanation," *Analysis*, vol. 10 (1949); reprinted in M. MacDonald, ed., *Philosophy and Analysis* (Oxford: B. Blackwell, 1954); A. Flew, "Motives and the Unconscious," *Minnesota Studies in the Philosophy of Science*, vol. 1 (Minneapolis: University of Minnesota Press, 1956); R. S. Peters, *The Concept of Motivation* (London: Routledge and Kegan Paul, 1958); A. C. MacIntyre, *The Unconscious* (London: Routledge and Kegan Paul, 1958); J. Ehrenwald, "Cause, Purpose and Meaning in Psychosomatic Medicine," *Journal of Experimental and Clinical Psychopathology* 11 (1950), 164-173; A. R. Louch, *Explanation and Human Action* (Berkeley and Los Angeles: University

of California Press, 1969); Roy Schafer, *A New Language For Psychoanalysis* (New Haven, Conn.: Yale University Press, 1976). Others have adopted a modified stance urging the value of the purely causal aspects of the theory. See M. Sherwood, *The Logic of Explanation in Psychoanalysis* (New York: Academic Press, 1969); P. Ricoeur, *Freud and Philosophy* (New Haven, Conn.: Yale University Press; and M. Eagle, "A Critical Examination of Motivational Explanation in Psychoanalysis," this volume.

2. Indeed, Freud complained late in life about the lack of any revision of the theory of dreams: "The analysts behave as though they had no more to say about dreams, as though there was nothing more to be added to the theory of dreams." S. Freud, *New Introductory Lectures on Psycho-Analysis. The Standard Edition of the Complete Psychological Works of Sigmund Freud*, 22 (1933 [1932]), 8. (Unless otherwise specified, all citations to Freud hereafter are to the *Standard Edition* [SE].) For a contemporary example of the degree to which the psychoanalytic dream theory remains where Freud left it in 1900, see Nagera, ed., *Basic Psychoanalytic Concepts on the Theory of Dreams* (New York: Basic Books, 1969). See also R. Fliess, *The Revival of Interest in the Dream: A Critical Study of Post-Freudian Psychoanalytic Contributions* (New York: International Universities Press, 1953), for a summary of what developments there have been in psychoanalytic dream theory since Freud.

3. Michael Scriven, for example, at times a severe critic of the theory, nonetheless considers Freud's dream theory to be a "brilliant conception." See M. Scriven, "The Experimental Investigation of Psychoanalysis," in Hook, ed., *Psychoanalysis, Scientific Method, and Philosophy* (New York: New York University Press, 1959), p. 250.

4. From the preface to third (revised) English edition of *The Interpretation of Dreams*, SE, 4 (1931) xxxii, written by Freud in 1931: "This book, with the new contribution to psychology which surprised the world when it was published, remains essentially unaltered. It contains, even according to my present-day judgment, the most valuable of all the discoveries it has been my good fortune to make. Insight such as this falls to one's lot but once in a lifetime."

5. See the review by Talcott Parsons in *Daedelus* 103 (1973), 91-96.

6. Freud, *Interpretation of Dreams*, p. 96.

7. Freud, *Introductory Lectures on Psycho-Analysis*, SE, 15 (1916 [1915-1916]), 106.

8. Ibid., p. 94.

9. Freud's "psychic determinism" is a postulate he relies on throughout the whole of psychoanalytic theory, not merely as a justification for trying to find meaning in dreams. A slip of the tongue, for example, could not in principle be explained adequately in terms of fatigue or other physical predispositions, even if those dispositions were sufficient causes: "Even though it may have been given a physiological explanation," the slips would "remain a chance event from the psychological point of view." Freud, *Introductory Lectures*, p. 32. Contrary to what Freud sometimes thought, such a postulate of psychic determinism does not follow from a determinist world view and cannot be supported by it alone. Thus, Freud's claim that anyone who believes that parapraxes are simply accidental "has thrown overboard the whole *Weltanschauung* of science," (*Introductory Lectures*, p. 32), or the more contemporary claim that the interpretation of dreams as wish fulfillments "is based on a deterministic assumption that everything has a cause and an effect" (B. B.

Wolman, *The Unconscious Mind* [Englewood Cliffs, N.J.: Prentice-Hall], p. 22), is simply wrong. For a more explicit separation of "psychic determinism" from ordinary scientific determinism, see Wesley Salmon, "Psychoanalytic Theory and Evidence," in Hook, *Psychoanalysis, Scientific Method and Philosophy*, pp. 252-267.

10. Freud, *Introductory Lectures*, p. 85.

11. Freud, *Interpretation of Dreams*, p. 512.

12. Ibid., p. 506.

13. Freud, *Introductory Lectures*, p. 120. Freud's more typical formulation is to treat the latent dream thoughts as "carriers" of the meaning: "It is from these dream thoughts and not from a dream's manifest content that we disentangle its meaning." Freud, *Interpretation of Dreams*, p. 277. R. M. Jones comes to a conclusion regarding dream thoughts similar to that discussed in the text in "Dream Interpretation and the Psychology of Dreaming," *Journal of the American Psychoanalytic Association* 13 (1965), 304-319.

14. One may have noticed that there is a fourth motivational explanation in the exposition of Freud's dream theory presented here, namely, that we have motives for selectively reporting our dreams. I have ignored such motives because they are not part of the psychoanalytic explanation of dreams but are given to explain our act of relating a dream in a particular way at a later time. Furthermore, discussion of such motives would involve an analysis of the important idea of *resistance*, an idea having far-reaching implications throughout psychoanalytic theory, not just for dreams.

15. There is a long-standing dispute among classicists as to precisely what Aristotle meant by "practical syllogism" in the scattered writings in which he used the expression. The sense of practical syllogism that I intend is that sense synonymous with certain contemporary accounts of what it means to explain actions by reasons. For an explicit defense of this view of practical syllogisms, see M. Nussbaum, "Practical Syllogisms and Practical Science," in *Aristotle's De Motu Animalum* (Princeton N.J.: Princeton University Press, 1977).

16. I have been influenced most heavily in the account that follows by D. C. Dennett, "Mechanism and Responsibility," in Honderich, ed., *Essays on Freedom of Action* (London: Routledge and Kegan Paul, 1973); and Donald Davidson, "Action, Reasons and Causes," *Journal of Philosophy* 60 (1963), 684-700.

17. One may make explicit the basic presupposition of rationality implicit in practical syllogisms by transforming the schema presented here from a schema of reasoning into a schema of explanation. While a reasoning agent will not often say to himself, "I am rational," as he reasons about some particular action, an explanation schema must include such a premise if it is to conform to the deductive model of explanation. Such an explanation schema would be:

$$\frac{\begin{array}{l} D(q) \\ B(p \supset q) \\ [D(q) \cdot B(p \supset q)] \supset p \end{array}}{p}$$

Where "$D(q)$" in the text example means "x desired that the wine be chilled," "$B(p \supset q)$" means "x believed that if he opened the window, then the wine would be chilled," and "$[D(q) \cdot B(p \supset q)] \supset p$" means "if x desired that the wine be chilled, and if x believed that, if he opened the window, the wine would be chilled, then x opened the window," and "p" means "x opened the window."

The third premise is a basic presupposition of rationality, for it asserts that the agent is rational in a very fundamental sense of "rational," namely, that he is a creature who uses his actions as means to achieve the objects of his desires. Some more stringent senses of rational are explored in a later section of this article. An even more stringent sense is developed in M. S. Moore, "Some Myths About 'Mental Illness,'" *Inquiry* 18 (1975), 233-265 (reprinted in *Archives of General Psychiatry* 32 (1975), 1483-1497), to take into account the obvious fact that an agent will often have more than one set of desires and beliefs bearing on any action.

We notice these presuppositions of rationality most when they are in question, as for the mentally ill or for those who suffer from weakness of will. In this regard, see M. S. Moore, "Legal Conceptions of Mental Illness," in B. Brody and T. Engelhardt, eds., *Mental Illness: Law and Public Policy* (Dordrecht: Reidel; 1980).

18. Whether motivational explanation is a species of causal explanation has been a much disputed matter in contemporary philosophy. One may trace the dispute by beginning with chapter 4 of Gilbert Ryle's *The Concept of Mind* (London: Hutchinson, 1949). For further discussions of this problem, see the articles by R. S. Peters, J. O. Urmson, and D. J. McCracken, presented at a symposium entitled "Motives and Causes," *Proceedings of the Aristotelian Society* 26 (1952), 139-194; R. S. Peters, *The Concept of Motivation* (London: Routledge and Kegan Paul 1958); P. Winch, *The Idea of a Social Science* (London: Routledge and Kegan Paul, 1958); A. I. Melden, *Free Action* (London: Routledge and Kegan Paul, 1961); and the excellent summary of arguments in Davidson, "Actions, Reasons and Causes." See also G.E.M. Anscombe, *Intention* (Ithaca, N.Y.: Cornell University Press), particularly secs. 5–15; A. I. Goldman, *A Theory of Human Action* (Englewood Cliffs, N.J.: Prentice-Hall), pp. 72-85; and the articles by R. S. Peters and Steven Toulmin, under "Reasons and Causes," in Borger and Cioffi, eds., *Explanation in the Behavioural Sciences* (Cambridge: Cambridge University Press, 1970). I will assume without argument here that motives are a species of causal explanation.

19. This is not to say that we never act for "mixed motives." Of course we do, just as many events in the world (other than actions) are caused by several factors. There are two sorts of mixed-motive cases: (1) where each belief/desire set was sufficient (overdetermination cases); and (2) where each set was necessary. Irrespective of what sort of mixed motives one has when one acts, it remains true that of all the belief/desire sets we may have that would rationalize an action, only those that (jointly or singly) cause it are the motives for that action.

20. E. Jones, "Rationalization in Everyday Life," *Journal of Abnormal Psychology* 3 (1908).

21. The reason for adding this last condition will become apparent only later in the discussion. Briefly, it is added to make explicit that only behavior independently established as an intentional action can be explained by motives; thus, the account of motivation developed herein is not subject to the counterexamples of wayward causal chains used against certain theorists of action or intentionality. See notes 106-108 and the corresponding text.

22. Ernst Nagel, "Methodological Issues in Psychoanalytic Theory," in S.

Hook (ed.), *Psychoanalysis, Scientific Method, and Philosophy* (New York: New York University Press, 1959) pp. 38-56, at p. 47.

23. Freud, "The Unconscious," in *Collected Papers*, Vol. IV (New York: Basic Books, 1959) pp. 98-136. See *id*. at 104. "In psycho-analysis there is no choice for us but to declare mental processes to be in themselves unconscious, and to compare the perception of them by consciousness with the perception of the outside world through the sense-organs; we even hope to extract some fresh knowledge from the comparison. The psycho-analytic assumption of unconscious mental activity seems to be an extension of the corrections begun by Kant in regard to our views on external perception. Just as Kant warned us not to overlook the fact that our perception is subjectively conditioned and must not be regarded as identical with the phenomena perceived but never really discerned, so psychoanalysis bids us not to set conscious perception in the place of the unconscious mental process which is its object. The mental, like the physical, is not necessarily in reality just what it appears to us to be. It is, however, satisfactory to find that the correction of inner perception does not present difficulties so great as that of outer perception — that the inner object is less hard to discern truly than is the outside world."

24. The analogy to Kant is pursued in Ilham Dilman, "The Unconscious," *Mind*, Vol. 68 (1959), pp. 446-473, at p. 456.

25. B. F. Skinner, "Critique of Psychoanalytic Concepts and Theories," in H. Feigl and M. Scriven (eds.), *The Foundations of Science and the Concepts of Psychology and Psychoanalysis* (Minneapolis: University of Minnesota Press, 1956) pp. 77-87, at pp. 85-6.

26. Michael Scriven, "A Study of Radical Behaviorism," in Feigl and Scriven (eds.), supra n.25, pp. 88-130.

27. David Levin, "Picturing the Freudian Unconscious," *The Psychoanalytic Review*, Vol. 68 (1981), pp. 255-263, at p. 259.

28. *Id*. at 258. For some related explication of Merleau-Ponty's notion of body (or "flesh"), see Paul Ricoeur, *Freud and Philosophy* (New Haven: Yale University Press, 1970) at p. 382.

29. J. Laird, "Is the Conception of the Unconscious of Value in Psychology," *Mind* 31 (1922), 434-435.

30. G. C. Field, "Is the Conception of the Unconscious of Value in Psychology," *Mind* 31 (1922), 413-414.

31. S. Freud, "A Note on the Unconscious in Psychoanalysis," SE, 12 (1912), 263.

32. Freud, *Introductory Lectures*, p. 22.

33. S. Freud, "The Unconscious," SE, 14 (1915), 167.

34. Freud was not above attacking a logical argument by psychologizing. He felt that the criticism depended "either on convention or on emotional factors." S. Freud, *The Ego and the Id*, SE, 24 (1923), 16. By the latter, he meant our inability to accept the fact that man "is not even master in his own house" (*Introductory Lectures*, p. 285), which, when added to the Copernican and the Darwinian insights, was just too much for man's ego to bear. Freud felt that "the general revolt against our science" arises from this emotional prejudice about man's importance in the universe. Ibid.

35. Freud, *Introductory Lectures*, p. 277.

36. Freud, "The Unconscious," p. 167. Contemporary psychoanalytic theorists have also claimed Humpty Dumpty's freedom "to make a word mean what

we want it to mean." See David Rapaport, "On the Psychoanalytic Theory of Motivation," in *Nebraska Symposium on Motivation* (Lincoln: University of Nebraska Press, 1960), in which the author gives an elaborate definition of 'motive' as a theoretical construct.

37. In looking back at his "discovery of the unconscious," Freud said, "Everywhere I seemed to discern motives and tendencies analogous to those of everyday life." S. Freud, *On the History of the Psychoanalytic Movement*, SE, 14, 11. See also Freud, "The Unconscious," p. 168: "All the categories which we employ to describe conscious mental acts, such as ideas, purposes, resolutions and so on, can be applied [to unconscious mental acts]. Indeed, we are obliged to say of some of these latent states that the only respect in which they differ from conscious ones is precisely in the absence of consciousness."

38. For an expansion of this argument against redefining words commonly referring to mental states as theoretical concepts referring only to abstract entities, see M. S. Moore, "Responsibility for Unconsciously Motivated Action," *International Journal of Law and Psychiatry* 2 (1979), 323-347.

39. F. A. Siegler, "Unconscious Intentions," *Inquiry* 10 (1967), 251-267, at p. 257.

40. The claim of "privileged access" often is taken to be much stronger than that of noninferential and nonobservational knowledge; often those that I call claims of incorrigibility and claims of self-intimation are included as claims of privileged access. See W. P. Alston, "Varieties of Privileged Access," *American Philosophical Quarterly* 8 (1971), for a lucid differentiation of a wide variety of epistemic claims under the label of privileged access.

41. Some authors, such as Alston, "Varieties of Privileged Access," and R. Audi, "The Limits of Self-Knowledge," *Canadian Journal of Philosophy* 4 (1974), 253-267, would distinguish incorrigibility from infallibility, and both from indubitability. An even weaker sense of incorrigibility is explored in R. Rorty, "Incorrigibility as the Mark of the Mental," *Journal of Philosophy* 67 (1970). The three distinct claims discussed here will suffice for my purposes, and I shall ignore these further nuances of this much-explored question.

42. The term *self-intimating* is Gilbert Ryle's. See generally, R. Audi, "The Epistemic Authority of the First Person," *Personalist* 56 (1975), 5-15.

43. Siegler, "Unconscious Intentions," at p. 256.

44. *Id*.

45. Quoted in Ilham Dilman, "Is the Unconscious a Theoretical Construct?" *The Monist*, Vol. 56 (1972), 313-342, at p. 325.

46. For example, T. R. Miles, *Eliminating the Unconscious* (London: Pergamon Press 1966); A. Pap, "On the Empirical Interpretation of Psychoanalytic Concepts", in Hook, *Psychoanalysis, Scientific Method and Philosophy*.

47. "The assumption of an unconscious is...a perfectly legitimate one, inasmuch as in postulating it we are not departing a single step from our customary and generally accepted mode of thinking. Consciousness makes each one of us aware only of his own states of mind; that other people, too, possess a consciousness is an inference which we draw by analogy from their observable utterances and actions, in order to make this behaviour of theirs intelligible to us. . . . The assumption of a consciousness in them rests upon an inference and cannot share the immediate certainty which we have of our own consciousness.

"Psychoanalysis demands nothing more than that we should apply this process of inference to ourselves also — a proceeding to which, it is true, we are not constitutionally inclined. If we do this, we must say: all the acts and manifestations which I notice in myself and do not know how to link up with the rest of my mental life must be judged as if they belonged to someone else: they are to be explained by a mental life ascribed to this other person." Freud, "The Unconscious," p. 169.

48. Freud, *Introductory Lectures*, p. 436.

49. For somewhat similar interpretations of psychoanalysis, see B. F. McGuiness, "I Know What I Want," *Proceedings of the Aristotelian Society* 57 (1957), 205; Flew, "Motives and the Unconscious"; MacIntyre, *Unconscious*, chap. 4; L. W. Beck, "Conscious and Unconscious Motives," *Mind* 75 (1966), 155; and particularly, I. Dilman, "Is the Unconscious a Theoretical Construct?" *Monist* 56 (1972), 313-342. As pointed out by Morris Eagle, one would not want to say that the actual recapturing of memories of certain mental states is a necessary condition to the existence of those states, for this would disallow far too many states that we are reasonably certain exist (because of other evidence). See M. Eagle, "Validation of Motivational Formulations: Acknowledgments as a Criterion," in Rubinstein, ed., *Psychoanalysis and Contemporary Science* (New York: International Universities Press, 1973).

50. The inadequacies of the criterial theory of meaning I have discussed at length in Moore, "The Semantics of Judging," *Southern California Law Review* 54 (1981), 151-294.

51. The word is capitalized to distinguish this characteristic from the more familiar "intention" "intentional" of ordinary speech. The idea derives from Franz Brentano, one of Freud's early teachers, who held that "every mental phenomenon is characterized by what the scholastics of the Middle Ages called the Intentional Inexistence of an object and which we would call. . . the reference to a content, a direction upon an object." F. Brentano, *Psychologie vom Empirischen Standpunkt*, book 2 (1874), chap. 1. A selection from this work is translated in R. Chisholm, *Realism and the Background of Phenomenology* (1960). Modern philosophy views Intentionality as a characteristic of mental *language*, not of underlying mental phenomena. Roderick Chisholm's explication of the concept is in terms of three criteria: (1) a sentence is Intentional if it uses a name or description in such a way that neither the sentence nor its contradictory implies either that there is or there is not anything to which the name or expression truly applies: "I hope for a sixty-foot sailboat," for example, does not imply there is a sixty-foot sailboat; (2) a sentence is Intentional if it contains a propositional clause whose truth or falsity is not implied by the sentence as a whole, or its contradictory: "I hope that it will rain," for example, does not imply that "it will rain" is true or false; and (3) a sentence is Intentional if codesignative names or descriptions cannot be substituted and yet preserve truth: I may, for example, order the largest room in some inn. Even if the largest room is identical with the dirtiest room in the inn, one cannot substitute the second description for the first; I did not order the dirtiest room in the inn. R. Chisholm, *Perceiving: A Philosophical Study* (1957), pp. 170-171. Many have urged that Intentionality is *the* distinguishing mark of our discussion of minds, and further, that this kind of discussion cannot be reduced to discussion of an extensional kind. See, e.g., D. C. Dennett, *Content and Consciousness* (1969), chap. 2.

52. For this distinction, as well as its relation to the Intentional/non-Intentional distinction, see Cornman, "Intentionality and Intensionality," *Philosophical Quarterly* 44 (1962). An extensional language is one in which two things (at

least) must be true: its logical connectives must be truth functional; and one must be able to substitute numerical identicals without change of truth value. Such are thought to be necessary requirements for a scientific language, because they allow scientific laws to be formulated without regard to varying descriptions of the particular things covered. Whatever can truthfully be said of the morning star can also truthfully be said of the evening star, because they are one and the same thing: Venus. As we have seen with regard to "intention," this substitution-preserving truth is not possible for the mental predicates we use for describing and explaining the actions of persons. Such vocabulary is accordingly said to be intensional, in that substitution-preserving truth now depends on sameness of meaning (intension) of descriptions. If we are not talking about the evening star itself, but about George's *beliefs* about the evening star, the fact that "evening star" and "morning star" name the same thing is no guarantee that the one description may be substituted for the other and still preserve truth. For the classic treatment of this, see W. V. Quine, "Reference and Modality," in *From a Logical Point of View* (1961). Because of this unamenability to the tools of modern logic, many philosophers, such as Quine, give up on there being a science of the mental in intensional terms. See. W. V. Quine, *Word and Object* (1960), chap. 6.

53. Only if one imposed a strong demand that the objects of a person's desires be *consistent* would the incorrigibility thesis be a general argument against there being unconscious mental states. Yet it is just with regard to unconscious mental states that we are most willing to countenance unresolved conflict.

54. Richard Peters, *The Concept of Motivation* (London: Routledge and Kegan Paul, 1958) p. 61.

55. A good example of this sort is the obsessive woman who repeatedly rang for her maid for no apparent reason. Her action was intentional, and the action is not intelligible to us as being performed for its own sake: one usually calls for one's maid only in order to get something else. Yet when asked why she performed this ritual, the woman could only answer that she didn't know (Freud, *Introductory Lectures*, pp. 261-263). When Freud suggests an unconscious motive for such an action, we are quite receptive to his suggestions in that regard because the action does seem to call out for a reason and the agent has none to give.

56. MacIntyre recognizes this, noting that when Freud called "some piece of mental activity unconscious, it is suggested both that it is carried on without conscious intention, that it is unknowing, and that it is such that it is unknown, at least to the agent, and perhaps to others as well." *The Unconscious*, p. 42.

57. See N. S. Sutherland, "Motives as Explanations," *Mind* 68 (1959), 145-159. There is, of course, a sense in which one "has" a motive just because one is in a situation whereby one stands to gain an intelligible advantage from such an act. Such 'motives' are called 'possible motives' by the law of evidence, where it is generally true that the prosecution may show that the accused had a possible motive for the crime as circumstantial evidence that he did the criminal act, and the accused may show that he had no possible motive for doing it as circumstantial evidence to the contrary. See Wigmore, *Evidence*, 3d ed., 1 (1940), 118. Such motives are *possible* motives precisely because they are not true motives at all. One "has" such motives simply because one is in a certain situation; that one has such possible motives says nothing at all about the individual's desires, beliefs, or mental states. Such cases accordingly do

not present a problem for the statement presented here, asserting that one does not simply have (true mental state) motives as one has pains or future intentions.

58. Imagine how easy a life plan would be for one who is always correct in his beliefs about his own desires! See, generally R. Audi, "The Limits of Self-Knowledge," *Canadian Journal of Philosophy* 4 (1974), 253-267.

59. Nagel, "Methodological Issues in Psychoanalytic Theory," at p. 45.

60. *Id*.

61. *Id*.

62. Perhaps what Nagel had in mind here is that the subject *believes* that the object of his wishes is impossible of attainment; that, accordingly, the actor could not have believed that his acts will get him what he wants; and that without the latter belief the wish cannot have been the motive for his adult behavior. This argument does not show that "unconscious wish" or "unconscious motive" are nonsense; only that often unconscious wishes are *nonmotivational* causes of behavior in Freud's theory.

63. See S. Schiffer, *Meaning* (Oxford: Oxford University Press, 1972), chap. 1, for a discussion of this and other senses of 'meaning'.

64. See note 57.

65. For an introduction, at least, to the difficult idea of 'rational belief', see R. J. Ackerman, *Belief and Knowledge* (New York: Doubleday, 1972), chap. 3. Theodore Mischel has argued that psychoanalytic explanations are irrational because the beliefs that would have to be posited to complete the subject's practical syllogisms would be irrational beliefs. T. Mischel, "Concerning Rational Behaviour and Psychoanalytic Explanation," *Mind* 74 (1965), 71-78. Examples to the contrary are provided by Robert Audi, "Psychoanalytic Explanation and the Concept of a Rational Action," *Monist* 56 (1972), 444-464. See also P. Alexander, "Rational Behaviour and Psychoanalytic Explanation," *Mind* 71 (1962), 326-341; H. Mullane, "Psychoanalytic Explanation and Rationality," *Journal of Philosophy* 68 (1971), 413-426.

66. The example is from Anscombe, *Intention*, and A. J. Watt, "The Intelligibility of Wants," *Mind* 81 (1972), 553. On intelligibility, see also A. Kenny, *Action, Emotion and Will* (London: Routledge and Kegan Paul), pp. 94-98; and Peters, *Concept of Motivation*, passim.

67. This is the sense that Carl Hempel explores in his article, "Rational Action," in Care and Landesman, eds., *Readings in the Theory of Action* (Indiana, 1968).

68. For example, Anscombe, *Intention*; and Goldman, *Theory of Human Action*.

69. The literature seems to be directed toward two points: (1) 'desire' (and its related terms) does not refer to a datable mental event, and (2) 'desire' does not name a cause of behavior. See T. F. Daveney, "Wanting," *Philosophical Quarterly* 2 (1961), 135; Melden, *Free Action*, pp. 65-70; and Charles Taylor, *The Explanation of Behavior* (New York: Humanities Press, 1974), chap. 2.

70. Thus Melden, for example, recognizes that his "starting point is an agent who acts as he does for reasons, because of the desires he has." *Free Action*, p. 157.

71. The example is from C. Hempel, "The Logic of Functional Analysis," in C. Hempel, *Aspects of Scientific Explanation* (New York: Free Press, 1965), pp. 297-330. See also J. L. Cohen, "Teleological Explanations," *Proceedings of the Aristotelian Society* 51 (1955), 255-292; E. Nagel, *The Structure of Science* (New

York: Harcourt Brace, 1961), pp. 401-428, 520-535; and L. Wright, "Functions," *Philosophical Review* 82 (1973), 139-208. The analysis of this section follows closely that provided in M. S. Moore, "Definition of Mental Disorder," in Spitzer and Klein, eds., *Critical Issues in Psychiatric Diagnosis* (New York: Raven Press, 1978).

72. Peters, *Concept of Motivation*, p. 21.

73. Hempel, *Aspects of Scientific Explanation*, pp. 237-238.

74. Freud, *Interpretation of Dreams*, p. 630.

75. Ibid., p. 268.

76. Ibid., p. 267.

77. Ibid., p. 234.

78. S. Freud, *The Origins of Psychoanalysis (1887-1902)* (New York: Basic Books, 1954), letter 108.

79. Freud's apparent reason for adopting this postulate of a wish to sleep was to maintain the parallel he thought existed between neurotic symptoms and dreams. Freud thought that "a symptom is not merely the expression of a realized unconscious wish; a wish from the preconscious which is fulfilled by the same symptom must also be present" (*Interpretation of Dreams*, p. 569). Accordingly, if dreams were to be "overdetermined" in this way, Freud needed to postulate some preconscious wish as motivating the dream along with the unconscious wish from childhood. Dreams as well as neurotic symptoms could then be seen as "compromise formations" between opposed wishes belonging to different topographical systems.

80. Ibid., p. 571.

81. Freud uses all such terms in speaking of the desire to sleep. See "The Theory of Dreams," in *Collected Papers*, 4 (137, 139) ("the intention to sleep"); *Interpretation of Dreams*, pp. 233-234 ('wish', 'purpose', and 'motive').

82. Freud, *Interpretation of Dreams*, p. 123. See also Freud's *Introductory Lectures*, pp. 128-129, and the *New Introductory Lectures*, pp. 16, 129-130, for further explicit discussion of "the function of dreaming."

83. E. L. Hartmann, *The Functions of Sleep* (New Haven, Conn.: Yale University Press, 1973).

84. Freud, *Interpretation of Dreams*, p. 573.

85. M. H. Hollender, "Is the Wish to Sleep a Universal Motive for Dreaming?" *Journal of the American Psychoanalytic Association* 10 (1962), 323-328. Hollender's insightful article is critical of the wish-to-sleep notion because he is unwilling to make the hypothesis stated here.

86. R. M. Jones, "The Psychoanalytic Theory of Dreaming — 1968," *Journal of Nervous and Mental Disease* 147 (1968), 587-604.

87. See W. Dement, "Experimental Dream Studies," *Science and Psychoanalysis* 7 (1964), 132, who, in his attempt to restate the psychoanalytic theory of dreams, mixes the two idioms as thoroughly as did Freud: "If by certain processes the instigated dream can then deal with the stimulus, it forestalls arousal and facilitates a return to deeper sleep, thus promoting the continuation of sleep which, it is assumed, the organism needs and desires. This is what is usually meant by the 'guardian of sleep' function of the dream, the motivating power of which is the wish to sleep, which in turn is assumed to arise out of a physiological need for sleep as well as perhaps an additional psychological need for sleep in the sense of withdrawing from the daily struggles and frustrations of the waking life."

88. James Strachey, "Introduction" to Freud's *Interpretation of Dreams*, p. xix.

89. See Dement, "Experimental Dream Studies"; and more recently, Fisher and Greenberg, *The Scientific Credibility of Freud's Theories and Therapy* (New York: Basic Books, 1977), chap. 2. See also R. M. Jones, *The New Psychology of Dreaming* (New York: Grune and Stratton, 1970), pp. 20-22.

90. Freud, *New Introductory Lectures*, p. 29. Freud was here dealing not with counterexamples to the wish to sleep but with counterexamples to the unconscious wish fantasized as fulfilled in the dream.

91. This functional interpretation applies equally well to the third wish Freud sometimes posited to explain dreams. The unconscious wish from childhood (the first wish), Freud thought, created tension that the dreaming subject, because he wished to sleep (the second wish), wished to discharge (the third wish). This "wished-for instinctual satisfaction" or discharge of psychic tension (*New Introductory Lectures*, p. 19) is a third wish Freud sometimes posits. Like the wish to sleep itself, however, Freud needs only to assert that the *function* of dreams is to discharge such tension, and by such discharge, keep the dreamer asleep (which itself promotes health). There is no more evidence of a "wish for discharge" than there is of a wish to sleep; whereas everything Freud seemingly wanted to assert can in both cases be conveyed in the language of function. Those who test the guardian-of-sleep hypothesis quite rightly construe this part of it as "discharge *function*" of dreams, not as a wish for discharge. See, e.g., Fisher and Greenberg, *Scientific Credibility*, pp. 46-62; B. Lerner, "Dream Function Reconsidered," *Journal of Abnormal Psychology* 72 (1967), 85-100. See also L. Breger, "Function of Dreams," *Journal of Abnormal Psychology Monograph* 72 (1967), 5, who interprets Freud as holding that "the function of dreams is to provide discharge for unconscious impulses" before rejecting the hypothesis as incompatible with the evidence.

92. Freud, *Interpretation of Dreams*, pp. 118-119.

93. Ibid., p. 117.

94. Ibid., p. 120.

95. Jones, "Dream Interpretation and Psychology of Dreaming," pp. 314-315, also notes that not a single dream reported in *Interpretation of Dreams* is explained by reference to such a wish.

96. Roy Schafer, *A New Language for Psychoanalysis* (1976).

97. Ibid., p. 139 (citing certain action theorists, such as Anscombe, for whom reasons are crucial in understanding intentional action).

98. Ibid., p. 148. See generally chap. 7, entitled "Claimed and Disclaimed Actions." In addition to his misconception of action, Schafer's position here results to some extent from the (potential) therapeutic efficacy of getting patients in analysis to view their dreams, slips, etc., as actions they performed. Freud also on occasion adopted such a therapeutic viewpoint. (See "Moral Responsibility for the Content of Dreams," in *Collected Papers*, 5, 155, where Freud urges that we view dreams as actions for which we are responsible: "Obviously one must hold oneself responsible for the evil impulses of one's dreams. In what other way can one deal with them?") A concept (re)defined because of its therapeutic efficacy is, of course, beside the point if one wants to know whether a dream is an action according to our ordinary conception of an action.

99. See E. D'Arcy, *Human Acts* (Oxford: Clarendon Press, 1963). The incorporation of consequences in descriptions of actions has been, for obvious reasons, of much concern to lawyers. See J. Austin, *Lectures on Jurisprudence*

(London, 1873), p. 427; J. Salmond, *Jurisprudence*, 11th ed. (London, 1957), pp. 400-402.

100. See Anscombe, *Intention*, pp. 84-89. ("A great many of our descriptions of events effected by human beings are *formally* descriptions of executed intentions.")

101. This feature of conventionally complex action descriptions was taken by many, following the later Wittgenstein, to provide the key to understanding human action as such. See, e.g., A. I. Melden, "Action," *Philosophical Review* 65 (1956), 523; Winch, *Idea of Social Science*, particularly pp. 24-33, 45-54; and Peters, *Concept of Motivation*, passim. Louch forcefully counters this analysis as an adequate analysis of *action* (as opposed to some species of complex action) in chap. 9 of his *Explanation and Human Action*.

102. See A. Danto, "Basic Acts," *American Philosophical Quarterly* 2 (1965), 141.

103. One might be tempted to say that one does do an even more basic action here, namely, moving all those muscles necessary to move one's arm. Yet significantly, this is not the way we think of this act. Most of us, without special training, do not know how to move "just those muscles" as a basic act — we can do so only as a complex act, i.e., we do so *by moving our arm*. (On this, see Melden, *Free Action*.) The notion of a basic act depends importantly on what an agent *knows* how to do directly, i.e., without doing something else first.

104. Notice that it would be awkward to make 'dreaming' into a complex action verb to cover such cases.

105. L. Wittgenstein, *Philosophical Investigations* (London: Basil Blackwell, 1958), p. 161e.

106. Goldman, *Theory of Human Action*, especially pp. 49-63.

107. The philosophy-of-action literature is rich with attempts to get around this problem. See R. Chisholm, "The Descriptive Element in the Concept of Action," *Journal of Philosophy* 61 (1964), 613-625 (first noticing the problem); Goldman, *Theory of Human Action*, pp. 61-63 (requiring that belief/desire sets cause basic acts "in a certain characteristic way," of which, Goldman claims, we are intuitively aware); D. Davidson, "Freedom to Act," in T. Honderich, ed., *Essays on Freedom of Action* (London: Routledge and Kegan Paul, 1973) (surveying others' attempts before despairing "of spelling out . . . the way in which attitudes must cause actions"); I. Thalberg, *Perception, Emotion and Action* (New Haven, Conn.: Yale University Press, 1977), pp. 56-62; D. F. Pears, "The Appropriate Causation of Intentional Basic Actions," *Critica* 7 (1975); C. Peacocke, "Deviant Causal Chains," *Midwest Studies in Philosophy* 4 (1979), 123-155.

108. See, e.g., Pears, "Appropriate Causation."

109. S. Freud, "Moral Responsibility for the Content of Dreams," in *Collected Papers*, 5, 154-157.

110. See Irving Thalberg, "Freud's Anatomies of the Self," in Richard Wollheim (ed.), *Freud: A Collection of Critical Essays* (Garden City, N.Y.: Anchor Books, 1973); Ronald de Sousa, "Rational Homunculi," in Amelie Rorty (ed.), *The Identities of Persons* (Berkeley: University of California Press, 1976).

111. I have elsewhere argued against the fragmentation-of-self notion in Freudian metapsychology. See M. S. Moore, "The Unity of Self," in Michael Ruse (ed.), *Nature Animated* (The Netherlands: D. Reidel Publishing Co., 1982). Compare Morris Eagle, "Anatomy of the Self in Psychoanalytic Theory" in the same volume.

112. To show this conclusively, one would have to work out a full-fledged theory of action and show that dreaming does not fit within it. If one gives up on refining a causal theory of action, one might revert to an epistemic criterion, suggested by Wittgenstein's remark that human actions are marked "by the absence of surprise." (*Philosophical Investigations*, p. 162e). Arthur Danto, for example, once claimed both that one has privileged access to one's basic actions and that these actions are self-intimating: "When one moves one's arm, one knows this, knows the thing itself, and not on the basis of some kind of evidence" ("What We Can Do," *Journal of Philosophy* 60 [1963]). Dreaming might then be defined as an "unconscious action," if one's memory allowed one to know noninferentially that one tried to produce a dream. Rarely, however, does Freud even attempt to have his patients recapture in their memory that they *tried* to produce a dream. (Robert Shope comes to a similar conclusion in his "Freud's Concepts of Meaning," *Psychoanalysis and Contemporary Science* 2 (1973), 276-303.) Rather, Freud and more contemporary analysts simply assume that if they have discovered unconscious wishes explaining an event, then that event can be viewed as an action. For an elaboration on this possibility, see M. S. Moore, "Responsibility and the Unconscious," *Southern California Law Review* 53 (1980), 1563-1675, particularly at pp. 1590-1602.

113. Freud, *Interpretation of Dreams*, p. 151.

114. The "Metapsychological Supplement" is in the *Standard Edition*, 14, 222-235.

115. Ibid., p. 229.

116. Ibid., p. 226-231.

117. Wittgenstein, for one, so interpreted what Freud had done: "If I take any one of the dream reports... which Freud gives, I can by the use of free association arrive at the same results as those he reaches in his analysis—although it was not my dream. And the association will proceed through my own experiences and so on. The fact is that whenever you are preoccupied with something with some trouble or with some problem which is a big thing in your life—as sex is, for instance—then no matter what you start from the association will lead finally and inevitably back to that same theme. Freud remarks on how, after the analysis of it, the dream appears so very logical. And of course it does. You could start with any of the objects on this table—which certainly are not put there through your dream activity—and you could find that they all could be connected in a pattern like that; and the pattern would be logical in the same way. One may be able to discover certain things about oneself by this sort of free association, but it does not explain why the dream occurred." L. Wittgenstein, *Lectures and Conversations* (Berkeley and Los Angeles: University of California Press), pp. 50-51. See generally Robert Steele, "Psychoanalysis and Hermeneutics," *Int'l Review of Psycho-Analysis* 6 (1979), 389-411, for a systematic development of this view of Freud's dream theory.

118. "Suppose I have a picture-puzzle, a rebus, in front of me. It depicts a house with a boat on its roof, a single letter of the alphabet, the figure of a running man whose head has been conjured away, and so on. Now I might be mislead into raising objections and declaring that the picture as a whole and its component parts are nonsensical. A boat has no business to be on the roof of a house, and a headless man cannot run. Moreover, the man is bigger than the house, and if the whole picture is intended to represent a landscape, letters of the alphabet are out of place because such objects do not occur in nature. But obviously we can only form a proper judgment of the rebus if we put aside

criticisms such as these of the whole composition and its parts and if, instead, we try to replace each separate element by a syllable or word that can be represented by that element in some way or other. The words which are put together in this way are no longer nonsensical but may form a poetical phrase of the greatest beauty and significance. A dream is a picture-puzzle of this sort." Freud, *Interpretation of Dreams*, pp. 227-228.

119. Ibid., p. 41. Jones, "Dream Interpretation and Psychology of Dreaming," documents Freud's explanatory (as well as his interpretive) intent in dream theory.

120. Freud, *Interpretation of Dreams*, p. 136.

121. Ibid., p. 308.

122. Ibid., p. 339.

123. Ibid., p. 490.

124. Ibid., pp. 470-471.

125. Ibid., p. 141.

126. Ibid., p. 339.

127. Ibid., p. 267.

128. The reasons given here for reconstruing "the motives of distortion" as functions do *not* include the lack of intelligibility of distortion as a motive; the phenomena of resistance and self-deception show us that often in waking life we do perform actions with distortion as our (unconscious) motive. In such cases the avoidance of pain is both the function served by our behavior and the motive that causes it. See notes 72 and 73, and the corresponding text.

129. Freud, *New Introductory Lectures*, p. 81.

130. See Freud, "Moral Responsibility for Content of Dreams"; Schafer, *New Language For Psychoanalysis*. See also Theodore Dreiser's *An American Tragedy*, wherein the psychoanalyst surrogate, the Reverend McMillan, holds Clyde responsible for the killing of Roberta because it was the outgrowth of wicked desires. It is also true that psychoanalytic explanations in terms of unconscious motives are often said to *decrease* our responsibility, not increase it. See, e.g., John Hospers, "Dreaming and Free Will," *Philosophy and Phenomenological Research* 10 (1950), 313-330; D. Blumenfeld, "Free Action and Unconscious Motivation," *Monist* 56 (1972), 426-443. Showing why this seemingly contradictory implication does not hold is the subject of another article. Briefly, it confuses psychic determinism with scientific determinism (of the "hard" variety), or it confuses motives with compulsions. See Moore, "Responsibility for Unconsciously Motivated Action," pp. 323-347; and M. S. Moore, "Responsibility and the Unconscious," *Southern California Law Review* 53 (1980) 1563-1675, for a discussion of these and related topics.

131. See the articles by Moore cited in note 130. Flew is also clear about this in his "Motives and the Unconscious." For a contrary view, see H. Fingarette, "Psychoanalytic Perspectives on Moral Guilt and Responsibility," *Philosophy and Phenomenological Research* 16 (1955), 18. Fingarette's conclusion is that "the wish is, in a sense, *morally* the act." He arrives at such a conclusion by noting, correctly, that we may feel as guilty about a wish as about an act; and by claiming, incorrectly, that we *are* responsible morally if we *accept* responsibility (which we do when we feel guilt at the wish).

132. See P. Alexander, "Cause and Cure in Psychotherapy," *Aristotelian Society. Supplementary Volume* 29 (1955), 25-42, who interprets the theory causally and thus construes the therapy as indoctrination.

Explanation and Causation in the Biomedical Sciences

Kenneth F. Schaffner*

INTRODUCTION

There is a cluster of issues intertwined with 'explanation' in the biomedical sciences, including prediction, causation, historicity, teleology, organization, and the autonomy of biology. In this essay I shall focus on the problem of explanation in rather general terms, though in the context of the biomedical sciences. In another place I have considered more specific, special types of explanation, such as historical, functional, and teleological explanations, and must refer the reader elsewhere for this discussion.[1]

Webster's New World Dictionary defines explanation as "the act or process of explaining," and in turn defines the verb *to explain* as "1: to make plain or understandable, 2: to give the reason for or cause of, 3: to show the logical development or relationships of..."[2] Each of these three facets of this definition will play a role in the accounts of explanation to be developed in the remainder of this article.

An explanation is usually given in response to a question or a

*This material is based on research supported by the National Science Foundation and by the National Endowment for the Humanities. I would like to thank John Coulehan, M.D., Peter Machamer, Sewal Wright and Jack D. Myers, M.D., for comments on an earlier draft of this article.

problem, whether this be implicit or explicit. It will be useful to mention some typical questions that arise in the biomedical sciences as a prelude to an analysis of 'explanation'.

Consider the following queries:

1. Why does the presence of lactose in its environment result in the synthesis of the enzyme B-galactosidase in *E. coli*?[3]
2. Why does an increase in the percentage of CO_2 in respired air result in an increase in the depth of respiration in humans?[4]
3. Why does the pattern of color coats in mice in the F_2 generation follow a 9:3:4 ratio $\left(\frac{9}{16}\right.$ = agouti [a greyish pattern]; $\frac{3}{16}$ = black; $\frac{4}{16}$ = albino$\left.\right)$?[5]
4. Why do 2-6 percent of American blacks have a sickle-cell gene?[6]
5. Why do individual cells of the slime mold *Dictostelium discoideum* aggregate and develop into an integrated multicellular organism?[7]
6. What is the function of the thymus in vertebrates?[8]

These are representative types of requests for explanations in the biomedical sciences. The first example admits of a causal microlevel deterministic explanation and has already been discussed extensively in several previous papers of mine.[9] The second example is an illustration of a complex causal system with feedback which will be discussed in some detail toward the end of this essay. The third example involves a partially stochastic or statistical explanation, but it also has causal components involving biosynthetic pathways. The fourth example typically is a request for an evolutionary explanation. The fifth example is causal and *roughly* deterministic, and involves the development of organization. The last example is a request for a functional analysis with an explanatory capacity.

All of these examples have explanations that involve the *general* issues on which I shall focus in this essay. Some of the examples, however, will require further analysis for a *complete* account of the types of explanation associated with them, and therefore cannot feasibly be analyzed here.[10]

Analyzing 'explanation' in science has been a major concern of philosophy of science during the past thirty years. In the past ten years there have been significant additional developments on this topic. My approach to explicating 'explanation' in the biomedical sciences will begin with an overview of some of this history, including recent developments, and then move to more specific analysis of these general problems in the context of biological explanation.

GENERAL MODELS OF EXPLANATION IN SCIENCE

I will begin with a brief summary of several of the classical extant models of scientific explanation. Basically these fall into categories of deductive-nomological, or D-N model; the deductive-statistical, or D-S, model; the inductive-statistical, or I-S, model; and the statistical-relevance, or S-R, model.

The deductive-nomological, or D-N, model is probably the ideal form of scientific explanation. There are foreshadowings of it in Aristotle's *Posterior Analytics* and *Physics*, and it is discussed, though not under that name, in Mill's *A System of Logic*. In the mid-1930s Sir Karl Popper discussed this type of explanation in his *Logik der Forschung*.[11] Today it is closely associated with the names of Hempel and Oppenheim, who about thirty years ago argued its cause in an extremely clear and influential article.[12] Hempel has also been its principal elaborator and defender.[13]

Schematically, the deductive-nomological model can be presented as

$$L_1 \ldots L_n$$
$$C_1 \ldots C_k$$

$$\overline{}$$
$$E$$

where the Ls are universal laws and the Cs represent initial conditions. Collectively these constitute the "explanation." E is a sentence describing the event to be explained, and is called the "explanandum." In this model, E follows *deductively* from the conjunction of the law, or nomological premises (from the Greek word *nomos*, which means law) and the statements describing the initial conditions. E here may be a sentence describing a specific particular event. In contrast, if the initial conditions are interpreted in a suitable general way, for example, as boundary conditions, E may be a law, such as Snell's law in optics or the Hardy-Weinberg law in population genetics.

The D-N model of explanation has generated a number of criticisms. One type of criticism arose from Hempel's initial view that an adequate explanation of X should give sufficient information to show that "X was to be expected—if not definitely as in the case of D-N explanation, then at least with reasonable probability."[14] This defensible notion led Hempel and Oppenheim to a *thesis of structural identity of explanation and prediction*, which Hempel later distinguished into two subtheses:

1. every adequate explanation is potentially a prediction.
2. every adequate prediction is potentially an explanation.[15]

Both of these subtheses have been extensively criticized in the literature on scientific explanation. Suffice it to outline two of the criticisms using three now-classic counterexamples.

Scriven's well-known syphilis-paresis example argues against subthesis 1. He writes:

> We can explain but not predict whenever we have a proposition of the form "the only cause of X is A..." — for example, "the only cause of paresis is syphilis." Notice that this is perfectly compatible with the statement that A is often not followed by X — in fact very few syphilitics develop paresis. Hence when A is observed we can predict that X is *more* likely to occur than without A, but still extremely unlikely. So we must, on the evidence, still predict that it will *not* occur.[16]

Hempel's response to this objection is to rejoin that "precisely because paresis is such a rare sequel of syphilis, prior syphilitic infection surely cannot by itself provide an adequate explanation of it [any more than we can] explain a man's winning the first prize in the Irish Sweepstakes by pointing out that he had previously bought a ticket, and that only a person who owns a ticket can win the first prize."[17] I will not attempt to resolve this dispute at this point. Note, however, that syphilis does (by our intuitions) *seem* to *explain* the paresis in some sense — the real question is whether a somewhat different model of explanation might account for the force of this intuition legitimately.

The second subthesis was also criticized by Scriven using his "barometer" example. Scriven noted that though we could *predict* a storm from a dropping barometer reading, we would not want to say that the falling barometer reading *explained* the storm.[18]

Hempel, citing the similar example of Koplik spots, which presage measles but do not explain the appearance of the disease, agreed, and now does not appear to subscribe to this second subthesis.[19]

Adequate deductive-nomological explanations can be found in the biomedical sciences, and certain limiting notions of causal explanations are instances of this type of explanation. Because of the number and variability of initial conditions, as well as genetic and environmental variations, however, partially or completely stochastic processes are widespread in the biomedical sciences.[20] In such cases the premises will involve one or more statistical "laws."

When the premises involve *statistical* generalizations, however, the type of logic in the model may change. If the generalizations are operated on deductively to generate an explanation sentence, as in population genetics with infinite populations, for example, we have an instance of deductive statistical, or D-S, explanation, and the logic is still deductive. Far more interesting to us, however, will be those situations in which we wish to explain an event in which the sentence describing that event only follows *with probability* from a set of premises. For example, to use one of Hempel's illustrations, if we wish to explain John Jones's recovery from a streptococcus infection, we might be told that he had been given penicillin. There is, however, no general *universal* exceptionless law that requires *all* individuals who have been given penicillin to recover from such an infection.

At most we can schematize the logical relation, and this instance of the I-S model, as:

> The statistical probability of recovery from severe streptococcal infections with penicillin administration *is close to 1*.
> John Jones has severe streptococcal infection and was given penicillin.

> John Jones recovered from the infection.

Here the double line does not stand for a *deductive* inference but means rather: "makes practically certain (very likely)."[21] The double line accordingly represents *inductive* support, whence the appellation "inductive statistical model."

The general form of the I-S model is schematized as follows using probability formalism:

$P(R/S \& P)$ is close to 1

$$\frac{S_j \& P_j}{R_j} = [\text{makes practically certain (very likely)}]$$

Most readers will realize, for reasons already mentioned, that a very large percentage of explanations in the biomedical sciences have this inductive-statistical character.

The I-S model has several peculiarities not usually associated with the D-N model. For example, it should be obvious that if John Jones were severely allergic to penicillin, the probability of his recovery would not have been close to 1 — he might well have died because of anaphylactic shock. This consideration points us toward the need to place John Jones, or any individual entity that is named in an I-S explanation, into the *maximally specific* reference class about which we have available data.[22] Hempel maintains that any "information... which is of potential explanatory relevance to the explanation event..." must be utilized in "formulating or appraising an I-S explanation."[23]

Reflection on some of these considerations and on certain counterexamples to the D-N model has led Wesley Salmon to propose an alternative to the models discussed thus far. For example, Salmon proposed that the following argument fulfills Hempel's requirements for a D-N explantion:

John Jones avoided becoming pregnant during the past year, for he has taken his wife's birth control pills regularly, and every man who regularly takes birth control pills avoids pregnancy.[24]

It is clear, however, that the above is *not* an explanation—men simply do not become pregnant.

Salmon's first approach to explicating explanation involved asserting that an explanation is *not an argument* and thus does not require us to appeal to either deductive or inductive logic in analyzing the relation between premises and conclusion.[25] Rather, according to Salmon, an explanation of the sentence, "Why does this X, which is a member of A, have the property B?" is "a set of probability statements." These represent the probability of members of various *epistemically homogeneous subclasses* having a particular property A, say, A & $C_2, \ldots$, and also possessing another property B. Also necessary to the explanation is "a statement specifying the compartment to which the explanandum event belongs."[26]

Thus, the S-R model is really a partition of a class into epistemically homogeneous subclasses, made on the basis of any available statistically relevant information. A property C_1 "explains" because it is *statistically relevant* to X having the property B if it has A.

In addition to the difference with Hempel over the nonargument status of an explanation, Salmon also contends that there is no reason that a probabilistic statement involving a *very low* probability cannot be utilized in an explanation. If the statistically relevant class, for example, the class of atoms of radioactive U^{238} that will decay into lead, is such that the probability of decay is very low, that is all that can be said in response to an explanation of why this atom of U^{238} decayed into lead.

SALMON ON CAUSAL EXPLANATION IN THE S-R MODEL

In elaborating the S-R model, Salmon found that he had to amplify it to accommodate theoretical explanations.[27] Further explication of this notion appears to have led him to a rather significant emphasis on causal explanations of the statistical generalizations that constituted the explanans of the initial S-R model. In his more recent essay, Salmon wrote:

> If we wish to explain a particular event, such as death by leukemia of GI Joe, we begin by assembling the factors statistically relevant to that occurrence — for example, his distance from the atomic explosion, the magnitude of the blast, and the type of shelter he was in. . . . We must also obtain the probability values associated with the relevancy relations. *The statistical relevance relations are statistical regularities, and we proceed to explain them. Although this differs substantially from things I have said previously, I no longer believe that the assemblage of relevant factors provides a complete explanation —or much of anything in the way of explanation.* We do, I believe, have a bona fida explanation of an event if we have a complete set of statistically relevant factors, the pertinent probability values, *and* causal explanations of the relevance relations. Subsumption of a particular occurrence under statistical regularities— which, we recall, does not imply anything about the construction of deductive or inductive arguments — is a necessary part of any adequate explanation of its occurrence, but it is not the whole story. The causal explanation of the regularity is also needed. This claim, it should be noted, is in direct conflict with the received view, according to which the mere subsumption— deductive or inductive—of an event under a lawful regularity constitutes a complete explanation. One can, according to the received view, go on to ask for an explanation of any law used to explain a given event, but that is a different explanation. I am suggesting, on the contrary, that if the regularity invoked is not a causal regularity, then a causal explanation of that very regularity must be made part of the explanation of the event [emphasis added].[28]

Causal explanation has assumed (or perhaps reassumed) a central role in the analysis of scientific explanation.[29] The pervasiveness of causal components in the six representative examples outlined earlier indicates that these developments may be quite useful for our inquiry. Our intuitions about causality are notoriously unclear, however, and a considerable amount of research on explications of this concept has been done in recent years. It will accordingly be useful to attend to some of that work as a prelude to proposing a general model of explanation in the biomedical sciences and locating causal explanation in relation to that model.

CAUSALITY AND CAUSAL EXPLANATION: HART, HONORÉ, AND MACKIE

Analyses of the nature of causality and the question of whether there is a univocal sense of 'cause' extend back to the pre-Socratic philosophers and attained their definitive ancient exposition in the contributions of Aristotle. Hume and Kant devoted substantial portions of their work to these questions, and the debates continue to the present day. An analysis of causal explanation, both in lay and scientific contexts, can be found in two excellent, relatively recent books to which I shall refer in this section: H.L.A. Hart and A.M. Honoré's *Causation in the Law* (1959) and John Mackie's *Cement of the Universe* (1974). These works are of particular interest to us for several reasons. First, they both are sufficiently general so that they can be considered as not limited to mathematical physics as the paradigm science. This is useful since causation in the biomedical sciences, as Ernst Mayr and George Gaylord Simpson have suggested, may well vary from the models found in the physical sciences.[30] Second, both Hart and Honoré and Mackie discuss extensively the role of generalizations in causal analyses, a topic that is especially relevant in the philosophy of biology in light of Smart's arguments against laws and theories in biology.[31]

Hart and Honoré also attempt to disentangle causes from conditions in a philosophically general way, and Mackie provides an analysis of complex generalizations that will turn out to be particularly useful for the biomedical sciences. In these pages I shall indicate in a brief summary fashion which elements of these authors' views are particularly useful, and why. Detailed arguments for and against these theses are offered elsewhere.[32]

There are a number of cogent and valuable points concerning causality made by Hart and Honoré and Mackie. Though both points of view are suspicious (and in Mackie's case, denying) of the need for generalizations in connection with a number of causal claims, it seems to me that arguments provided elsewhere indicate that the role of generalization in causation is merely more complex.[33] The generalizations function in a complicated network, sometimes as background theories and often in connection with *comparative* or *contrasting* causal claims. In addition, a thesis concerning the narrowness of generalizations in the biomedical sciences argued for in a recent essay of mine[34] seems to be quite congruent with Mackie's stress on singular causal assertions, though it disagrees with his interpretation.

Hart and Honoré's interpretation of the distinction between causes and conditions, and Mackie's (and Anderson's)[35] notion of a causal field are heavily *pragmatic*, and suggest that *explanations* that utilize causal generalizations will also be significantly affected by pragmatic considerations as to which factors to cite, how much fine structure is required, and how far a causal chain (or chains) needs to be articulated.

Mackie's notions of *inus* conditions and gappy universals (or generalizations) are also valuable contributions to our understanding of causality. Mackie introduced these notions in the following way, commencing his presentation by reviewing the work of John Stuart Mill.

Mill recognized the complication of plurality of causes by which several different assemblages of factors, say, *ABC* as well as *DGH* and *JKL*, might each be sufficient to bring about an effect *P*. Let us now understand these letters to represent types rather than tokens. Then, if (*ABC* or *DGH* or *JKL*) is both necessary and sufficient for *P*, how do we describe the *A* in such a generalization? Such an element is for Mackie an *insufficient* but *non-redundant* (necessary) part of an *unnecessary* but *sufficient* condition—a complex expression for which Mackie uses an acronym (*inus*) based on first letters of the italicized words.[36] Using this terminology, then, what is usually termed a cause is an *inus* condition.

But our knowledge of causal regularities is seldom *fully* and *completely* characterized: we know some of the *inus* conditions but rarely all possible ones. Causal regularities are, according to Mackie, *"elliptical* or *gappy* universal propositions."[37] One can represent this, using Mackie's formalism, by invoking (following Anderson) a causal field of background conditions, *F*, that focuses our attention on some specific area and/or subject of inquiry, and by noting that:

In F, all $(A \ldots \overline{B} \ldots$ or $D \ldots \overline{H} \ldots$ or $\ldots)$ are followed by P and, in F, all P are preceded by $(A \ldots \overline{B} \ldots$ or $D \ldots \overline{H} \ldots$ or $\ldots)$.[38]

The bar above *B* and *H* indicates that these types are functioning as negative causes in this generalization.

In addition to my view that these notions are valuable, however, I believe that they need both further development and further relaxation. *Inus* conditions that function in gappy generalizations require more intrastructure and explicit connection with other causal factors in order to provide sufficiently detailed models in the biomedical sciences. In a later section I shall develop one possible representation using the techniques of regression equations and path analysis that may provide the additional intrastructure.

Equally important in the biomedical sciences is the need to relax the concept of causality so that it covers not only deterministic causality but also stochastic or *probabilistic causality*. The biomedical sciences contain such notions as Mendelian random variables, the statistical diffusion processes of evolutionary theory, epidemiological "risk factors," and incompletely determined physiological processes with stochastic residual factors. In addition, judgments in the more clinical subjects are highly probabilistic. In recent years several philosophers of science have begun a close examination of 'probabilistic causality'. The philosopher who has done most to connect this notion with scientific explanation is Wesley Salmon. Earlier I discussed Salmon's S-R model and indicated that he has now moved considerably beyond that model. I now turn to a discussion of Salmon's new theory of explanation and its connection with probabilistic causality, as a prelude to further inquiries into generalizing explanation by Skyrms and van Fraassen, and to the development of a path-analytic causal model of explanation.

SALMON'S NEW THEORY OF CAUSAL EXPLANATION

In his new theory of causal explanation, Salmon suggests that "by employing a *statistical conception of causation* along the lines developed by Patrick Suppes and Hans Reichenbach, it is possible to fit together harmoniously the causal and statistical factors in explanatory contexts" [emphasis added]. [39] For Salmon, the basic features of such a statistical conception of causation involve interdigitated notions of (1) statistical relevance, (2) causal processes, (3) causal interactions, and (4) common cause.

A concept of 'statistical relevance' can be formulated in several different ways, and Reichenbach, Good, and Suppes in their accounts use various characterizations of the notion in connection with probabilistic causality.[40] A simple and straightforward definition of the notion is given by Salmon:

> A property C is said to be *statistically relevant* to B within A if and only if $P(B/A \& C) \neq P(B/A)$.[41]

An event (or property) C is, as was noted above, *explanatory* of B because it is statistically relevant.[42] In this elaborated causal model of Salmon's, however, C will be analyzed as having probabilistic *causal* relevance to event B.[43]

Partially in order to eliminate some standard problems, such as the classic barometer counterexample, Reichenbach's screening-off relationship is also introduced by Salmon to provide a stronger (*comparative*) notion of statistical relevance.[44] Screening off is characterized as follows:

> Formerly, we may say that D screens off C from B in reference class A if (and only if) $P(B/A \& C \& D) = P(B/A \& D) \neq P(B/A \& C)$.[45]

Screened-off causes are not explanatory; they are equivalent to what Suppes terms "spurious causes."[46]

Causal processes are understood by Salmon to be similar to what Russell called a causal line, and roughly are processes extended in space and time that propagate influences.[47] A ray of light or a moving material particle are instances of causal processes. For Salmon, it is crucial to distinguish causal processes from *pseudoprocesses*, such as a shadow moving across a landscape, and he proposes that the distinction can be made by using Reichenbach's notion of a "mark."[48] A mark is a modification imposed (or *imposable*, to strengthen the notion in a counterfactual manner) on a causal process. Causal processes can carry "marks," whereas pseudoprocesses cannot. Salmon employs what he terms an "at-at" theory of causality to avoid "the sort of mysterious power Hume warned us against."[49] In the *"at-at"* theory, "a causal process. . . gets from one place to another by being *at* the appropriate intermediate points *at* the appropriate instances of time."[50] Marks are similarly propagated without any *additional* interactions needed to regenerate the mark.

Causal processes are also distinguished by Salmon from *causal interactions*. In order to characterize in what causal interactions consist, Salmon utilizes and expands further the Reichenbach notion of "common cause."[51] A *common cause* is roughly an event that explains prima facie coincidence, such as a blown fuse explains all the lights simultaneously going out in a room.

The common-cause notion requires, for detailed explication, the concepts of a 'conjunctive fork' and an 'interactive fork'. A conjunctive fork *ACB*, where *C* is the common cause, is defined by Salmon, following Reichenbach as:

$$P(A\&B/C) = P(A/\,C) \times P(B/C)$$
$$P(A\&B/\overline{C}) = P(A/\overline{C}) \times P(B/\overline{C})$$
$$P(A/C) > P(A/\overline{C})$$
$$P(B/C) > P(B/\overline{C})\ ^{52}$$

A conjunctive fork is open to the future but not the past, and can be used to characterize temporal asymmetry. It is important to note that *C*, in effect, "screens off" *A* and *B* from each other. The concept of common cause introduces a desirable explanatory asymmetry into event sequences, permitting identification of an explanatory *C* even though $P(B/A) > P(B)$. Thus *C* screens off *A* from being potentially identifiable as a "cause" of *B* in an account of statistical causation.

Though conjunctive forks are important in explicating the notion of common cause, Salmon argues that "there are. . . certain sorts of causal *interactions* in which the resulting effects are more strongly correlated with one another than is allowed in Reichenbach's conjunctive forks [emphasis in original]."[53] This will occur where there are *constraints*, in addition to *C*, which relate *A* to *B*, taken conjointly, such that the probabilistic independence of *A* and *B* fails. Salmon cites Compton scattering of a photon and an electron as a case in point. He notes:

In the conjunctive fork, the common cause *C* absorbs the dependency between the effects *A* and *B*, for the probability of *A* and *B* given *C* is *equal to* the product of the probability of *A* given *C* and the probability of *B* given *C*. In the interactive fork, the common cause *C* does not absorb the dependency between the effects *A* and *B*, for the probability of *A* and *B* given *C* is *greater than* the product of the two separate conditional probabilities [emphasis in original].[54]

These notions are then used, in a rough manner and following von Bretzel, to characterize the notion of a 'causal interaction'.[55] Briefly, Salmon suggests that

when two [causal] processes intersect [spatiotemporally], and both are modified in such ways that changes in one are correlated with changes in another — in the manner of an interactive fork... — we have a causal interaction.[56]

These, then, are the elements of Salmon's theory of causal explanation, and indicate in a general way how causal processes are to be characterized and appealed to as statistically relevant explainers of explananda.[57] Causal explanation can, in Salmon's account, take either of two forms:

Either there is a direct causal connection from *A* to *B* or from *B* to *A*, or there is a common cause *C* which accounts for the statistical dependency. In either case, those events which stand in the cause-effect relation to one another are joined by a causal process. The distinct events *A*, *B*, and *C* which are thus related constitute interaction — as defined in terms of an interactive fork — at the appropriate places in the respective causal processes. The interactions *produce* modifications in the causal processes, and the causal processes *transmit* the modifications. Statistical dependency relations arise out of local interactions — there is no action-at-a-distance (as far as macro-phenomena are concerned at least) — and they are propagated through the world by causal processes [emphasis in original].[58]

Salmon contends that his account subsumes a covering-law model under it by analyzing explanations of laws by theories, say, as a subclass relation or a part-whole relation. He writes:

Kepler's laws of planetary motion describe a restricted subclass of the class of all motions governed by Newtonian mechanics. The deductive relations *exhibit* what amounts to a part-whole relationship, but it is, in my opinion, the physical relationship between the more comprehensive physical regularity and the less comprehensive physical regularity which has explanatory significance. I should like to put it this way. An explanation may sometimes provide the materials out of which an argument, deductive or inductive, can be constructed; an argument may sometimes exhibit explanatory relations. It does not follow, however, that explanations are arguments [emphasis in original].[59]

SALMON'S PROGRAM FOR EXPLICATING STATISTICAL CAUSATION

A number of elements of Salmon's new causal account of explanation have now been surveyed. Importantly, however, the essence of the new model, an explication of a "statistical conception of causation" has not yet been delineated. This notion was mentioned earlier as being the keystone, as it were, "fit[ting] together harmoniously the causal and statistical factors in explanatory contexts."[60]

In a searching examination of the three extant analyses of statistical causation in the work of Reichenbach, Good, and Suppes, Salmon recently argued that the elements of his own approach, as outlined above, can resolve several problems associated with probabilistic causality.[61] These problems he sees as (1) the difficulty of assigning a degree of strength to a causal chain on the basis of strengths of individual links in the chain (this primarily affects Good's account), (2) the difficulty of analyzing "cases in which an effect is brought about in an improbable fashion," and (3) the failure of screening off to handle "spurious causes" (in Suppes's sense).[62]

In this essay I shall not be able to discuss in any detail these issues.[63] Suffice it to say that regarding the first point Salmon suggests that the information contained in probability values that relate *individual* links in a causal chain must be preserved in any analysis of the strength of the chain. Replacing these individual values with a more holistic (for the whole chain) statistical relevance measure appears to throw away enough information so that the holistic values for the *joint* causal chain are strongly counterintuitive.[64]

The third issue is handled by, first, introducing the notion of an interactive fork, as above, and second, explaining the causal processes involved.

Salmon analyzes at great length and with a number of examples the second difficulty, which plagues all three extant accounts of probabilistic causality. This difficulty arises in those situations in which there is (at least) one alternative, comparatively improbable causal path to an effect. This problem is central for a probabilistic theory of causality, whether it be of the Reichenbach, Good, or Suppes form, or any statistically relevance-based account of probabilistic causality. Any such account will require something like Reichenbach's "causal betweenness" definition. Essentially,

> An event B is *causally between* the events A and C if these relations hold:
>
> $$1 > P(C/B) \quad > P(C/A) > P(C) > 0$$
> $$1 > P(A/B) \quad > P(A/C) > P(A) > 0$$
> $$P(C/A\&B) \quad = P(C/B)^{65}$$

These relations license the causal chain $A \rightarrow B \rightarrow C$, where the arrow ($\rightarrow$) denotes the probabilistic causation.

However, Reichenbach's, Suppes's and Good's proposals for constructing causal sequences run into this second problem of the improbable alternative causal path. Salmon writes that Glymour was the first to notice the problem for Reichenbach's concept of causal betweenness, and Suppes notes that his attention was first directed to this problem by his students Bolton and Rosen.[66] I shall not have space to discuss here Rosen's clear and forceful counterexample, but I shall summarize a similar example that Salmon views as fatal for any attempt to repair a statistical relevance-based account of probabilistic causality.[67]

Salmon introduces this example as follows:

We have an atom in an excited state which we shall refer to as the 4th energy level. It may decay to the ground state (zeroeth level) in several different ways, all of which involve intermediate occupation of the 1st energy level. Let $P(m \rightarrow n)$ stand for the probability that an atom in the mth level will drop directly to the nth level. Suppose we have the following probability values:

$$P(4 \rightarrow 3) = \frac{3}{4} \qquad P(3 \rightarrow 1) = \frac{3}{4}$$

$$P(4 \rightarrow 2) = \frac{1}{4} \qquad P(2 \rightarrow 1) = \frac{1}{4}$$

It follows that the probability that the atom will occupy the 1st energy level in the process of decaying to the ground state is $\frac{10}{16}$; if, however, it occupies the 2nd level on the way down, then the probability of its occupying the 1st level is $\frac{1}{4}$. Therefore, occupying the 2nd level is negatively relevant to occupation of the 1st level. Nevertheless, if the atom goes from the 4th to the 2nd to the 1st level, that sequence constitutes a causal chain, in spite of the negative statistical relevance of the intermediate stage.[68]

A comparatively improbable path such as $4 \rightarrow 2 \rightarrow 1$ energy levels will contain all the features contained in Rosen's and others' counterexamples, but because the energy-level transitions are at the level of what I shall term "stochastic bedrock," no additional detail or intermediate interpolatable causal events are possible.

Though I believe Salmon's counterexample can be outflanked by appropriate and careful conditionalization,[69] it is more to the point to note here that Salmon would rather propose an *alternative* nonstatistical relevance-based explication of probabilistic causality.

This different approach outflanks the problem by referring to causal processes. It is worth quoting Salmon on this *in extenso*:

An appropriate causal description of the atom, it seems to me, can be given in the following terms. Our particular atom in its given initial state (e.g., what we called the 4th energy level) persists in that condition for some time, and as long as it does so it retains a certain probability distribution for making spontaneous transitions to various other energy levels $\left(\text{i.e., } P(4 \rightarrow 3) = \frac{3}{4}; P(4 \rightarrow 2) = \frac{1}{4}\right)$. Of course, if incident radiation impinges upon the atom, it may make a transition to a higher energy by absorbing a photon, or its probability of making a transition to a lower energy level may be altered due to the phenomenon of stimulated emission. But in the absence of outside influences of that sort, it simply *transmits* the probability distribution through a span of time. Sooner or later, it makes a transition to a lower energy level (say the 2nd), and this event, which is marked by emission of a photon of characteristic frequency for that transition, transforms the previous process into another—namely, that atom in the state characterized by the 2nd energy level. This process carries with it a new probability distribution $\left(\text{i.e., } P(2 \rightarrow 1) = \frac{1}{4}; P(2 \rightarrow 0) = \frac{3}{4}\right)$. If it then drops to the 1st level, emitting another photon of suitable frequency, it is transformed into a different process which has a probability of 1 for a transition to the ground state. Eventually it drops into the ground state [emphasis in original].[70]

Salmon stresses that his preferred approach is *not* a statistical relevance account:

It is to be noted that the relation of positive statistical relevance does not enter into the foregoing characterization of the example of the decaying atom. Instead, the case is analyzed as a series of causal processes, succeeding one another in time, each of which transmits a definite probability distribution—a distribution which turns out to give the probabilities of certain types of interactions. Transmission of a determinate probability distribution is, I believe, the essential function of causal processes with respect to the theory of probabilistic causality. Each transition event can be considered as an intersection of causal processes, and it is the set of probabilities of various outcomes of such interactions which constitute the transmitted distribution.

It is not clear that this account is in conflict with an (appropriately) conditionalized) statistical relevance explication, and for my purposes I prefer to construe the two analyses as triangulating on the same model (which will be elaborated in further detail below). It is clear, however, that Salmon's preferred explication has a core notion of a "series of causal processes... each of which transmits a definite probability distribution."[71] This core notion requires further characterization if it is to serve as a basis for a probabilistic theory of causality. One direction in which both approaches might be further developed and integrated into a general account of explanation will now be considered.

DISTINGUISHING STATISTICAL CORRELATIONS FROM PROBABILISTIC CAUSATION

Salmon's explications of probabilistic causal explanation are valuable and, in general (with the minor caveats cited above), point in what I believe is the correct direction. As mentioned, in the biomedical sciences probabilistic causality may be found in genetics, in evolutionary theory, and in epidemiology. Insofar as events are not completely determined by known causes in complex physiological systems, an important residuum of stochasticity enters. (A detailed example of stochastic residuality will be provided later.) Salmon's analysis, however, can be usefully supplemented by several generally accepted epidemiological indicators of *causal* as opposed to *spurious* relations. It seems to me that these indicators can also usefully function in a general screening process that evaluates prima facie causal connections in the biomedical sciences.

The following nine criteria have been proposed by Hill in his recent book (and in earlier editions of this work) and with minor variations in categorization, appear to have been widely accepted by epidemiologists.[72] They are not sufficient in themselves, and they also assume the concept of a trial with controls (equivalent to a statistical interpretation of the generalized method of difference and Claude Bernard's method of comparative experimentation).[73] (Incidentally, these notions do not appear explicitly in Salmon's analysis, which is effectively restricted to probability values with 0 variance, though no doubt Salmon could easily extend his theory to incorporate the complicating effects of probability *distributions*.)[74]

Hill suggests that when examining an epidemiological association to determine whether it is causal, we consider: (1) *the strength of the association*, by which he means the relative incidence in the two compared populations in which the alleged causal factor is present and absent; (2) *consistency*, namely, has the effect "been repeatedly observed by different persons, in different places, different circumstances and times?";[75] (3) *specificity*, or the one-to-one association of the cause with the effect. This is a desirable condition, but it is very often violated and is only a weak desideratum; (4) *the relationship in time*, or "which is the cart and which is the horse?"[76] Causation that is "backwards in time" is eliminated by this condition;[77] (5) *the biological gradient*, or dose-response curve, in which one looks for evidence that an increase in the causal factor generates a (not-necessarily) linear increase in the effect; (6) *biological plausibility* or agreement with current biological knowledge. This, it is acknowledged, depends on the underlying laws and theories of the day which may be erroneous, but in general it is an important constraint; (7) *coherence of the evidence*. This is a feature that is narrower than plausibility but similar to it. Coherence refers to the interplay of factors associated with the disease (or system) in question. Thus, in considering whether cigarette smoking causes lung cancer, attention is paid to diverse links, such as the temporal rise in the two variables over time, the sex difference (now, unfortunately, attenuating), the histopathological evidence from the bronchial epithelium of smokers, and the isolation of factors in smoke that are carcinogenic for the skin of laboratory animals; (8) *the experiment*, by which Hill refers to another contrast case, such as where preventive action is taken to ameliorate a health hazard, and the incidence of the disease falls. In general, this would refer to any manipulation of the variable of a system and its consequent effects; and (9) *reasoning by analogy*. This is a weak factor, but Hill has in mind that with the known effects of the drug thalidomide and the disease rubella we would be ready to accept slighter but similar evidence with another drug or another viral disease in pregnancy.[78]

These features, which evaluate the causal status of an association, do not necessarily increase the frequency (or the probability in the first-order sense of the term), but they do increase the security of a causal claim. They thus tend to decrease the variance and make a causal claim more stable.

The pretheoretical analysis of causal claims is thus complex and, as noted earlier, has pragmatic features as well. Some of these themes appear again in very recent explications of scientific explanation.

COMPARATIVE DIMENSIONS OF SCIENTIFIC EXPLANATION

Several recent contributions have begun to stress what I shall term the *comparative* dimensions of scientific explanation. I noted earlier that both Hart and Honoré and Mackie cited scientific generalizations as being particularly useful in certain comparative contexts where potential competing explanations were possible. Quite recently, several authors (including Skyrms, van Fraassen, Schaffner, and Gardenfors) have underscored the comparative aspects of explanations.[79] In this section I shall have space only to outline Skyrms's brief account of various desiderata for scientific explanations. The comparative account, I shall argue in this and the succeeding sections, (1) provides a natural place for probabilistic causal explanation of the type discussed in the previous section, (2) permits one to resolve certain long-standing paradoxes of scientific explanation, (3) allows for further elaboration of a causal probabilistic model especially appropriate for the biomedical sciences, and (4) gives a good preliminary explication of the various examples of explanation with which we began this chapter.

SKYRMS'S DESIDERATA FOR SCIENTIFIC EXPLANATION

In his recent book *Causal Necessity,* Brian Skyrms proposes four desiderata for a scientific explanation. His desiderata are expressed in terms of a specific canonical form, which he characterizes as follows:

I will be interested in explanations having a certain canonical form. Let us assume that what is to be explained is that a certain system is in a certain physical state S^*. Let $\{S_i\}$ be an exhaustive set of mutually exclusive possible states of the system of which S^* is a member. (Where the system is capable of an infinite number of alternative states, we assume some natural finite partition.) Let us also suppose that we have a set $\{E_j\}$ of competing explanatory accounts for the system's being in State S^*. (I do not assume that these accounts are mutually exclusive or exhaustive.) I also assume that for each account $\{E_j\}$ and each possible state $\{S_i\}$, we have the conditional probability of the account on the state, $Pr(S_i$ given $E_j)$. (It will be useful to assume that the set of explanatory accounts always contains a null explanatory account, E_{null} (a tautology will do): $Pr(S_i$ given $E_{null}) = Pr(S_i)$.) These conditional probabilities are not current epistemic probabilities. We don't try to explain a system's being in a state unless we know that it is in that state. Rather, we are interested in the *prior* objective conditional probabilities.[80]

In terms of this canonical form, Skyrms proposes the following four desiderata:

The first desideratum for an explanatory account is truth.
  The second desideratum is that the connection between the explanatory account and the explanandum be lawlike.
  The third desideratum of an explanatory account is explanatory power, the degree to which an explanatory account renders the state to be explained more likely than other alternative states. An explanatory account might render S^* overwhelmingly likely, in the most favorable case; or it might render S^* more likely than all of the alternatives taken together, that is, more likely than not; or it might render S^* more likely than each of its competitors; and so forth.

Degrees of explanatory power are relevant to the force with which the explanation resolves the puzzlement: why S^* rather than something else?

The fourth desideratum of an explanatory account is comparative strength, the degree to which the explanatory account renders the explanandum more probable than do competing explanatory accounts. If $Pr(S^*$ given $E_i) > Pr(S^*$ given $E_j)$, then I shall say that E_i is a stronger explanation of S^* than E_j. In the degenerate case where the only competitor for an explanatory account is the null explanation, the demand for comparative strength reduces to the demand for positive statistical relevance (i.e., that $Pr(S^*$ given $E) > Pr(S^*)$.[81]

Skyrms's outline as presented above is clear and suggestive. It could be elaborated in several different directions. Two such elaborations, one involving the techniques of "path analysis" and another involving graphically represented regression analysis, will be presented in the following section. In another place I have indicated how these desiderata merge with and are satisfied by an independent model of scientific explanation presented recently by van Fraassen, but I cannot reproduce that account here because of space limitations. It seems to me that Skyrms's desiderata and various comparative accounts of explanation offer answers to several traditional conundra in the area of scientific explanation, such as the famous Scriven paresis example. As Skyrms puts it, if one pays attention to the second comparative aspect of explanation represented by his fourth desideratum, the explanatory force of the syphilis as an etiological agent becomes clear as an instance of statistical relevance. Skyrms writes that "Scriven's famous paresis example focused attention on positive statistical relevance, which we can see as a special case of [desideratum] (4) comparative strength,"[82] and adds, locating several authors within his own schema, that

the importance of statistical relevance for explanation has also often been stressed by Salmon. Jeffrey, on the other hand, and following him Railton, stress the importance of [desideratum] (2) the lawlike nature of the conditional probabilities involved, and they argue that one may have an acceptable scientific explanation even in the absence of comparative strength and explanatory power.[83]

A MODEL OF PROBABILISTIC CAUSAL EXPLANATION

SUMMARY OF CONCLUSIONS TO THIS POINT

Thus far we have argued that scientific explanation involves appeal to generalizations, albeit rather narrow generalizations in some cases. These generalizations often have a causal character, though it is important to construe causation broadly to encompass the Reichenbach, Good, Suppes, and Salmon sense of *probabilistic* causation. Causation has been shown to be a complex and multifaceted concept, often involving pragmatic aspects. Explanations, it has been argued, are usually (even if tacitly) doubly comparative: the explanandum is compared with a contrast class, and the explanans is compared in strength with alternative, often competing explanans. As such, explanation also involves *evaluations* of the relevance relation connecting explanans and explanandum. In addition to these features of (causal) explanation, it should be restressed that the biomedical sciences often involve appeals to multifactorial (and usually interlevel) causation in explanations.

THE CONCEPTS OF PATH ANALYSIS

These various features of explanation in the biomedical sciences can be brought together in the form of a provisional model that utilizes the notions of *path analysis*. Path analysis is a technique developed by the eminent geneticist Sewall Wright in the 1920s, and which has, in the past two decades, been largely appropriated by the economists in econometrics and by sociologists, though there have also been continued applications in genetics and in physiology, and more recently in epidemiology.

The path-analysis approach has its limitations and is premised on a number of assumptions that must be satisfied if the method is to be correctly used.[84] In general, background knowledge must be appealed to, to identify a set of causal factors responsible for an effect. The weak causal *ordering*, namely the identification of which factors are causes and which are effects, can often be accomplished on the basis of known temporal features, well-known background theories in the sciences, and the type of considerations developed by Hill, as discussed earlier. (This weak causal ordering will be formally captured by the *recursive* character of the system's equations.) The relation(s) between causes and effect(s) must be *linear*, but this restriction can be relaxed by employing an appropriate transformation of variables to accommodate parabolic, cubic, exponential and fairly arbitrarily complex relations.[85] The causal system is assumed *closed*, though here an "error" factor can be explicitly appealed to which covers unknown "residual" causal factors. The causal factors and their ordering is usually represented by a diagram in which unidirectional arrows represent causal influence and double-headed arrows (noncausal) represent correlations. A simple example of both types from Li is shown in figure 1*a* and 1*b*.[86]

In figure 1*a*, X and Z are causes affecting Y. The numbers .60 and .80

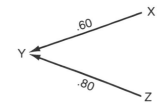

Fig. 1*a*. Uncorrelated causes.

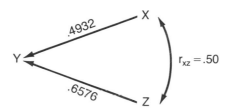

Fig. 1*b*. Correlated causes. Both illustrations reprinted, by permission, from Li, "Concept," p. 195.

are *path coefficients* and represent a measure of the degree of causal influence of X and Z on Y, respectively, which we shall write p_{YX} and p_{YZ}, following standard conventions. These path coefficients are defined as the portion of the standard deviation of Y that is the result of variation in the affecting variable. The affecting variables can be "probabilistic" variables, for example, by *reversing* the directions of the arrows in figure 1*a* one can interpret Y as an individual producing two gametes, represented by X and Z. Subject to the chance of segregation in meiosis, the path coefficients can be shown to be equal to $\sqrt{1/2}$ for a random individual (see Li, *Population Genetics*, p. 174).

Since it is important to be clear about this central notion of path coefficient in connection with probabilistic causality, several comments of a somewhat technical character are in order. On a first reading, the reader may wish to skip the following section.

MATHEMATICAL ANALYSIS OF PATH COEFFICIENTS

If we write the usual multiple-regression equation for Y in figure 1 as a function of X and Z we obtain:

$$Y - \overline{Y} = B(X - \overline{X}) + C(Z - \overline{Z}),\tag{1}$$

where the bar over the variables signifies the mean of the random variable under consideration, and the constants B and C are obtained by the standard method of least squares.

(Recall that a regression equation in this case can be pictured as a plane directed through a "cloud" of points in a three-space, where the "cloud" clusters around and along the regression plane that is chosen by minimizing the square of the distance of the "cloud's" points from the regression plane. A confidence region for the regression line or plane can be specified by either classical or Bayesian procedures, and such confidence limits [say, at 95 percent] can similarly be mapped into confidence limits for the path coefficients. I shall discuss these probabilistic features in more detail later.)

Now, the constants in equation (1), namely B and C, will be sensitive to the physical units employed in measuring the variables. This sensitivity can be eliminated by using so-called standardized variables. Rewriting (1) as

$$\frac{Y-\overline{Y}}{\sigma_Y} = \frac{B\sigma_X}{\sigma_Y}\frac{(X-\overline{X})}{\sigma_X} + \frac{C\sigma_Z}{\sigma_Y}\frac{(Z-\overline{Z})}{\sigma_Z}, \tag{2}$$

we obtain an equation that is independent of the physical units involved. This equation is further simplified notationally by writing

$$b = \frac{B\sigma_X}{\sigma_Y} = p_{YX}, \quad = \frac{C\sigma_Z}{\sigma_Y} = p_{YZ} \tag{3}$$

and

$$x = \frac{X-\overline{X}}{\sigma_x}, \text{ etc., yielding} \tag{4}$$

$$y = p_{YX}\, x + p_{ZX}z. \tag{5}$$

The expression p_{YX} is the *path coefficient* for the direct path from X to Y. The coefficient is thus a type of regression coefficient, and p_{YX} represents in a precise numerical manner the "portion of the standard deviation of Y due to the variation" in X. If X and Z are *un*correlated as in figure 1*a*, then the path coefficients are numerically equal to the traditional standardized *correlation* coefficients between X and Y and Z and Y, respectively. If, however, X and Z are correlated as in figure 1*b*, this identification does not hold, though the *path*-coefficients method can still be used. Thus, *in general*, path-analysis coefficients ought *not* to be identified with correlation coefficients between the variables, as Glymour appears to do.[87]

Path coefficients, unlike correlation coefficients, can have values that exceed plus or minus one. Negative correlations in path analysis refer to the effect of *reducing* a variance. Values that fall outside the range -1 to $+1$ are in part artifacts resulting from correlations back of the affecting variables for which they compensate.[88]

The equation $y = p_{YX}x + p_{YZ}z$, given earlier, can be written in more general notation as

$$X_0 = p_{01} X_1 + p_{02} X_2 + \ldots + p_{0m} X_m + p_{0u} X_u \tag{6}$$

where $X_1 \ldots X_m$ are the causal factors affecting X_0, and where X_u is an uncorrelated residual variable. When all standard deviations are scaled to 1, all correlation coefficients are reduced to product moments, and it is possible to express the general equation (6) as

$$r_{0q} = p_{01} r_{1q} + p_{02} r_{2q} + \ldots + p_{0m} r_{mq} + p_{0q} r_{uq} = \sum_{i=1}^{u} p_{0i} v_{iq}. \tag{7}$$

This is the *basic equation of path analysis*. It has two important, more specific forms, one being:

$$r_{01} = p_{01} + p_{02} r_{12} + \ldots + p_{0m} r_{1m}, \tag{8}$$

in cases where the affecting variable V_1 is an immediate factor. If the factor being examined is the affected factor itself, i.e., V_0, we have the second specific form:

$$v_{00} = p_{01} r_{01} + p_{02} r_{02} + \ldots + p_{0m} r_{0m} + p_{0u}^2 = 1$$

or

$$v_{00} = \sum_{j=1}^{m} p_{0j} r_{0j} + p_{0u}^2 = 1 \qquad (j \neq u). \tag{9}$$

These equations will be used in an illustration in the next subsection.

It must be remembered that these values such as p_{01} or p_{YX}, are *estimators* of the true influence (say, β). It would take us beyond the scope of this article to discuss the probabilistic details of regression coefficients, but several brief comments may be in order.[89]

First, it should be noted that a thoroughgoing Bayesian account of linear regression has been provided by D. V. Lindley.[90] Lindley shows that plausible uniform priors for the parameters in regression equations can be specified, and that the posterior expectation of β, namely b, equals $\Sigma(X_i - \overline{X})(Y_i - \overline{Y}) / \Sigma(X_i - \overline{X})^2$, in accordance with more classical results. As was noted earlier, b is a least-squares estimator of β, and is also a maximum-likelihood estimator of β. Confidence limits, in the 95 percent range, for example, can be specified for β by using a t-distribution. In addition, a Bayesian analogue of a significance test, used to determine if a significant regression effect exists, can be provided by referring to another well-known distribution (F) and performing an analysis of variance using an F-test.[91]

PATH COEFFICIENTS, STATISTICAL RELEVANCE, AND PROBABILISTIC CAUSALITY

Path analysis is a representation of causal influence in complex cases. Consider the limiting case of total determination by the identified causes, where there is no residual error term but where there are fluctuations, represented by the fact that the estimates, such as b, have a finite nonzero variance demanded by a probabilistic system. In this case we may note that the *squares* of the path coefficients, termed the degree of determination, or d, capture the notion of the causes' degree of influence on the effect assuming all factors have been identified so as to eliminate correlations back of the affecting variable. In figure 1a, $(.60)^2 = 36$ percent of Y's variation is determined by the variation in X, and $(.80)^2 = 64$ percent is determined by the variation in Z.[92] If the variables X and Z are *correlated* as in figure 1b, then the expression for the percentage of influence is more complex but still precise, and can be shown to be given by

$$1 = p_{YX}^2 + p_{YZ}^2 + 2p_{YX}p_{YZ}r_{XZ} \tag{10}$$

where r is the correlation coefficient. In such a case, Li notes:

We say X *directly* determines $(.4932)^2 = 24.32\%$ of Y's variation while the *joint effect* of X and Z determine $2 (.4932) (.6576) (.50) = 32.43\%$ of Y's variation [emphasis in original].[93]

The path coefficient, then, is a highly refined measure of statistical relevance of various causal factors' influence on an effect. Appropriately backgrounded by prima facie causal identifications and orderings, path analysis provides a highly developed methodology for representing complex multifactorial probabilistic causation.

APPLICATION TO MORE COMPLEX INTERACTIONS

In addition to the two simple cases of two independent causes (figure 1a) and two correlated causes (figure 1b), path analysis can be applied to more complex causal interactions that will be of biomedical

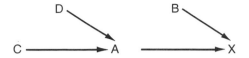

Fig. 2. A chain of independent causes.

interest. One type of interaction is a *chain* of independent causes, such as depicted in figure 2.

For such a chain, it can be shown that the effect of C on X, for instance, is equal to the product of the path coefficients of C on A and A on X, or

$$p_{X \cdot C} = p_{X \cdot A} \cdot p_{A \cdot C} \qquad (11)$$

and, in addition,

$$d_{X \cdot C} = d_{X \cdot A} \cdot d_{A \cdot C} \cdot \qquad (12)$$

Thus, if C determined 25 percent of A's variance ($d_{A \cdot C} = .25$) and A determined 75 percent of X's variance ($d_{X \cdot A} = .75$), C would directly determine $(.25)(.75) = .1875$ of A's variance. In this chain, B could play the role of a residual unknown determinant, or set of determinants, and be set equal to an E, or "error," factor.

In addition to chains of complex causes, the notion of a *common cause* (with or without correlations between common causes) can be elegantly represented in path analysis. Path analysis can be used to represent clearly the source of correlation resulting from common causes affecting variables as, for example, in figure 3.

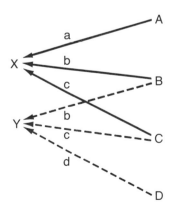

Fig. 3. Common independent causes. Reprinted by permission, from Li, *Population*, p. XX.

Using the general equation of path analysis (8), it can be shown that the correlation between X and Y produced by the common causes B and C is given by:

$$r_{XY} = p_{X \cdot B} p_{Y \cdot B} + p_{X \cdot C} p_{Y \cdot C}. \tag{13}$$

This result can be both formally proved and generalized to any set of common causes relating an X and Y:[94]

$$r_{XY} = \sum_i p_{X \cdot i} p_{Y \cdot i}. \tag{14}$$

(And since $r_{XY} = r_{YX}$, $r_{XY} = \sum p_{Yi} p_{Xi}$, in addition.)

Where correlations between the common causes exist, this is generalized to

$$r_{XY} = \sum_i p_{Xi} p_{Yi} + \sum_{i \neq j} p_{Xi} r_{ij} p_{Yi}.\text{[95]} \tag{15}$$

That path-analysis diagrams can represent probabilistic causation is developed in an argument sketched by Wright which contends that probabilities can be identified with path coefficients. It is worth quoting him on this point in full. He writes

If a variable, V_0, consists merely of one of a group of alternatives, with constant values $C_1, C_2, \ldots, C_m$, drawn with probabilities $P_1, P_2, \ldots, P_m$, respectively, these probabilities may be treated as frequencies.

$$\overline{V}_0 = \sum^m C_i P_i.$$

$$\sigma^2_0 = \sum^m (C_i - \overline{V}_0)^2 P_i.$$

Assume, however, that V_0 is drawn with probabilities $P_1, P_2, \ldots, P_m$ from a group of *variable* alternatives $V_1, V_2, \ldots, V_m$ with momentary deviations from their means, $\delta V_1, \delta V_2, \ldots, \delta V_m$, respectively. These variables may have different variances, δ_i^2, etc., and may be correlated (r_{i2}, etc.).

$$\overline{V}_0 = \sum P_i \overline{V}_i, \quad \delta \overline{V}_0 = 0.$$

The best estimate of the deviation of V_0 is $E(\delta V_0) = \Sigma^m P_i(\delta V_i)$. The probabilities appear here as path regression $c_{0i} = P_i$. The corresponding path coefficients may accordingly be written $P_{01} = P_1 \sigma_{1}/\sigma_0$. The identification of probabilities with path regressions in general, and with path coefficients where all contributing variables have the same variance is useful in analyzing the consequence of mating systems [emphasis in original].[96]

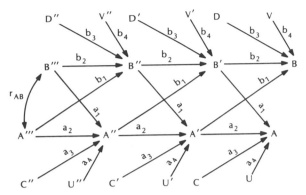

Fig. 4. Path diagram representing reciprocal interaction between two variables, *A* and *B*, with different lags between action and reaction. *C* and *D* represent known external factors that affect *A* and *B* respectively, and *U* and *V* represent the unknown residual factors. Reprinted, by permission, from Wright, "Treatment," p. 424.

Employing these results for independent causes, correlated causes, chains of causes, and common causes, a diagram of any complexity can be analyzed using path-analytical techniques. For cases with feedback, or reciprocal interaction, the analysis can be naturally extended, subject to certain general provisos dependent on the lag times. Wright has provided accounts of path analysis for both reciprocal interaction with lag and for instantaneous reciprocal interactions. His path diagram for the former type of interaction is provided as figure 4.

Of considerable biomedical interest is Wright's path analysis of respiratory homeostasis, to which I shall turn in the next section.

AN EXAMPLE IN THE BIOMEDICAL SCIENCES

When Wright initially developed and then, over the course of several decades, elaborated the concepts of path coefficients, he tended to exclude concepts of feedback and reciprocal interactions. Partially as a response to comments by Tukey and Turner and Stevens,[97] Wright decided to re-examine the applicability of path analysis to interactive systems.[98] Some of his results were depicted in figure 4.

Turner and Stevens, in their article, outlined a brief application of a path analysis to J. S. Haldane and J. G. Priestley's classical account of the regulation of human respiration. In general, this work provides the beginnings of an answer to our second example of a "why question": Why does an increase in the percentage of CO_2 in respired air result in an increase in the depth of respiration in humans?

Haldane and Priestley's general research objective was to investigate the function(s) of the "respiratory center" and to elucidate "the factor or factors determining the rate of lung-ventilation under normal conditions."[99] At the time of their research in 1905, essentially all investigators subscribed to the view that "the respiratory movements are regulated, partly by afferent nervous impulses reaching the [respiratory] center [located in the medulla], particularly through the vagus nerves, and partly by direct chemical stimuli resulting from the more or less 'venous' condition of the blood passing through the centre."[100] The specific contribution of the neural and chemical factors (and, of these chemical factors, whether oxygen deficiency and/or excess carbon dioxide were important) were not well understood and constituted the focus of Haldane and Priestley's experiments.

Much of Haldane and Priestley's data were obtained by experimenting on themselves (whence the reference to the scientists as J. S. H. and J. G. P. in their tables and in the discussion that follows).

Lung ventilation is affected both by the *frequency* of respirations and the *depth* of respiration. It had been known that small increases in the percentage of CO_2 in inspired air would result in a significant increase in lung ventilation (e.g., Haldane and Priestley found that an increase of 0.2 percent CO_2 resulted in a doubling of ventilation). This percentage of CO_2 was progressively increased by having J. S. H. and J. G. P. rebreathe their own exhaled air, whence the use of the term "respired air," with changes in frequency and depth of respiration noted. Their *general* conclusion, which built in part on both denervation and cross-circulation experiments by other investigators,[101] was that "under normal conditions the regulation of the lung-ventilation depends on the presence of CO_2 [PCO_2] in the alveolar air."[102] The *specific* contributions of frequency and depth of respiration, and the interaction via feedback of these effects on the cause or stimulus of PCO_2, is the focus of Turner, Stevens, and Wright's applications of path analysis.

Haldane and Priestley's experiment was subsequently analyzed in considerable detail by Wright, first in an article in *Biometrics* and then in volume 1 of his book *Evolution and the Genetics of Populations*. Wright began from a path-analysis diagram essentially equivalent to that

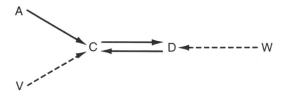

Fig. 5. Path diagram of relations in respiration.

depicted in figure 5, suggested by Turner and Stevens, with the important addition of the "residual" factors V and W.

Wright reviewed Turner and Stevens's analysis, and though in general agreement with their approach, found it important to augment in successive modifications the path diagram by several additional variables.[103]

The data used by Turner and Stevens, and reproduced from Wright's account, are as follows:[104]

% CO_2 in respired air: $\overline{A} = 3.106$, $\sigma_A = 1.6052$, $r_{DA} = .9814$.
% CO_2 in alveolar air: $\overline{C} = 5.810$, $\sigma_C = .5058$, $r_{DC} = .8132$.   (16)
Depth of respiration: $\overline{D} = 1224.5$, $\sigma_D = 431.7$, $r_{CA} = .8577$.

The path-analysis equations for the systems are given by Wright, along with this solution, as follows:[105]

$$r_{DA} = .9814 = p_{DC}r_{CA}, p_{DC} = 1.1442, c_{DC} = 977,$$
$$c_{CA} = 1 = p_{CA}\sigma_C/\sigma_A, p_{CA} = 3.1735, c_{CA} = 1,$$ (17)
$$r_{CA} = .8577 = p_{CD}r_{DA} + p_{CA}, p_{CD} = -2.3596, c_{CD} = -.00277.$$

Wright notes that calculation of other path coefficients, not examined by Turner and Stevens, led to difficulties. In particular, the calculation of the coefficients for the residual variable p_{DW} and p_{CV} yields:[106]

$$p_{DW} = \sqrt{(1 - p_{CD}p_{DC})(1 - p_{DC}r_{DC})} = .820$$
$$p_{CV} = \sqrt{(1 - p_{CA}r_{CA} - p_{CD}r_{CD})(1 - p_{CD}p_{DC})} = \sqrt{-.1284}$$ (18)

In this modification and elaboration of respiratory physiology, Wright first introduced a new variable X for alveolar CO_2 of which C is an "imperfect measure." This permitted Wright to eliminate the above-cited nonsensical result that the path coefficient p_{CV} in figure 5 was *imaginary* $(= \sqrt{-.1284})$. The path diagram and Wright's values for the various paths are reproduced in figure 6.

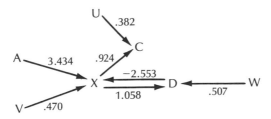

Fig. 6. Modified path diagram of variables in figure 5. Path diagram of same variables as in figure 11, except that C is represented as an imperfect measure of alveolar CO_2 content, deviating at random U from a quantity X, which stands in the average relation to A and D in these experiments. Reprinted, by permission, from Wright, "Treatment," p. 434.

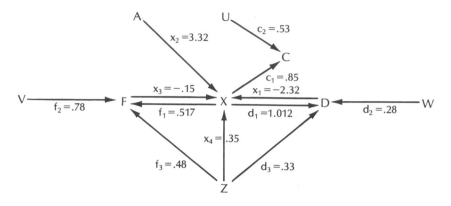

Fig. 7. Path diagram of relations of CO_2 concentration of respired air (A). CO_2 concentration of alveolar air — estimated (C) and unknown actual (X), depth of respiration (D), frequency of respiration (F), and residual factors U, V, W, and Z from data from one subject. Reprinted, by permission, from Wright, *Evolution*, p. 365.

The actual interactions between Haldane's and Priestley's study included one additional variable, F, the frequency of respiration. This can be included in an augmented path-analysis diagram, but its inclusion also required *another* additional residual factor, Z, which contributes positively to observed correlations between F, X, and D. The Z factor, Wright noted, "presumably consists primarily in variability in the amount of CO_2 released into the blood by metabolism throughout the body".[107] This new, rather complex set of homeostatic causal interactions is depicted in figure 7.

The path equations that yield these path-coefficient values are obtained partially from the application of the fundamental theorem of path analysis ([8] and [9]) and partially from the empirical data of Haldane and Priestley. Wright's summation of these data is shown in tables 1 and 2.

TABLE 1
ESTIMATED PATH COEFFICIENTS AND PATH REGRESSIONS OF FIGURE 7

Path Coefficients				Path Regressions
$c_1 = p_{CX} = 0.85$		$d_1 = p_{DX} = 1.012$		$c_{CD} = -0.00263$
$c_2 = p_{CU} = 0.527$		$d_2 = p_{DW} = 0.28$		$c_{CA} = 1$
$z_1 = p_{XD} = -2.328$		$d_2 = p_{DZ} = 0.33$		$c_{XF} = -0.0280$
$x_2 = p_{XA} = 3.323$		$f_1 = p_{FX} = 0.517$		$c_{DX} = 893$
$x_3 = p_{XF} = -0.15$		$f_2 = p_{FV} = 0.78$		$c_{FX} = 2.81$
$x_4 = p_{XZ} = 0.35$		$f_3 = p_{FZ} = 0.48$		

SOURCE: Wright, *Evolution*, p. 367.

TABLE 2
FORMULAS FOR CORRELATIONS BETWEEN VARIABLES OF FIGURE 7 AND VALUES
CALCULATED FROM THE DEDUCED PATH COEFFICIENTS

No.	Formulas	Value
1	$K = 1 - x_1 d_1 - x_3 f_1$	3.433
2	$r_{XA} = 0.8229/c_1$	0.968
3	$= x_1 r_{DA} + x_2 + x_3 r_{FA} = x_2/(1 - x_1 d_1 - x_3 f_1) = x_2/K$	0.968
4	$r_{DA} = 0.9793 = d_1 r_{XA}$	0.979
5	$r_{FA} = 0.5008 = f_1 r_{XA}$	0.501
6	$r_{XW} = x_1 r_{DW} + x_3 r_{FW} = x_1 d_2/K$	-0.190
7	$r_{DW} = d_1 r_{XW} + d_2$	$+0.088$
8	$r_{FW} = f_1 r_{XW}$	-0.098
9	$r_{XV} = x_1 r_{DV} + x_3 r_{FV} = x_3 f_2/K$	-0.034
10	$r_{DV} = d_1 r_{XV}$	-0.035
11	$r_{FV} = f_1 r_{XV} + f_2$	$+0.762$
12	$r_{XZ} = x_1 r_{DZ} + x_3 r_{FZ} + x_4 = (x_1 d_3 + x_3 f_3 + x_4)/K$	-0.143
13	$r_{DZ} = d_1 r_{XZ} + d_3$	$+0.186$
14	$r_{FZ} = f_1 r_{XZ} + f_3$	$+0.406$
15	$r_{XD} = 0.7718/c_1$	$+0.908$
16	$= x_1 + x_2 r_{DA} + x_2 r_{DF} + x_4 r_{DZ}$	$+0.912$
17	$= d_1 + d_2 r_{XW} + d_3 r_{XZ}$	$+0.911$
18	$r_{XE} = 0.3541/c_1$	$+0.417$
19	$= x_1 r_{DF} + x_2 r_{FA} + x_3 + x_4 r_{FZ}$	$+0.424$
20	$= f_1 + f_2 r_{XV} + f_3 r_{XZ}$	$+0.422$
21	$r_{DF} = 0.5295$	$+0.530$
22	$= d_1 r_{XF} + d_2 r_{FW} + d_3 r_{FZ}$	$+0.528$
23	$= f_1 r_{XD} + f_2 r_{DV} + f_3 r_{DZ}$	$+0.532$
24	$r_{XX} = 1 = x_1 r_{XD} + x_2 r_{XA} + x_3 r_{XF} + x_4 r_{XZ}$	0.995
25	$r_{DD} = 1 = d_1 r_{XD} + d_2 r_{DW} + d_3 r_{DZ}$	1.004
26	$r_{FF} = 1 = f_1 r_{XF} + f_2 r_{FV} + f_3 r_{FZ}$	1.005

SOURCE: Wright, *Evolution*, p. 366.

There are interesting physiological features embodied in the path
diagram. For example, Wright notes that "the relative effect
($X_3 = -.15$) of rate of respiration on alveolar CO_2 is almost negligible
in comparison with that ($X_1 = -2.328$) of depth of respiration."[108]
This diagram, however, is still not completely adequate for Wright, and
he develops it further. To review these further elaborations would,
however, not add anything of philosophical interest, though the elaborated diagrams are of considerable significance physiologically. As the
reader will realize from the earlier discussion of Haldane and Priestley's general objective, even as far as Wright goes, he presents only a
fragment of the complex causal network of lung physiology and, in
particular, does not consider neurophysiological interactions.[109]

It is of interest to note that Haldane and Priestley obtained data from *two* human subjects (as remarked earlier, these subjects were the scientists themselves, J. S. H. and J. G. P.), and Wright's analysis of their differing physiologies suggests there is a "great difference between the subjects." "Alveolar CO_2 content. . . seems to have been controlled about twice as much by frequency of respiration [F] as by depth [D] in the case of J. G. P. in contrast with virtually exclusive control by depth in the case of J. S. H."[110] This finding is not unexpected, given the thesis I have developed elsewhere concerning biomedical variability, and it indicates that path analysis can represent this biomedical individuality and even highlight it in appropriate cases.[111] Further comments will be made concerning the subgrouping of subjects in this regard. It may also be of interest to note that Turner and Stevens suggested, in connection with the kind of path analysis represented here, that

use might possibly be made of the estimated path coefficients in comparing individuals, in following the course of a pulmonary disease in a single individual, or in differential diagnosis of a disease.[112]

The respiratory homeostasis illustration of the techniques of path analysis shows how the various complex and multi-interactional forms of biomedical causation can be rigorously modeled. Note that the physiological parameters can be drawn from any level provided the parameter is appropriately quantifiable.[113] The physiological example is also of general interest to investigators of path analysis because the underlying mechanisms are much better understood than *formally* similar situations in the social sciences, where much of the emphasis on the application of path analysis has occurred.

It should also be noted that Wright's successive refinements and evaluations of his path-analysis models (figures 5, 6, 7) represent the comparative aspects of explanation. Contrast of the explananda is, as usual in scientific contexts where the explanandum tends to be fixed by the traditional literature, primarily implicit (but see any textbook of lung pathophysiology for specified contrast cases).[114] A comparison of the successive explanans (the second comparative aspect in explanation) is quite explicit both in Wright's path-analysis diagrams and in Haldane and Priestley's original discussion of the possible causes, e.g., neural and chemical (including PCO_2 and PO_2). Further, more formal statistical evaluation (for example, by a chi-squared test, an F-test, ANOVA methods, or by using nonparametric tests) are feasible for this approach, but cannot be pursued here.[115]

Finally, the stochastic element of causality or probabilistic causality is represented in path analysis in at least four ways: (1) in the fact that regression coefficients and path coefficients represent random variables with a mean and a variance, (2) in the residual values such as V_u (and p_{qu}), in general, and in W and V in figure 5, in particular, (3) by the fact that Mendelian random variables can be naturally modeled in path analysis (see Li for various examples),[116] and (4) through Wright's arguments, quoted earlier, that probabilities can be identified with path coefficients. Two of these, namely (1) and (2), are involved in the Haldane and Priestley example, which is primarily deterministic. In addition, (3) and (4) would be present in more clearly stochastic examples, such as those discussed in an earlier section.

The path-analytical model outlined earlier appears to represent, in a formally precise manner, a number of important features of biomedical explanation. As noted, it is limited by the requirement of linearity. It is also somewhat pedagogically opaque as a way of representing the strength of causal relations where path coefficients with negative values and absolute values greater than one are employed. The method also requires careful equation specification, especially in cases involving negative feedback, as well as fairly tedious and often approximate calculations. There are alternative, more conventional modes of representation that offer greater transparency of interpretation as well as freedom from the linearity requirement, but they tend to obscure the multifactorial, feedback interactive, and often partially stochastic features of biomedical causation.

A brief comment on one widely employed mode of causal representation in the biomedical sciences should be cited here for the sake of comparison. This involves the familiar tool of using two (and occasionally three) dimensional "scattergrams" and their associated curves. Following the convention of designating the abscissa as the independent variable(s), the effect of a variation in the independent variable(s) on the dependent variable measured along the ordinate can be ascertained. Data points are entered on the graph and will constitute the "scattergram." A curve can be fitted to these points, usually employing a least-squares, goodness-of-fit criterion. If the curve is linear, or if it is a member of a known, not-too-complex type of function (such as a parabola, hyperbola, or exponential relation), one can specify means and variances for the curve on the graph. One typical way of representing the data and the variation from the idealized functional relation is to compute the standard error of estimate, and to represent this visually on the graph as vertical (and occasionally horizontal) bars drawn through the curve at appropriately chosen points. The formal definition of the standard error is given by:

$$S.E. = \sqrt{\frac{\sum_{i=1}^{n}(y_i - y'_i)^2}{n - 2}}$$

where y_i is an actual data point, y'_i the predicted data point based on the linear or nonlinear curve, and n is the number of observations. (It should be pointed out that the curve so chosen is equivalent to a regression "line," and thus both the path-analytic approach and the graphical-curve-fitting approach share an important common core of assumptions.) The standard error, under certain general assumptions, is an estimate of the standard deviation and can be used to calculate a "prediction band" to any desired degree of confidence, say, 95 percent or 99 percent. (These general assumptions are that the $y_i - y'_i$ are independently and normally distributed with 0 means and the same standard deviation.)[117] Purely probabilistic relations such as Salmon considers (see earlier section) could also be represented graphically as a line chart, where the ordinate represents probability values between 0 and 1, and the abscissa either the unconditional or conditional occurrence of events.[118]

To illustrate this graphical mode, I will refer to more recent lung-ventilation experiments that are similar to those performed by Haldane and Priestley. These experiments were conducted on thirty-three subjects by Lambertsen and his associates; the data are depicted in figure 8(*a, b,* and *c*).[119] Lambertsen also found considerable variability among his subjects, as is noted in figure 9, which represents a cluster analysis of these subjects into four subgroups. (Again, the point concerning biomedical variability should be recalled in this connection.)

These curves are essentially linear, and Lambertsen suggests that the departure from linearity is the result of sampling error using alveolar PCO_2. Where arterial PCO_2 is used as the independent variable instead, "the PCO_2 respiratory minute volume response is essentially linear."[120] Many relationships in the biomedical sciences, however, are by no means linear and exhibit quite complex vocations. Figure 10, based on Bulow's work, indicates the effect of PCO_2 on lung ventilation in alert and in sleeping subjects. This graph reveals the strengths of the pictorial representation in capturing the high-fidelity complex variations, but it also indicates the limitations of prediction and explanation based on this representative mode, namely, that it is difficult to extrapolate to any but the most general trends. (Note also the lack of explicit

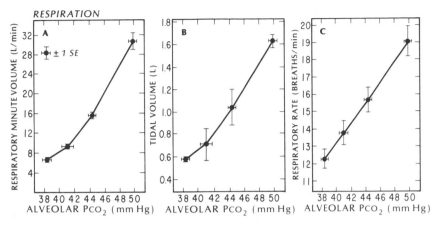

Fig. 8. Response of, *a*, respiratory minute volume, *b*, tidal volume, (which measures depth of respiration), and *c*, respiratory frequency, to increases in alveolar P_{CO_2} produced by breathing approximately 2%, 4%, and 6% CO_2 in 21% O_2 in N_2. (Average values in 33 normal subjects.) Magnitudes of largest effects on respiration are graphically equalized to show that effects of CO_2 on both frequency and depth of respiration are proportional to change in P_{CO_2}. Reprinted, by permission, from Lambertsen, "Chemical Control," p. 1779.

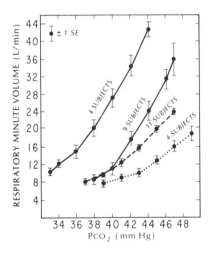

Fig. 9. Variability of respiratory response to low concentrations of inspired CO_2. Alveolar P_{CO_2} values determined by using end-tidal values. Same normal subjects and data employed for average curves of Fig. 8 are here placed in four groups to show that normal individuals may exhibit different patterns of respiratory response to CO_2. These may range from extreme reactivity of group *A* to low "sensitivity" shown by subjects of group *D*. Response of latter group is no greater than that seen in some patients with emphysema or in overdose of a narcotic such as meperidine. Reprinted, by permission, from Lambertsen, "Chemical Control," p. 1778.

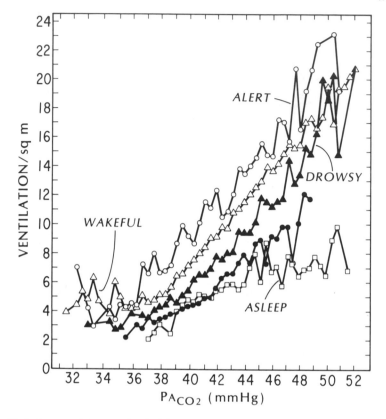

Fig. 10. Influence of degree of wakefulness on respiratory response to CO_2. Curves are based on more than 3,000 ventilation-Pco_2 points in normal subjects. State of wakefulness or degree of sleep was determined by analysis of EEG recordings. Curves represent mean findings plotted as differences from data obtained in state of tense alertness. Sleep leads to progressive decrease in reactivity to CO_2. Reprinted, by permission, from Lambertsen, "Chemical Control," p. 1779.

standard-error information, because no simple "linear" relationship is proposed.)

The path-analytical and the graphical modes of representing causation each has its strong and weak points. Graphical representations often overlook or suppress variability (though they need not do so), and cannot easily deal with more than two independent variables, unless one uses a *series* of graphs in which all but one (or two) variables are held constant.[121] This leads to a fragmented representation. Path analysis succinctly and unitarily represents arbitrarily complex causal interactions, but it requires careful equation specification as well as complex calculations to obtain the necessary coefficients.[122] Both modes of representation (and others not discussed, such as factor analysis) are consistent with and are more fine-structured realizations of the general explanation schema developed in the next section.

Before returning to the general issue of biomedical explanation, however, it would be appropriate to comment very briefly on the current status of various theories of respiratory regulation. It is now generally accepted that there are *two* reactive regions: one *central*, which is associated with but not identical to the respiratory center, and the other located in the *periphery* (in the aortic bodies above and below the aortic arch, and in the carotid bodies at the bifurcation of the common carotid arteries). Chemical stimuli resulting from low O_2, high CO_2, and acidity changes are known to be factors that influence respiration via chemical and neurally mediated actions on the two regions, though these are somewhat different effects in the two regions. There are several current competing general theories of respiratory regulation, some of which have quantitative components akin to regression equations, and some of which are primarily qualitative or at best comparative. *Comparative* is used here in the sense that these theories predict an increase or decrease in an effect resulting from change in a causal variable, but do not provide specific quantitative predictions. This is a complex and evolving subject that cannot be addressed here, and the interested reader should consult Lambertsen's excellent review for a sophisticated introduction and references. Suffice it to say, there appears nothing in these theories that would not be subjectible to the analysis discussed earlier and now to be amplified on.

WHAT DOES IT MEAN "TO EXPLAIN" IN THE BIOMEDICAL SCIENCES?

In answering the question, "What does it mean 'to explain' in the biomedical sciences?" we propose the following schema:

"to explain" means to increase the probability (in the sense of a posterior judgmental probability) of the explanandum (E_j) given the explanans (C_j). This increase will be a function of the relevance relation between C_j and E_j (often causal though regression analyses can subsume non-causal determinations), and the successful doubly-comparative judgmental evaluation (1) of C_j to E_j and its contrast cases $E_1 \ldots E_i$ and (2) of C_j with *its* contrast explanations $C_1 \ldots C_i$ with respect to E_j.

This schema can be more formally represented in a path analysis model or in a series of graphs representing multiple regression relationships, in which various path coefficients or partial regression coefficients will generally explain the proportion of the effect(s).[123] The causes will generally be either necessary or contributory and jointly sufficient. The role of necessary conditions in such a schema can be represented by a *comparison* case (distinguished from a competing *contrast* case) in which a causal antecedent is eliminated and the effect does not occur. Similarly Mackie's *inus* conditions can be introduced in such a path analysis diagram as well as in a graph in which a "control" is depicted. Which factors are construed as *causes* is partially pragmatic, but is conditioned by an evaluational procedure similar to that proposed by Hill above and augmented by appropriate statistical tests which will vary from situation to situation (dependent on distributions, number in a series, etc.). Which of the antecedent causal conditions are "conditions" and which are "causes" will also be a pragmatic judgment.[124]

I believe that Salmon's examples, which led him away from the Hempelian schema, can be accounted for in the proposed explication. Salmon was concerned about explanations in which the premises were true but irrelevant, and which explanations met all the criteria for good D-N explanations. The explanation of a man's non-pregnancy premised on his taking birth control pills, which was cited earlier, is such an example. In the analysis presented in these pages such premises are not explanatory: they do not increase the probability of the explanandum, nor does their denial alter that probability. Accordingly they do not qualify as explanations.

Salmon's assertions contra Hempel about low weight explanations are also assimilable within the present model. In general, one should prefer that explanation which offers the largest conjoint or net probability compared to its rivals. That probability could be low, but it would be the "best" explanation.

As noted in the discussion of Wright's modelling of Haldane and Priestley's results, usually what is exhibited is a not-completely-resolved-to-the-smallest-detail fragment of the causal network. Based on interests, needs, and the nature of the scientific inquiry each interaction in the "gappy" generalization can often be "exploded" into more detail, and additional causal variables exported out of the residuum. What conditions and causes are explicitly cited and how the causal "field" is described is again often partially pragmatic and partially idiosyncratic to specific examples.

This analysis is applicable to each of the six representative requests for explanations in the biomedical sciences with which I began this essay. The explanation of the synthesis of β-galactosidase by *E. coli* in

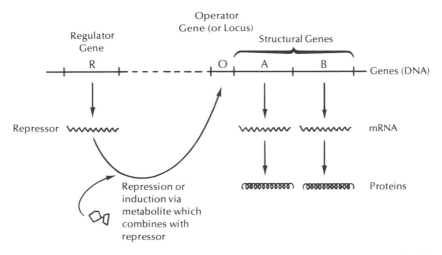

Fig. 11. Diagrammatic representation of the operon theory in 1961 (based on Jacob and Monod, 1961). The model is somewhat different from contemporary accounts since the repressor is not depicted as a protein, the messenger RNA is not synthesized as a unit for the regulated structural genes, and there is no "promotor" locus depicted. These modifications were made by Jacob, Monod, and their colleagues in the years after 1961. When there is lactose in its environment, *E. coli*, with the above genetic constitution, will receive a signal indicating the presence of the lactose. In the absence of a preferred metabolite, the lactose will combine with the repressor rendering it ineffective in binding to the operator site, permitting the enzyme RNA polymerase to transcribe mRNA, which is then translated into two proteins, permease and β-galactosidase. The latter protein is an enzyme that hydrolyzes lactose, a requirement for its digestion by the *E. coli*.

the presence of lactose is explained by the *lac* operon theory. This involves presenting something very much like a path-analysis diagram, though the path coefficients have not yet been calculated and there are likely to be qualitative elements as well. The various conditions for protein synthesis can be modeled in such a diagram (see figure 11).

Our second example concerning respiratory homeostasis has already been discussed extensively in the previous section.

The question concerning the 9:3:4 ratio of color coat in mice can be answered in two ways. One, a more superficial explanation, will involve a probabilistic path-analysis diagram for two gene pairs, with each pair assorting independently. In the explanation, one gene in a homozygous recessive state is epistatic to the other. Thus, a probability distribution in which *aa* is expected (where *A* is the color dominant over albino [*a*] and *B* is the agouti color dominate over black [*b*] four out of the sixteen times will account for the 4/16 albino ratio. The other color distributions follow similarly.[125]

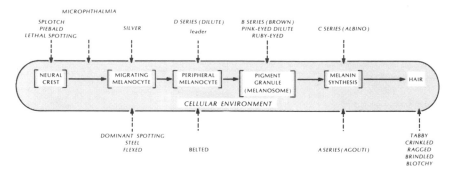

Fig. 12. Developmental stages at which coat color genes in the mouse are believed to act. The upper part of the figure shows genes that probably act directly on the pigment cells, and the lower part shows genes that may act on the environment of these cells. Reprinted, by permission, from Strickberger, *Genetics*.

A more fine-structure explanation of epistasis itself can be formulated. It involves a series of biosynthetic pathways in which an epistatic gene blocks further melanin syntheses. A diagram from Strickberger is provided as figure 12.[126] This figure is also amenable to path analysis, assuming correlation and regression values are experimentally available.

Our remaining representative requests for explanations, namely, the question concerning sickle-cell anemia, the question about slime-mold aggregation (*Dictostelium discoideum*), and the questions about the function of the thymus illustrate (1) historical (or genetic in the "genesis" sense), (2) organizational, and (3) functional types of explanations. I believe the theses of explanation developed in this article can be appropriately elaborated to accommodate each of these often-discussed types of explanation, but this will be done elsewhere.[127]

NOTES

1. Portions of this chapter will appear in an expanded form in my forthcoming book *Discovery and Explanation in the Biomedical Sciences*, in which I relate explanation to these issues. See also David Hull, *Philosophy of the Biological Sciences* (Englewood Cliffs, N.J.: Prentice-Hall, 1974) and Michael Ruse, *Philosophy of Biology* (London: Hutchinson, 1973).
2. David B. Guralnik, ed., *Webster's New World Dictionary* (Cleveland: William Collins, World Publishing Co., 1974), p. 493.
3. See F. Jacob and J. Monod, "Genetic Regulatory Mechanisms in the Synthesis of Proteins," *Journal of Molecular Biology* 3 (1961): 318-356.

4. See J. S. Haldane and J. G. Priestley, "The Regulation of Lung Ventilation," *Journal of Physiology* 32 (1905): 225-266.

5. See Monroe W. Strickberger, *Genetics*, 2d ed. (New York: Macmillan, 1976), p. 206.

6. A. Jacquard, *The Genetic Structure of Populations* (New York: Springer-Verlag, 1974).

7. W. F. Loomis, "Biochemistry of Aggregation in *Dictostelium*," *Developmental Biology* 70 (1979): 1-12.

8. See J.F.A.P. Miller, "Immunological Function of the Thymus," *Lancet* 2 (September 30, 1961): 748-749.

9. See K. F. Schaffner, "Logic of Discovery and Justification in Regulatory Genetics," *Studies in History and Philosophy of Science* 4 (1974): 349-385, and also K. F. Schaffner, "The Peripherality of Reductionism in the Development of Molecular Biology," *Journal of the History of Biology* 7 (1974): 111-139.

10. See my forthcoming book cited in note 1 above.

11. Karl R. Popper, *Logik der Forschung* (Vienna, 1935). Translated as *The Logic of Scientific Discovery* (London: Hutchinson, 1959).

12. C. G. Hempel and P. Oppenheim, "Studies in the Logic of Explanation," *Philosophy of Science* 15 (1948): 98-115.

13. See the essays in C. G. Hempel, *Aspects of Scientific Explanation and Other Essays in the Philosophy of Science* (New York: Free Press, 1965).

14. Hempel, *Aspects*, p. 368.

15. Ibid., p. 367.

16. M. Scriven, "Explanation and Prediction in Evolutionary Theory," *Science* 130 (1959): 477-482.

17. Hempel, *Aspects*, pp. 369-370.

18. Scriven, "Explanation."

19. Hempel, *Aspects*, pp. 374-375.

20. See K. F. Schaffner, "Theory Structure in the Biomedical Sciences," *Journal of Medicine and Philosophy* 5 (1980): 57-97.

21. See Hempel, *Aspects*, p. 383.

22. Ibid., pp. 394-403

23. Ibid., p. 400.

24. Wesley C. Salmon, *Statistical Explanation and Statistical Relevance* (Pittsburgh: University of Pittsburgh Press, 1970), p. 34.

25. Ibid., pp. 10-11.

26. Ibid., pp. 76-77.

27. W. C. Salmon, "Theoretical Explanation," in *Explanation*, ed. Stephan Körner (Oxford: Oxford University Press, 1975), pp. 118-145.

28. W. C. Salmon, "Why Ask 'Why?'? — An Inquiry Concerning Scientific Explanation," *Proceedings and Addresses of the American Philosophic Association* 51, 6 (August 1978): 683-705, 699.

29. For reasons discussed earlier, and to be developed further, in connection with the work of Skyrms and van Fraassen.

30. See Ernst Mayr, "Cause and Effect in Biology," in *Man and Nature*, ed. Ronald Munson (New York: Delta Books, 1971), pp. 101-116; and George G. Simpson, *This View of Life* (New York: Harcourt Brace and World, 1964).

31. J.J.C. Smart, *Philosophy and Scientific Realism* (London: Routledge and Kegan Paul, 1963).

32. See my essay "Causation and Responsibility: Medicine, Science, and the

Law," in *The Law-Medicine Relation*, ed. Stuart Spicker (Dordrecht: Reidel, 1981), 95-122.

33. Ibid.

34. See Schaffner, "Theory Structure."

35. See H. L. A. Hart and A. M. Honoré, *Causation in the Law* (Oxford: Oxford University Press, 1969); John Mackie, *The Cement of the Universe* (Oxford: Oxford University Press, 1974); and J. Anderson, "The Problem of Causality," *Australasian Journal of Philosophy* 16 (1938): 127-142.

36. Mackie, *Cement*, p. 62.

37. Ibid., p. 66.

38. Salmon, "Why," p. 699.

39. Ibid., p. 688.

40. Hans Reichenbach, *The Direction of Time* (Berkeley and Los Angeles: University of California Press, 1956). I. J. Good, "A Causal Calculus I-II," *British Journal of Philosophy of Science* 11 (1961): 305-318, and 12 (1962): 43-51. Errata 13 (1963): 88. Patrick Suppes, *A Probabilistic Theory of Causality* (Amsterdam: North-Holland 1970).

41. Salmon, *Statistical Explanation*, p. 42.

42. Ibid., pp. 76-77.

43. See W. C. Salmon, "Probabilistic Causality," *Pacific Philosophic Quarterly* 61 (1980): 50-74.

44. Reichenbach, *Direction*.

45. Salmon, *Statistical Explanation*, p. 55.

46. Suppes, *Probabilistic Theory*, passim.

47. Bertrand Russell, *Human Knowledge, Its Scope and Limits* (New York: Simon and Schuster, 1948), p. 459.

48. Hans Reichenbach, *The Philosophy of Space and Time* (New York: Dover, 1958), section 21.

49. Salmon, "Why," p. 690.

50. Ibid.

51. Reichenbach, *Direction*, section 19.

52. Salmon, "Why," p. 704.

53. Ibid., p. 692.

54. Ibid., p. 694.

55. P. von Bretzel, "Concerning a Probabilistic Theory of Causation Adequate for the Causal Theory of Time," *Syntheses* 35 (1977): 173-190.

56. Salmon, "Why," p. 696.

57. But see below for a further elaboration based on Salmon, "Probabilistic."

58. Salmon, "Why," pp. 699-700.

59. Ibid., p. 700.

60. Ibid., p. 688.

61. Salmon, "Probabilistic."

62. Ibid.

63. See my forthcoming *Discovery and Explanation*, chap. 7, for details.

64. Salmon, "Probabilistic," p. 55.

65. Reichenbach, *Direction*, p. 190.

66. Salmon, "Probabilistic," p. 57.

67. See Suppes, *Probabilistic Theory*, p. 41; and D. Rosen, "In Defense of a Probabilistic Theory of Causality," *Philosophy of Science* 45 (1978): 604-613.

68. Salmon, "Probabilistic," p. 65.

69. The procedure will go something like the following. What is needed is to represent formally the (to me) sound intuition that *if* the population of discourse is electrons taking the improbable path, each successive stage occupied still has a higher probability, thus conforming to the betweenness axiom. One suggestion obtained from Clark Glymour, in conversation, is to consider the probability of the *paths*, so that transition $4 \to 2 \to 1$ is written $P(4.2.1)$, subject to the following constraint:

$$P(4.2.1 / 4.2) > P(4.2.1 / 4) > P(4.2.1) > 0$$

This condition is necessary, and would have to be supplemented with appropriate additional condition(s) to restrict state 1 from being between 4 and 2.

70. Salmon, "Probablistic," p. 70.

71. Ibid.

72. Arthur B. Hill, *Principles of Medical Statistics*, 10th ed. (Oxford: Oxford University Press, 1977). See also Mervyn Susser, *Causal Thinking in the Health Sciences* (New York: Oxford University Press, 1973); and the U.S. Department of Health, Education, and Welfare's famous *Smoking and Health: Report of the Advisory Committee to the Surgeon General* (Washington, D.C.: Government Printing Office, 1964).

73. See Claude Bernard, *Introduction to the Study of Experimental Medicine* (New York: Dover, 1957 [originally published in 1865]), and my discussion of this method, suitably modified, in *Discovery and Explanation*, chap. 4.

74. The point that Salmon has no well-defined notion of a "trial" was first suggested to me in conversation with Teddy Seidenfeld. For an additional comment concerning Salmon's approach and its relation to regression analysis, see note 118 of this article.

75. Hill, *Principles*, p. 289.

76. Ibid., p. 292.

77. Since temporal asymmetry is assumed, this approach is weaker than Reichenbach's attempt in *Direction* to characterize a theory of time and to *derive* the appropriate asymmetry.

78. Hill, *Principles*, p. 294.

79. Brian Skyrms, *Causal Necessity* (New Haven, Conn.: Yale University Press, 1980), especially pp. 140-145. Bas C. van Fraassen, *The Scientific Image* (New York: Oxford University Press, 1980), especially chap. 5. Schaffner, "Causation and Responsibility." P. Gardenfors, "A Pragmatic Approach to Explanations," *Philosophy of Science* 47 (1980): 404-423.

80. Skyrms, *Causal Necessity*, pp. 140-141.

81. Ibid., pp. 141-142.

82. Ibid., p. 142.

83. Ibid., p. 143. Skyrms's reference to Salmon is to his *Statistical Explanation* monograph. The other references are R. Jeffrey, "Statistical Explanation vs. Statistical Inference," in *Essays in Honor of Carl G. Hempel*, ed. Nicholas Rescher (Dordrecht: Reidel,1969), pp. 104-113; and P. Railton, "A Deductive-Nomological Model of Scientific Explanation," *Philosophy of Science* 45 (1978): 206-226.

84. See D. Heise, "Problems in Path Analysis and Causal Inference," *Sociological Methodology* 1 (1969): 38-73, for an excellent discussion of the assumptions that need to be satisfied for path analysis to be applied. My only quarrel with Heise concerns his account of feedback, which should be compared with S. Wright, "The Treatment of Reciprocal Interaction, With or Without Lag, in Path Analysis," *Biometrics*, 16 (1960): 423-445, which is more general and most

important for biomedical systems. Heise's later book *Causal Analysis* (New York: John Wiley, 1975) discusses reciprocal interaction in depth and should be consulted by anyone interested in this subject. See also the references in note 98 of this article.

85. Not every variable can be accommodated by such a transformation, but the practice is not clearly limited by any general theorem of which I am aware.

86. See C. C. Li, "The Concept of Path Coefficient and Its Impact on Population Genetics," *Biometrics* 12 (1956): 190-210.

87. See Clark Glymour's excellent and stimulating discussion of path analysis in *Theory and Evidence* (Princeton, N.J.: Princeton University Press, 1980), chap. 7. Glymour is not incorrect in his account of path coefficients, but as noted in the text, his analysis is not the most general.

88. Compare S. Wright, "Path Coefficients and Path Regression: Alternative or Complementary Concepts?" *Biometrics* 16 (1960): 189-202, especially pp. 194-195.

89. See M. E. Turner and C. E. Stevens, "The Regression Analysis of Causal Paths," *Biometrics* 15 (1959): 236-258, for a discussion of estimators.

90. See Dennis V. Lindley, *Introduction to Probability and Statistics, Part 2. Inference*. (Cambridge: Cambridge University Press, 1970), especially chap. 8. In my forthcoming *Discovery and Explanation*, I defend a generalized Bayesian account of theory testing and evaluation, and being able to provide a Bayesian account of path coefficients is accordingly important.

91. See Lindley, *Introduction*, p. 212.

92. See Li, "Concept," p. 197.

93. Ibid.

94. See Ching Chung Li, *Population Genetics* (Chicago: University of Chicago Press, 1955), pp. 152-153.

95. Li, "Concept," p. 198.

96. Sewall Wright, *Evolution and the Genetics of Populations*, vol. 1 (Chicago: University of Chicago Press, 1968), pp. 315-316.

97. J. Tukey, "Causation, Regression, and Path Analysis," in *Statistics and Mathematics in Biology*, ed. O. Kempthorne et al. (Ames: Iowa State University Press, 1954), pp. 35-66. Turner and Stevens, "Regression Analysis."

98. Wright, "Treatment" (see note 84). Introduction of reciprocal interactions into path analysis raises a number of difficult issues. One fundamental problem is that recursivity, in the strict sense, is eliminated; this leads to the necessity of finding alternatives to least-squares estimation. H. A. Simon has developed the notion of "vector causality" to isolate this problem in his "Causal Ordering and Identifiability," in *Studies in Econometric Method*, ed. W. C. Hood and T. C. Koopmans (New York: John Wiley, 1953). For a general discussion of these problems and other solutions see H. M. Blalock, ed., *Causal Models in the Social Sciences* (Chicago: Aldine, 1971), especially pp. 1-4 and part 3. See also A. Koutsoyiannis's *Theory of Econometrics*, 2d ed. (London: Macmillan, 1977), part 3.

99. J. S. Haldane and J. G. Priestley, "The Regulation of Lung Ventilation," *Journal of Physiology* 32 (1905): 225-266, p. 225.

100. Ibid.

101. Ibid., pp. 253-254.

102. Ibid., p. 252.

103. Wright, "Treatment," pp. 433-444.

104. Ibid., p. 433.

105. Ibid., p. 434.

106. Details of how these coefficients are calculated are not made explicit in Wright. The interested reader may compare Wright's analysis of market supply and price in ibid., figure 10, p. 433, which yields the equation given in the same article on p. 431. Solutions are provided on p. 432. The subdiagram $D \overset{w}{\to} P \overset{x}{\underset{y}{\to}} Q$ is shown to lead to a solution $W = \sqrt{(1 - xy)(1 - xr_{PQ})}$, which is formally equivalent to the equation for p_{DW} with appropriate substitutions.

107. Ibid., p. 436. As will be noted, if the P_{CO_2} in the arterial blood is measured directly, cleaner (in the sense that non-linear threshold effects are eliminated) results are obtained, confirming Wright's speculations. This type of measurement was not available to Haldane and Priestley.

108. Ibid., p. 437.

109. See J. E. Cotes, *Lung Function*, 3d ed. (Philadelphia: Lippincott, 1975), pp. 5-7, for a discussion of Haldane's work in historical perspective. For a readable account of lung physiology, with all its complexities, see John F. Murray, *The Normal Lung* (Philadelphia: Saunders, 1976).

110. Wright, "Treatment," p. 434.

111. See Schaffner, "Theory Structure."

112. Turner and Stevens, "Regression Analysis," p. 254.

113. In moving between levels, care must be taken to avoid certain fallacies. See Susser, *Causal Thinking*, pp. 60-63.

114. See A. P. Fishman, ed., *Pulmonary Diseases and Disorders* (New York: McGraw-Hill, 1980).

115. For a discussion of some statistical tests of path-analysis models, see N. H. Nie, ed., *Statistical Package for the Social Sciences* (New York: McGraw-Hill, 1975), pp. 392-394.

116. See Li, *Population*, chap. 13.

117. See P. Hoel, *Elementary Statistics*, 4th ed. (New York: John Wiley, 1976), p. 231.

118. See ibid., chap. 4, for examples of line charts. As noted earlier, Salmon's examples are idealized probabilities in the sense that they assume 0 variance (or at least an unspecified variance). Accordingly it is difficult to map the Salmon examples into regression analyses, but the correlation may go as follows. Salmon is dealing with dichotomous events, i.e., A happens or it does not, which on the basis of a frequency class of the A's, can be given a probability value for A. Similarly, conditional probabilities could be represented by a line chart, the only difference being that the dependent-variable axis would represent conditional probability rather than unconditional probability. One could, on the basis of such a graph, also represent Reichenbach's betweenness condition, namely, that if the X-axis represents two triple sequences of dichotomous positive events, C, C/A, C/B and A, A/C, A/B, and if the Y-axis represents the unconditional or conditional probabilities as line charts, then the betweenness conditions mentioned earlier require that the slope of the line connecting the end points of the line charts always be positive. This is not terribly illuminating, however. More interesting methodologically would be a further development of Salmon's and others' concepts of probabilistic causality in the regression direction. Such an account is beyond the scope of this

article, but its outlines can be very briefly sketched. In place of dichotomous variables one employs continuous variables. For a simple causal sequence, say, $A \rightarrow B \rightarrow C$, one writes three recursive equations as in path analysis. These equations are assumed to fit, by a least-squares criterion, the data supporting this dependence. The scattergram will occupy a three-space. Alternatively, one could use two successive graphs for this system, with A as the independent variable and B dependent in the first graph, and with B independent and C dependent in the second. The probability of obtaining some specific value for B, given a value of A, for example, depends on the confidence interval one chooses for B and the scatter of the data points. In Salmon's approach the data points are reduced dichotomously to yield two classes, B and not-B, for a positive occurrence of A, and the probability is computed on the basis of these B and not-B frequencies. In the suggested expansion to continuous variables, the relation between A and B is still probabilistic, but the structure is much richer.

119. C. J. Lambertsen, "Chemical Control of Respiration at Rest," in *Medical Physiology*, vol. 2, 14th ed. V. Mountcastle (St. Louis: Mosby, 1980), pp. 1774-1827.

120. Ibid., p. 1778.

121. Representations of a family of interactions could be sketched, thus increasing the number of independent variables by one, but this family could be only partially represented in such an approach.

122. Assuming that a least-squares criterion was used and a standard error was computed for the graphical analysis, the graphical approach would require similarly difficult calculations. Computer programs such as SPSS can make these computations easier, however, for nonfeedback situations. More complex programs such as are employed in econometrics would be required if recursivity was to be eliminated.

123. This approach to explanation can also be captured at a quite general level, i.e., independent of the path analytic or graphical representations. See Schaffner "Causation" and also Chapter 7 of Schaffner, *Discovery and Explanation*.

124. See Schaffner, "Causation."

125. See Strickberger, *Genetics*, pp. 205-208.

126. Ibid., p. 213.

127. See Schaffner, *Discovery and Explanation*, chaps. 8, 9, and 10.

Puzzles about the Causal Explanation of Human Actions

Joseph Margolis

Discourse about causal relations appears to be conceptually anchored in two extremely different kinds of accounts: (1) relations are said to be causal if they are explainable by appeal to causal laws; and (2) relations are said to be causal if they are instances of agency or of some process thought to be suitably similar to agency. Merely to mention these alternatives is to collect an extraordinarily large nest of puzzles of a profound sort. We are, for example, hard-pressed to provide proper accounts of the nature of laws, causal laws, explanations, causal explanations; also, to provide a proper account of human, animal, and inanimate agency or causal process. But apart from such strenuous matters, it may be usefully noted that: (1) it is entirely possible that appeal to so-called natural laws need not directly bear on the causal explanation of a given phenomenon, simply because the laws in question need not be causal laws, laws formulating a direct causal relationship between paired phenomena (even if an underlying causal connection is presupposed); (2) to hold that explanatory models in science are specifically causal in nature may require appeal to more than the form of laws or to the form of explanations: (3) causal relations may, on the agency paradigm, be said to be perceived or identified (as by a successful human agent) directly and independently of reference to any causal law or causal explanation. Thus, for instance, the Boyle-Charles law for ideal gases, is, in Ernest Nagel's opinion, "not a causal law," primarily because it is expressed in terms of concomitant changes.[1] Nagel also observes, characterizing causal laws in general, that, among qualifying conditions to be met, "the relation [involved must be] an invariable or uniform one, in the sense that whenever the alleged cause occurs so does the alleged effect."[2] Whatever weakness or vagueness may be charged to this or similar conditions (which Nagel concedes), it is reasonably clear that not all familiar laws are causal laws; furthermore, it is doubtful that *any* laws have *ever* been formulated that, in the relevant sense, exhibit a strict invariance; statistical laws could not be causal laws, on the condition posed; and any more rigorous formulation along these lines of what it is to be a causal law would even further dampen the likelihood of providing convincing instances.

There are problems also with the alleged logical form of causal explanations. For instance, Carl Hempel holds that

causal explanation is a special type of deductive-nomological explanation; for a certain event or set of events can be said to have caused a specified "effect" only if there are general laws connecting the former with the latter in such a way that, given a description of the antecedent events, the occurrence of the effect can be deduced with the help of the laws.[3]

On Hempel's view, a deductive-nomological explanation "may be construed as an argument in which the explanandum is deduced from the explanans."[4] But this raises questions of at least two sorts. First of all, it may be that there are laws linking antecedent and subsequent events that are not causal laws: Hempel's condition is formulated only as a necessary constraint; what makes such a regularity a causal regularity is not supplied. Secondly, since explanations invoking statistical laws cannot be deductive, explanations employing statistical laws cannot, on Hempel's view, be causal explanations, yet one supposes that there must be some. Thirdly, the mere form of the deductive-nomological model may be defective as an explanatory model, since there are formulable cases that would meet the conditions of the model without being admissible as explanations—*a fortiori*, without being causal explanations. For example, Sylvain Bromberger offers the example of a flagpole's shadow being cast over a particular length, depending on the elevation of the sun: we explain the length of the shadow by reference to the sun's position, the height of the flagpole, and the laws governing the behavior of light; but though we may also infer the height of the flagpole from the shadow's length and the position of the sun, we would not view the inference as explanatory of the flagpole's height. Asymmetrical temporal relations, Wesley Salmon insists, "are crucial in this example."[5] Fourthly, as Salmon also points out, the argument model tends to lead us to suppose that, where determinism is abandoned, as modern physics seems to require, we still suppose that statistical explanation must make the explanandum at least highly probable. Yet, as he adds,

an explanation is not an argument that is intended to produce conviction; instead, it is an attempt to assemble the facts that are relevant to the occurrence of an event. There is no more reason to suppose that such a process will increase the weight we attach to such an occurrence than there is to suppose that it will lower it.[6]

On Salmon's view, shifting to statistical explanation, we move to a suitable explanation insofar as we achieve "a relevant partition of an inhomogeneous reference class into homogeneous subclasses"; that is, roughly, "a reference class [the class of events to which the explanandum belongs, and which, on some rule, yields reliable statistics] is homogeneous if there is no way, even in principle, to effect a statistically relevant partition without already knowing which elements have the attribute in question and which do not. . . . Each member of a homogeneous reference class is a random member."[7] Clearly, the notion of a statistical explanation requires an adjustment in the concept of causality, since invariances no longer obtain. Following Hans Reichenbach,[8] Salmon favors an agency model—though one not requiring human agency; as he remarks:

Producing is, of course, a thoroughly causal concept; thus, the relation of interaction to orderly low entropy state becomes the paradigm of causation on Reichenbach's view, and the explanation of the ice cube in the thermos of water is an example of the most fundamental kind of causal explanation.[9]

Still, it is not unfair to note that the "production" Salmon and Reichenbach speak of involves a combination of considerations: (1) analogy between human or animal agency and the alleged "production"; and (2) stipulation in accord with certain favored theories of physical science. The reason for the quibble is straightforward. We cannot, except on the theory and the analogy favored, be said to perceive the "production" in question. But, in the case of human agency, we cannot even understand the rationality of an agent, the linkage between perception, intention, desire, belief, action, and the like *without conceding that human agents produce states of affairs and changes in states of affairs and that, in behaving intentionally and with some regular success, they can perceive and understand that they and others have caused such states and changes to occur.* The concept of a human agent, therefore, is, necessarily, the concept of a causally efficacious agent.

Animal agency and the agency of inanimate processes are, by an increasingly attenuated (but not for that reason inappropriate) analogy, construed as sources of causal efficacy. As the analogy of agency is weakened, the affirmation of causality depends on the explanatory importance of such processes—for instance, the appearance of a low entropy state. But, though questions may always arise about whether this or that agent did or did not produce this or that effect, these questions make no sense unless we concede standard sorts of cases in which we normally do exert agency in a causal way and in which we normally see or know that we or others are exerting such agency. Thus, a human agent is a creature capable of (1) causal agency, and (2) perceiving particular instances of causal agency.

Now, the single most important point bearing on human agency and the causal explanation of human action is that the perception or knowledge that *S* has exerted agency or produced an action does not require any knowledge, or even any formulated belief or sketch of a belief, of any *law*, deterministic or statistical, under which the causal process is to be explained. It may well be that there is a sense—conceivably, a trivial sense—in which to know that an agent produced an action intentionally is to be able to explain it: for instance, it may be that merely to redescribe a given action as an action one intended to produce *is* to explain it.[10] But, however generously we construe explanation, it is not necessary that, in treating an instance of human agency as causally efficacious, we make reference in any way at all—explicit or remote—to causal laws of any kind. Granting this, it is but a step to see that causal relations, at least instances of human agency or sufficiently similar animal agency, may not even presuppose that there are relevant covering laws—*a fortiori*, covering causal laws—under which they fall, or may not presuppose that they are or must be explainable under covering laws of some sort.

The possibility is admittedly heterodox. But consider that *if* causality is ascribed on the model of agency, then, assuming *A* to designate a human action, there is no apparent reason for holding that the following pair of propositions must be incompatible:

1. *A* caused *B*;
2. there is, in principle, no formulable causal law under which "*A* caused *B*" can be explained.

It may well be true that there are causal laws (of some sort) covering *some* human actions and their effects; and it is very clear that, as the analogy between human agency and the causal agency of inanimate physical events and processes is invoked, the ascription of causal efficacy to factors of the latter sort is made to depend upon the accessibility, at least in principle, of covering causal laws. To mention one influential author, Donald Davidson concedes that "singular causal statements" may be known to be true without any knowledge of any relevant covering law. Still, he also maintains, in the spirit of David Hume and John Stuart Mill, that *if* causality obtains, then there must be a covering law under which the singular causal connection falls.[11]

Davidson offers not the slightest defense for this position—all the more worth stressing, since he holds that causal connections behave extensionally, whereas causal explanations (all explanations) behave intensionally. That is, *on* Davidson's thesis—that causal laws are linguistic formulations of some sort—there appears to be a considerable lacuna in the argument that holds that the admission of the first proposition (given above) entails the falsehood of the second.[12] Of course, if the distinction of a causal law is made sufficiently informal, it may be that the affirmation of a covering law may be trivialized; but it is difficult to countenance such a tolerant line, given the usual emphasis on nomic universals as the paradigms of covering laws and the care with which suspect statistical laws are admitted to be genuine laws (rather than mere epistemically defective approximations of "true" laws). In any event, on the strongest and most characteristic view, there appears to be no genuine argument of a compelling sort that shows a logical connection between the truth of the first proposition and the truth of the denial of the second. J.J.C. Smart's sanguine view about eliminating all referring import from genuine nomic universals pretty well suggests that the stricter the constraints on what would count as a causal law, the less obvious it is that propositions 1 and 2 could be connected in the manner sketched.[13] The thesis that they are so connected, however, suggests as well that a strongly reductive program—physicalism, for instance—gains plausibility precisely in that it dismisses the agency paradigm of causality and assimilates human agency to the processes of inanimate forces; for, as already remarked, the ascription of causal efficacy to inanimate events and processes is normally made to depend on physical theories that promise (competitively) to yield covering causal laws by reference to which the phenomena in question may be suitably explained. Others, of course, on independent grounds—Karl Popper, for instance—reject the possibility of formulating valid natural laws.[14] Popper does not deny that would-be laws must be formulated as universals; but if they were genuinely fixed and if they obtained in the manner Smart favors, we should, Popper thinks, be committed to an untenable form of essentialism. Effectively, therefore, Popper construes explanations in terms of universal laws of nature as mere phases of some inexhaustible

effort to plumb the "depth" of a domain—in a sense, "hardly susceptible of logical analysis."[15] He modifies essentialism "radically," therefore; though, ironically, he seems to preserve an attenuated form of the
covering-law model of explanation.

There is no doubt that appeal to the phenomenon of human agency
as providing the fundamental model of causality strikes many as rather
naive. But it is not altogether implausible. It is, in fact, peculiarly
congruent with the familiar admission that singular causal statements
may be known to be true without knowledge of relevant covering laws.
In what more convincing setting could the thesis be sustained than in
that in which we ourselves deliberately and intentionally effect
changes in our surroundings? Thus, the advantages of the agency
model deserve to be collected. The following claims are, then, favored
by that model as opposed to the covering-law model: (*a*) *Particular
causal processes, notably those involving human actions, may be directly
perceived or known to occur, without reference at all to covering laws;*[16] (*b*)
*without denying that there are causal laws covering some particular causal
processes, notably inanimate causal processes, the affirmation of a human
action's causing an event does not as such entail that that process fall under any
covering law.*

It would appear that these claims may be greatly strengthened. Since
we have already favored a heterodox view of causality, we may as well
see how extreme an account may be plausibly advanced without
violating any known conceptual constraint. Certainly, we should want
to see whether, (*c*) *for some subset of human actions, there is, in principle, no
formulable causal law under which pertinent causal sequences can be
explained.* Thus far, we have merely shown that (*b*) is a strongly
reasonable claim; (*c*), if true, would require a fundamental shift in our
theory of explanation—in fact, it would argue a distinction between
the physical sciences and the "human studies" (*Naturwissenschaften*
and *Geisteswissenschaften*) that would challenge the familiar assumptions of the unity of science. Also, *if* (*c*) obtained and if we conceded,
along the lines sketched, that inanimate causal processes do entail
covering laws, then it is reasonably clear that (*d*) *actions satisfying (c)
cannot be reduced to mere physical processes*—for instance, along the lines
of Herbert Feigl's familiar use of the notion "physical."[17] Furthermore,
the most extreme claim that we could hope to make, conceding (*c*) and
(*d*) and affecting the issue of the unity of science, would be (*e*) *actions
satisfying (c) and (d) cannot be identified in the causal processes in which they
enter, in a purely extensional way.* This goes entirely contrary to Davidson's neat distinction—shared by a great many—that, although contexts of causal explanation (being linguistic) behave intensionally,

causal processes (obtaining in nature) behave extensionally. Arthur Danto speaks of the causal connection as "semiintensional," but he means by that, precisely, that the causal process *is* open to explanation under a covering law.[18] But that is not the sense here required. The sense of (*e*) required is that human actions—some human actions at least—cannot be assigned a causal role except under some description, consistently with (*b*), that is, without reference to any causal law at all; and that, once assigned a causal role, these human actions may be treated extensionally (shall we say, "semiextensionally"?) in the sense that if an action causes some event or change of state, it does so under any description that picks out that very same action and event. Claims (*a*) through (*e*), therefore, constitute a very different picture of the causal nature of human agency from that which obtains in standard theories of physical causality. The striking thing is that, even at this stage of the argument, our set of claims enjoys a certain prima facie reasonableness.

Now, the key consideration regarding the causal explanation of human action is this: the paradigm of human action is free action, action performed in such a way that it is presupposed that the human agent is at the moment of acting capable of refraining from acting thus and capable of performing an alternative action.[19] It is (1) precisely because a human agent is, as already noted, a creature essentially capable of causal agency and (2) because human agency is such that agents can perceive or know that they and others produce effects in the causal way, that (3) the paradigms of human agency are free actions. How else should we understand human agency unless at least as including the deliberate or intentional production of certain effects? It is because human agents act *to* produce intended effects that we concede, without reference to covering laws, that they may perceive themselves and others as succeeding in bringing such effects about, and they may come to know that their intentional actions have such effects. This means, of course, that the admission of the causal efficacy of human actions is incompatible with the admission that all causal processes fall under covering laws, where covering laws are deterministic in the strictest sense. For the notion of free action supposes that, at any time *t* at which an agent acts of his own volition, by choice, deliberately, intentionally, for a purpose or the like, he is capable of refraining from that action or of performing another action of some sort: if determinism signifies that real possibility is exhausted by whatever is actual, then human freedom is incompatible with determinism.[20]

But the admission of free action has further consequences. For one thing, (4) human actions can be identified *initially* only in intentional terms, that is, in terms of the intentional states of the agent. This (4) is misleading, however. It is *not* true that every human action is or needs to be describable in terms of an agent's actual *intentions*; but human actions must be described *intentionally*. For example, a man may be doodling in a kind of trance or shifting from foot to foot without being aware of doing so: to characterize what he is doing as occurring "in a kind of trance," "without being aware of doing so" *is* to characterize (at least incipiently) what he is doing in intentional terms but not in terms of his actual intentions. This seems to be an empirical point. Yet Davidson maintains that "action does require that what the agent does is intentional under some description, and this in turn requires, I think, that what the agent does is known to him under some description."[21] This either confuses the difference between intentional descriptions and descriptions in terms of an agent's intentions or else it begs the question about the individuation of actions — probably it does both.[22] But if an action must be initially identified in intentional terms, then it is impossible to identify a *free* action *initially* except under some cognitively favored description, that is, intensionally. For example, concede Davidson's case of one and the same action identified under four alternative descriptions: *flipping the light switch, turning on the light, illuminating the room, alerting a prowler.*[23] If the agent may be said to have acted freely *in* flipping the light switch or in turning on the light or in illuminating the room, he cannot be said — *initially at least* — to have acted freely in alerting a prowler who happened to be in the house. *If* what he did is one and the same action under the four descriptions proffered, then *if* he acted freely *in* what he did, that action, now described as alerting a prowler, was indeed a free action. He did *not*, by choice, act *to* alert a prowler; by choice, he acted *to* flip the light switch, *to* turn on the light, *to* illuminate the room. But *what* he did, *initially* identified under the description of choice or intended action, is (on pain of contradiction) a free action under any description that picks out the same action. So the admission of (4) entails that, (5) for free actions, particular actions can be identified initially only intensionally (partially, but only partially, the sense of [(e)] of a previous tally); and hence, (6) that free actions can be re-identified only on intensional grounds, that is, by reference to rules, institutions, conventional practices, traditions, or the like. There are, for example, no compelling extensional grounds that would oblige us to regard what occurred under the four descriptions provided as one and the same *action*. For one thing, one might well hold, along the lines developed by Alvin Goldman, that there were four different actions, three "generated" in different ways from the original (probably "basic") action of flipping the light switch.[24] In that case, even if the agent could be said to have performed an action in alerting a prowler, even if he acted freely in flipping the light switch, he did not act freely in alerting the prowler. Alternatively, one may deny that the agent performed any action at all *in* alerting the prowler: alerting the prowler may (on a suitable theory) have been the mere *effect* of what he did in the way of performing a free action.

There is no settled way of individuating actions. Certainly, admitting Goldman's strategy as a viable one, there is no way of individuating actions in terms of the spatiotemporal boundaries of purely physical events or their causal consequences that does not beg the question. This, of course, goes against Davidson.[25] The important thing to bear in mind is simply that the admission of (5) and (6) does not entail that the causality of human agency cannot be treated extensionally; it entails only that, (7) although causal contexts behave extensionally, the identification and re-identification of free actions *that function* causally cannot be managed in a purely extensional way. Doubtless, we may concede that constraints regarding the same spatiotemporal boundaries and the same effects serve as extensionally relevant limits *on* the re-identification of the same action; but it does not follow that human actions may be *initially* identified in terms of such constraints or other *physical* constraints like them. Clearly, the expectation that it would follow is likely to be linked, as in Davidson's case, to some form of reductionism.[26]

Human actions, then, qua causes, may be said to behave, as all causal connections do, extensionally: whatever causes a given effect, causes it. The trouble is that human actions, particularly free actions, cannot be identified or re-identified except in intensional terms. So the extensional feature of causality *is inoperative where the explanation of free action is concerned, except under intensional identificatory constraints*. But if this is so, and if causal agency does not entail covering laws (*b*), then we have very effectively begun to shape a defense for (*c*), that free actions cannot be explained under covering laws at all.

It is, in fact, the discovery of (7)—that the identification and re-identification of free actions cannot be managed except intensionally— that must surely be the key to the often seriously marred insistence of so many post-Wittgensteinian theorists of action who deny that human action may be explained in causal terms.[27] They have, some-how, confused the issue of causal explanation with an essential condition on which human action may be causally explained. They are right to press the point, because its admission enables us to grasp the very distinction of the causal explanation of human action; but they wrongly suppose that it actually precludes such explanation. The motivation is obvious: having assumed that causal explanation must involve covering laws and phenomena identifiable in a "purely extensional way," perhaps even deterministic laws, the post-Wittgensteinians simply opted for construing the explanation of human action—particularly free actions—as properly noncausal in nature.[28] But if claims (a)—(e) were vindicated, or some set of claims very much like them, then it would be possible to concede the conceptual insight of the post-Wittgensteinians—that the identification of human actions must be made in intentional terms; in particular, that certain actions, notably free actions, cannot be identified or re-identified except intensionally—at the same time we admit that human action is explainable in causal terms.[29]

In contrast, emphasis on the problem of identification and re-identification shows both the implausibility of *identifying human actions with physical events* and the effect on the causal explanation of actions of rejecting such an identity. Consider that Davidson's favored specimen of a free action is a particularly simple one like flipping a light switch. Here, there *is* some temptation to identify human actions with physical events. In fact, Davidson asserts explicitly: "our primitive actions, the ones we do not by doing something else, mere movements of the body— these are all the actions there are. We never do more than move our bodies: the rest is up to nature."[30] The notion of a primitive action is closely related to that of a basic action, as employed by Danto and Goldman: basic actions are taken to be identical with bodily movements—hence, to be identifiable in a purely extensional way (as physical events) and to permit the conventional covering-law explanation. Danto is particularly explicit about this.[31] But apart from the difficulty of specifying *which* actions are or must be basic actions,[32] there is no clear way of showing either that (i) for more complex actions—particularly those that have a large cultural import—actions can be traced to some putatively basic action that initiated the "generated" series; (ii) (in Davidson's sense) once we have accounted for how we move our bodies (as in primitive actions), the rest (presumably, whatever would causally explain such complex actions) is "up to [physical] nature"; or (iii) the causal explanation of basic actions constitutes or entails a causal explanation of seemingly more complex, culturally qualified actions—which, on Davidson's view, would be identical with primitive actions and, on Goldman's view, would (in various ways) be "generated" from basic actions. For example, suppose one of President Nixon's speeches caused even his closest cohorts to press for his resignation. What *bodily movements* could serve as the basic actions with which his speaking could be identified? How could his action of uttering *significant words* be explained by an explanation of how he produced a certain sequence of *sounds*? Most important, how could the explanation of the effect, upon the culturally informed *decision* of his cohorts, of *his having spoken in the role of beleaguered president* possibly be reduced to the explanation of the bodily movements taken to be the basic actions underlying his speech?

There is no room here to attempt to refute the intended reductionism.[33] But we must see that the viability of the explanatory claim about basic actions presupposes some form of mind/body reductionism. That thesis has not yet been satisfactorily formulated: in the case of actions of the complexity of Nixon's speech, the weakness of the reductive program is peculiarly obvious.[34]

A very useful economy suggests itself, therefore. Let us leave to one side—as not proved—the identity thesis. The fact is that, even if it were valid, appeal to it would not clarify the way in which we explain human actions causally without some explicit strategy showing *how* to move from the explanation of intensionally identified actions (5) to the explanation of purely physical movements. Of course, *if* a relationship other than identity obtains between the mental or psychological and the physical, we may well explain the *bodily movements* that are, by that alternative relation, associated with *human actions*, without at all explaining the actions thus linked.[35] If we remain agnostic, therefore, about the relationship between the mental and the physical, we may at least regard it as question-begging or as unresponsive to claim that, in explaining the putative basic actions on which complex, culturally significant actions somehow depend, we are explaining the latter as well. There is no need to deny that the *bodily movements* (agnostically conceded to be) "linked" to human actions, particularly free actions, fall under covering causal laws in the manner already sketched; also, granting the linkage, there is no need to deny that, in some fair sense, the explanation of those bodily movements forms at least a *part* of the explanation of free actions. But the essential issue of explaining the causal role of intensionally qualified actions—and, correspondingly, of intensionally qualified effects—remains a mystery.

The point that is entirely missed by all those who anticipate reducing complex actions to basic or primitive actions (à la Davidson), or who anticipate linking them to the basic actions from which they are "generated," as far as providing an adequate causal explanation is concerned (à la Goldman), is simply that the explanation of free actions, cultural phenomena in general, tends not to focus at all or to emphasize the causation of the bodily movements with which particular actions and the like are linked. What causal account can be given of the production of Dante's *Commedia*? What explains the event of Hitler's rise to power? What explains the hysterical compulsion of Emma, in Freud's *Scientific Project*? Even the most fundamental *actions* that could be linked with these complex matters are never, in any obvious way, identified as basic bodily movements of any sort; the relevant actions (however "basic") are already richly informed by intentional considerations *that cannot be identified except in the context of an enveloping culture*. Broadly speaking, when we explain human actions, particularly free actions and phenomena identified as culturally important, we explain phenomena that are distinguished functionally. To explain a free action is to explain a functionally distinctive phenomenon, the function of which is specifiable in and only in a cultural context. So if (7) is admitted, that is, if free actions can be identified and reidentified only intensionally, it seems reasonable to insist as well that (8) the causal explanation of free actions is essentially concerned with the explanation of functionally specified phenomena, where to specify an action functionally, that is, in culturally relevant terms, is to specify the intensional properties of that action. In short, to explain a free action is to explain a phenomenon that is not initially identifiable except in intensional terms, *and* it is to explain as well the causal relations in which, qua possessing intensionally qualified intentional properties, the free action actually enters. Thus, the cultural disciplines need never deny the relevance of causal accounts in purely physical terms—of, that is, bodily movements somehow "linked" to free actions or to related cultural phenomena. But *in* explaining such phenomena, those disciplines are primarily concerned to explain how it is, say, that a human being steeped in certain literary traditions, religious, philosophical, and political doctrines, produces a poem of such invention and significance as the *Commedia*; how it is that, in a certain historical setting in Germany, an amoral monster was able to captivate an entire population and to move people to unheard-of acts of violence; and how it is that, having suffered certain traumata at an early age, a young woman finds herself now able to go into shops alone.

The reason the purely physical explanation of human actions is largely beside the point—though, of course, hardly irrelevant—is quite straightforward. In conceding that (8) free actions and cultural phenomena are functionally distinguished, we implicitly concede as well that *there are indefinitely many alternative ways in which a culturally (or functionally) characterized action or phenomenon may be "linked" to some bodily event*.[36] Imagine, for instance, that Dante composed the *Com-

media by writing with his toes; or imagine that Hitler's recorded speeches were synchronized (undetected) with his (seemingly) live ranting. There is absolutely no reason to believe that, under such circumstances, *which* basic bodily movement happened to be the one by which the culturally significant actions of Dante and Hitler were manifested bears in any important explanatory way on the causal account of those actions. True enough, *some* account of physical causation must be relevant, that is, some account of how the action was actually "conveyed" or "manifested." But that tells us nothing of *what happened* in the pertinent sense (of what was thus conveyed); *and* substantial differences among possible physical movements suited to the phenomena in question are likely to have little or no bearing on the explanation of the particular phenomena themselves. Once conceded, the argument is a *reductio* of the basic-action model. For *if* free actions must be intensionally specified, and if what is causally important in the explanation of free action bears directly on properties that can be specified only intensionally, then, without mounting a full-scale argument, we have good grounds for resisting any version of the identity thesis.

If this much be conceded, then, admitting (7) and (8), we have made a very strong gain on vindicating claim (c), that is, that for some subset of human actions, there is, in principle, no formulable causal law under which pertinent causal sequences can be explained. Claim (c) does not follow, of course. But *if* we could strengthen the claim that the intensionally specified intentional properties of cultural life are precisely not the sort of thing that either could be convincingly treated as exhibiting lawlike regularities or must be so construed, we should have strengthened the reasonableness of (c) as well. The supporting grounds, are, as it happens, hardly difficult to muster. First of all, authors like Herbert Feigl and Wilfrid Sellars regularly admit that intentional features (in Brentano's sense) are "irreducible to a physicalistic description."[37] Secondly, if we construe intentional features (now, including intensionally qualified intentional features) as the *actual*, distinguishing traits, properties, capacities of human persons, then the irreducibility conceded turns out (contrary to Feigl's and Sellars's purpose) to undermine the prospects of mind/body reductionism.[38] Some treat intentionality entirely in terms of the intensional. But even if that claim were conceded (which is unconvincing[39] — at least for the reason that languageless animals appear to have mental states),[40] the admission of linguistic *abilities* (as distinct from the abstraction, language) would restore our problem. If this much is conceded, then we may simply press the obvious: that there appear to be no laws of human history, no laws of historical change as such.[41] This is not to deny that there *may* be political, economic, sociological, psychological, psychopharmacological laws, or laws of similar sorts. On the theory thus far advanced, such laws could not be more than statistical laws. But more than that, they would have to be laws that were intentionally informed in the peculiar way cultural phenomena are informed. What must be emphasized is that there need not be any causal laws of such sorts in order to provide an intelligible causal explanation of particular human actions (*b*); *and* that it may be quite impossible to formulate relevant covering laws for at least much that we are prepared to countenance as requiring causal explanation (*c*).

Claim (*c*) would be strengthened if the *causal* explanation of human actions were, characteristically, or at least in a wide range of important cases, given in terms of historically relevant factors—factors that appear not to be of the sort for which covering laws may be discovered. Thus, to explain how it was that Hitler mobilized Germany in the way he did, one might have to resort to historically qualified sensibilities among the Germans—possibly along the lines by which Erich Fromm tries to show the sadomasochistic and dependency traits of the sub-population that rallied to Hitler's call.[42] One could not hope to explain the transformation of capitalist Germany into the peculiar totalitarian form of the expanding Nazi empire by way of any laws of historical phases of development. And the explanation in terms of a combination of economic and psychological regularities, however reasonable, neither has the clear force of subsuming the phenomenon under a genuinely statistical law nor demonstrates that all cultural phenomena fall under covering laws.

The issue seems (but only seems) to be stalemated. The crucial feature affecting all such explanations is already in our hands. It is (7), that the identification and re-identification of free actions cannot be managed except intensionally. In short, *if* there are culturally pertinent (*Geisteswissenschaftlichen*) laws, they would have to be formulated in terms of statistical regularities ranging over large sets of phenomena from different historical contexts. But that would mean, first, that particular human actions and the like could initially be causally explained in terms of the intensionally qualified properties belonging to it and its peculiar cultural or historical milieu; and, second, that the lawlike uniformities allegedly ranging over culturally or historically distinct sets of *such* phenomena would themselves require that functional similarities, *under some transculturally favored intensional qualification*, could be ascribed to *behavior thus intensionally qualified* (that is, historically and culturally distinctive) within different societies. First, then, (let us say), we explain how, in terms uniquely appropriate to the cultural life of Germany, it was that Hitler transformed the German people; *then*, assuming, say, that Hitler's ability and the ability of other historical figures constitute instances of a certain general charismatic power, we attempt to formulate the *laws* of personal charisma.[43]

What this shows is the reasonableness of (c), that is, for some subset of human actions, there is, in principle, no formulable causal law under which pertinent causal sequences can be explained. The reason is a multiple one: first, because any arguably valid laws of the required sort both express and presuppose uniformities that cannot be collected in a "purely extensional way" ([5], [6])—and hence, that cannot be tested except via the intensional criteria by which they were first collected; second, because the phenomena in question are functionally specified—and hence, whatever is assigned a causal role in a "purely extensional way," bodily movements, for instance, casts little or no light on the explanation of the culturally pertinent phenomena in question; and third, because the underlying phenomena on which the would-be culturally relevant laws depend are themselves first explained in terms of intensional distinctions prevailing in their own historical milieus. But, *if* culturally pertinent laws are logically weak in the manner marked, then there would appear to be no likelihood that the causal phenomena to be first explained *could*, as such, be subsumed under covering laws. But that, precisely, *is* claim (c).

In matters of this sort, we normally cannot hope to provide a knockdown argument. Still, the claim may be tightened further. What needs to be stressed is simply that the intensionally qualified uniformities that we appeal to in explaining human actions, particularly free actions and related cultural phenomena, are nothing more than the system of traditions, institutions, doctrines, practices, rules, culturally induced habits, and the like that (i) psychologically inform in various ways the behavior of particular human agents belonging to a given culture; and (ii) *are themselves subject to causal change*. Traditions, institutions, and the rest, therefore, cannot be treated as, or as directly yielding, causal laws. Yet we do explain in the causal sense *particular* actions and the particular consequences of human action by reference to such general but severely circumscribed regularities. In fact, the very idea that a human agent, performing a free act, acts intentionally—in accord with a purpose or plan of action, by choice, on the basis of appraising available alternatives—makes no sense unless the intentional properties that inform his behavior are suitably groomed by the organized and organizing cultural milieu in which he develops. Hence, (4) to be a human agent is to behave in ways explainable in the causal sense by reference to the intensionally qualified institutions of one's own culture. Since, as has been said, such institutions are themselves subject to causal change (through the inventive agency of human beings), the relevant form of explanation— what we may call explanation under *covering institutions* — cannot be subsumed under the model of explanation by covering law. Claim (*c*), therefore, seems to be true, without endangering the prospect or intelligibility of causal explanation itself.[44]

NOTES

1. Ernest Nagel, *The Structure of Science* (New York: Harcourt, Brace and World, 1961), chap. 4.
2. Ibid., p. 74.
3. Carl G. Hempel, "The Logic of Functional Analysis," in *Aspects of Scientific Explanation* (New York: Free Press, 1965), pp. 300-301.
4. Ibid., p. 299.
5. Wesley C. Salmon, "Statistical Explanation," in *Statistical Explanation and Statistical Relevance*, eds. Wesley C. Salmon et al. (Pittsburgh: University of Pittsburgh Press, 1971), pp. 71-72.
6. Ibid., pp. 64-65.
7. Ibid., p. 43.
8. Hans Reichenbach, *The Direction of Time* (Berkeley and Los Angeles: University of California Press, 1956).
9. Salmon, "Statistical," p. 68.
10. See R. S. Peters, *The Concept of Motivation* (London: Routledge and Kegan Paul, 1958).
11. Donald Davidson, "Causal Relations," *Journal of Philosophy* 64 (1967): 700-701.
12. See Donald Davidson, "Mental Events," in *Experience and Theory*, eds. Lawrence Foster and J. W. Swanson (Amherst: University of Massachusetts Press, 1970).
13. J.J.C. Smart, *Philosophy and Scientific Realism* (London: Routledge and Kegan Paul, 1963), chap. 3.
14. Karl R. Popper, "The Aim of Science," in *Objective Knowledge* (Oxford: Clarendon, 1972), pp. 196-197.
15. Ibid., p. 197.
16. Curt J. Ducasse, "Critique of Hume's Conception of Causality," *Journal of Philosophy* 63 (1966): 141-148.
17. See Herbert Feigl, *The "Mental" and the "Physical." The Essay and a Postscript* (Minneapolis: University of Minnesota Press, 1958, 1967); see also Joseph Margolis, *Persons and Minds* (Dordrecht: D. Reidel, 1977).
18. Arthur C. Danto, *An Analytical Philosophy of Action* (Cambridge: Cambridge University Press, 1973), p. 98.
19. One of the most perceptive accounts of this aspect of human action appears in J. L. Austin, "Ifs and Cans," in *Philosophical Papers*, ed. J.O. Urmson and G.J. Warnock (Oxford: Clarendon, 1961).
20. See Roderick M. Chisholm, "Human Freedom and the Self," in *Freedom and Morality*, ed. John Bricke (Lawrence: University of Kansas Press, 1976).

21. Donald Davidson, "Agency," in *Agent, Action, and Reason*, eds. Robert Binkley, Richard Bronaugh, and Ansonio Marras (Toronto: University of Toronto Press, 1971), p. 12.

22. I have explored the issue of individuation further, in "Action and Causality," *Philosophical Forum*, in press.

23. Donald Davidson, "Actions, Reasons and Causes," *Journal of Philosophy* 60 (1963): 686-700. On the issue of explanation and identity of actions, see Joseph Margolis, "Puzzles about Explanations by Reasons and Explanation by Causes," *Journal of Philosophy* 67 (1970): 187-195; and a review ("Action and Causality") of Alvin Goldman's *A Theory of Action*, in *Metaphilosophy* 5 (1974): 348-364.

24. See Alvin Goldman, *A Theory of Action* (Englewood Cliffs, N.J.: Prentice-Hall, 1970).

25. See Donald Davidson, "The Individuation of Events," in *Essays in Honor of Carl G. Hempel*, eds. Nicholas Rescher et al. (Dordrecht: D. Reidel, 1969); and Margolis, *Persons and Minds*, chap. 13.

26. See Davidson, "Mental Events."

27. See, for instance, A.I. Melden, *Free Action* (London: Routledge and Kegan Paul, 1961).

28. Davidson, "Agency," p. 8.

29. This is the thesis of Margolis, "Action and Causality."

30. Davidson, "Agency," p. 23.

31. See Danto, *Analytical Philosophy*, pp. 97-115; and Goldman, *Theory*.

32. See Myles Brand, "Danto on Basic Actions," *Nous* 2 (1968): 187-190; and Frederick Stoutland, "Basic Actions and Causality," *Journal of Philosophy* 65 (1968): 467-475.

33. The full argument is the theme of Margolis, *Persons and Minds*.

34. Davidson does, of course, subscribe to a version of the identity theory; but it is fair to say that the thesis is merely announced, not at all defended. See Davidson, "Mental Events"; for a sustained criticism of Davidson's view, see Margolis, *Persons and Minds*, chap. 11.

35. In *Persons and Minds*, I develop such an alternative relation, embodiment, along the lines of a nonreductive materialism.

36. See Hilary Putnam, "Minds and Machines," *Dimensions of Mind*, ed. Sidney Hook (New York: New York University Press, 1960); and Jerry A. Fodor, *Psychological Explanation* (New York: Random House, 1968).

37. Feigl, *The Mental*, pp. 50-51. See Wilfrid Sellars, "Philosophy and the Scientific Image of Man," in *Science, Perception, and Reality* (London: Routledge and Kegan Paul, 1963); and Wilfrid Sellars, "A Semantic Solution of the Mind-Body Problem" *Methodos* 5 (1953): 45-84.

38. The full account appears in Margolis, *Persons and Minds*, chap. 1.

39. See James Cornman, "Intentionality and Intensionality," *Philosophical Quarterly* 12 (1962): 44-52.

40. See Margolis, *Persons and Minds*, chap. 9-10.

41. See Karl R. Popper, *The Poverty of Historicism* (London: Routledge and Kegan Paul, 1957).

42. Erich Fromm, *Escape from Freedom* (New York: Rinehart, 1947).

43. See H.H. Gerth and C. Wright Mills, trans. and eds., *From Max Weber: Essays in Sociology* (New York: Oxford University Press), chap. 9-10.

44. I pursue this thesis further in "Nature, Culture, and Persons," *Theory and Decision* 13 (1981): 311-329.

The Foundations of Psychoanalysis

Adolf Grünbaum

STATEMENT OF THE CONTROVERSY AS TO CLINICAL TESTABILITY

Hans Eysenck (1963: 220) has maintained that "we can no more test Freudian hypotheses 'on the couch' [used by the patient during psychoanalytic treatment] than we can adjudicate between the rival hypotheses of Newton and Einstein by going to sleep under an apple tree." And, in Eysenck's view, although clinical data from the couch may be heuristically fruitful by suggesting hypotheses, only suitably

*Parts of an earlier version of this article were presented at the Conference on Confirmation held at the Minnesota Center for Philosophy of Science, June 17-20, 1980. Other parts were delivered at the International Symposium on the Philosophy of Sir Karl Popper, which took place at The London School of Economics, July 14-16, 1980. A first draft of the section entitled "Is the Tally Argument Viable?" was read at the Conference on Methods in Philosophy and the Sciences, held in New York, November 17, 1979.

The author is indebted to the Fritz Thyssen Stiftung for support of his research. He is also grateful to Michael Roth, Benjamin Rubinstein, and Rosemarie Sand for helpful reactions to some parts of the earlier version. Peter Urbach made comments at the London Symposium on the excerpt that was presented there. The stimulus of these comments prompted some further articulations herein.

designed *experimental* studies can perform the *probative* role of *tests*. Against this denial of clinical testability, Clark Glymour (1974: 304) has argued that "the theory Sigmund Freud developed at the turn of the century was strong enough to be tested [cogently] on the couch." Furthermore, Glymour proposes to illuminate Eysenck's disparagement of clinical data, but then to discount it, in the following dialectical give-and-take:

> It stems in part, I think, from what are genuine drawbacks to clinical testing; for example, the problem of ensuring that a patient's responses are not *simply* the result of suggestion or the feeling, not without foundation, that the "basic data" obtained from clinical sessions — the patient's introspective reports of his own feelings, reports of dreams, memories of childhood and adolescence — are less reliable than we should like. But neither of these considerations seems sufficient to reject the clinical method generally, although they may of course be sufficient to warrant us in rejecting particular clinical results. Clinicians can hopefully be trained so as not to elicit by suggestion the expected responses from their patients; patients' reports can sometimes be checked independently, as in the case of memories, and even when they cannot be so checked there is no good reason to distrust them generally. But I think condemnations like Eysenck's derive from a belief about clinical testing which goes considerably beyond either of these points: the belief that clinical sessions, even cleansed of suggestibility and of doubts about the reliability of patients' reports, can involve no rational strategy for testing theories. [1974: 287]
>
> I think that Eysenck's claim is wrong. I think there is a rational strategy for testing important parts of psychoanalysis, a strategy that relies almost exclusively on clinical evidence; moreover, I think this strategy is immanent in at least one of Freud's case studies, that of the Rat Man. Indeed, I want to make a much bolder claim. The strategy involved in the Rat Man case is essentially the same as a strategy very frequently used in testing physical theories. Further, this strategy, while simple enough, is more powerful than the hypothetico-deductive-falsification strategy described for us by so many philosophers of science. [1974: 287-288]

Despite this epistemological tribute to Freud's couch, Glymour issues a caveat:

> I am certainly not claiming that there is good clinical evidence for Freud's theory; I am claiming that if one wants to test psychoanalysis, there is a reasonable strategy for doing so which can be, and to some degree has been, effected through clinical sessions. [1974: 288]

More recently, Glymour (1980) told us more explicitly why we should countenance the rationale that animated Freud's clinical investigation of psychoanalytic hypotheses during the treatment of his Rat Man patient Paul Lorenz.[1] Glymour points to at least three important specific episodes in the history of physical science in which he discerns just the logical pincer-and-bootstrap strategy of piecemeal testing that he also teased out from Freud's analysis of Paul Lorenz. Thus, he says, "unlikely as it may sound . . . the major argument of the Rat Man case is not so very different from the major argument of Book III of Newton's *Principia*" (1980: 265). And he stresses that this argument employs a logical *pincer* strategy of more or less *piecemeal* testing *within* an overall theory, instead of the completely global theory appraisal of the hypothetico-deductive method, which altogether abjures any attempt to rate different components of the theory individually as to their merits in the face of the evidence.

Precisely because he sees the piecemeal procedure as thus able to *allocate* praise or blame *within* the total theory, Glymour considers this method a salutary and effective antidote to the intratheoretic epistemological promiscuity that is endemic to the fashionable holism championed by Duhem and Quine (1980: 145-152). If you have been smarting under the holist dogma, which has it that intratheoretic epistemic bewilderment is the inevitable fate of rational man, Glymour beckons you to be undaunted and of stout heart: the logical pincer method affords deliverance by *vindicating* the actual contrary conduct of science and common sense, which is to accept or reject those particular component hypotheses that are at issue in scientific debate or daily life at a given time.

Yet Glymour (1980: 151) acknowledges that there is a "kernel of truth" in holism's emphasis on the *network* character of the linkages between the component hypotheses of a theory. And this kernel is such that the pieces of a theory must be *assessed* together prior to selecting particular ones for acceptance or rejection, because this selection "must depend on what else we believe and what else we discard" (p. 152). In short, one lesson drawn by Glymour from the pincer strategy is that the viable residue of the holist legacy need not saddle us with philosophical defiance of scientific practice and good sense.

Besides commending Freud's clinical study of the Rat Man for its rationale, Glymour likewise attributes a fair degree of scientific rigor to a *few* of Freud's other investigations. But he couples these particular appreciative judgments with a largely uncomplimentary overall evaluation, deploring the very uneven logical quality of the Freudian corpus. Indeed, Glymour (1980: 265) thinks he is being "gentle" when he deems Freud's 1909 case study of Little Hans to be "appalling." He finds that "on the whole Freud's arguments for psychoanalytic theory are dreadful," marred by the frequent—though by no means universal—substitution of "rhetorical flourish" for real argument, and a "superabundance of explanation" rather than cogent evidence (p. 264).

Yet clearly these quite fundamental dissatisfactions with Freud's all too frequent lapses do not militate against Glymour's espousal of the clinical testability of such central parts of psychoanalytic theory as the specific etiology of the psychoneuroses, at least in the etiological versions that Freud enunciated before 1909.

Just this championship of the *probative* value of data from the analytic treatment sessions is philosophical music to the ears of those who echo Freud's own emphatic claim that the bulk of psychoanalytic theory is well founded empirically. For, as Ernest Jones reminded everyone in his "Editorial Preface" to Freud's *Collected Papers*, the clinical findings are "the real basis of Psycho-analysis. All of Professor Freud's other works and theories are essentially founded on the clinical investigations" (Jones 1959, 1: 3). Thus most advocates of this theoretical corpus regard the analyst's many observations of the patient's interactions with him in the treatment sessions as the source of findings that are simply *peerless*, not only heuristically but *also* probatively. We are told that during a typical analysis, which lasts for some years, the analyst accumulates with each patient a vast number of variegated data that furnish evidence relevant to Freud's theory of personality no less than to the dynamics and outcome of his therapy. The so-called "psychoanalytic interview" sessions are claimed to yield genuinely probative data because of the alleged real-life nature of the rich relationship between the analyst and the analysand. Even an analyst who recently declared it to be high time that Freudians "move from overreliance on our hypothetical discoveries to a much-needed validation of our basic theoretical and clinical concepts" (Kaplan 1981: 23) characterizes "the naturalistic observations within the psychoanalytic treatment situation" as "the major scientific method of psychoanalysis" (p. 18). Hence, the clinical setting or "psychoanalytic situation" is purported to be the arena of *experiments in situ*, in marked contrast to the contrived environment of the psychological laboratory with its superficial, transitory interaction between the experimental psychologist and his subject. Thus, the analysts A. M. Cooper and R. Michels (1978: 376) tell us that "increasingly this [psychoanalytic] inquiry has recognized the analytic situation itself as paradigmatic for all human interactions." (p. 376). Indeed, the psychoanalytic method is said to be uniquely suited to first eliciting some of the important manifestations of the unconscious processes to which Freud's *depth* psychology pertains.

This superior *investigative value* of the analyst's clinical techniques is thus held to make the psychoanalytic interview at once the prime testing ground and the heuristic inspiration for Freud's theory of personality as well as for his therapy. Some leading orthodox analytic theoreticians have been concerned to *exclude* the so-called "meta-psychology" of Freud's psychic energy model, and *a fortiori* its erst-while neurobiological trappings, from the avowed purview of clinical validation. Therefore, it is to be understood that the term "psychoana-lytic theory of personality" is here construed to *exclude* the meta-psychology of psychic energy with its cathexes and anticathexes. In any case, most analysts have traditionally been quite sceptical, if not outright hostile, toward attempts to test Freudian theory experimen-tally *outside* the psychoanalytic interview.

Just such an assessment was enunciated again quite recently by Lester Luborsky and Donald Spence (1978). They do issue the sobering caveat that "psychoanalysts, like other psychotherapists, literally *do not know* how they achieve their results" (p. 360). But they couple this disclaimer with the tribute that analysts "possess a unique store of clinical wisdom." Moreover, Luborsky and Spence emphasize that *"far more is known now* [in psychoanalysis] *through clinical wisdom than is known through quantitative* [i.e., controlled] *objective studies* [emphasis in original]" (p. 350). In short, they claim that—in this area—clinical confirmation is presently superior to experimentally obtained valida-tion. And they deem findings from the psychoanalytic session to have such epistemic superiority not only therapeutically but also in the validation of Freud's general theory of unconscious motivations (pp. 356-357). Similarly, clinical validation is claimed for Heinz Kohut's currently influential variant of psychoanalysis, which supplants Freud's Oedipal conflict by the child's *pre*-Oedipal narcissistic struggle for a cohesive self as the major determinant of adult personality structure (Ornstein 1978; Goldberg 1978).

Having extolled "clinical wisdom" vis-à-vis experimental studies, Luborsky and Spence (1978: 356) declare that "Freud was probably right" in his terse negative response to the psychologist Saul Rosenzweig, when the latter sent him experimental results that Rosenzweig took to be supportive of Freud's theory of repression (Rosenzweig 1934). Though Freud was then in his late seventies and ill with cancer, he took only a short time to react to this unsolicited claim of confirmation. Quite soon thereafter, he wrote Rosenzweig with almost patronizing disenchantment:

I have examined your experimental studies for the verification of the psycho-analytic assertions with interest. I cannot put much value on these confirma-tions because the wealth of reliable observations on which these assertions rest make them independent of experimental verification. Still, it can do no harm. [quoted in MacKinnon and Dukes 1964: 703; the German original is repro-duced on p. 702]

Just what was Freud's rationale for feeling entitled to dismiss Rosenzweig's experimental investigation in the way he did?

Note at once that Freud's dissatisfaction was *not* that Rosenzweig's experiment failed to qualify logically as a genuine test of the psychoanalytic conception of repression. Thus, Freud's objection was *not* that sheer evidential *irrelevance* rendered the experimental results probatively unavailing. Nor did he level the weaker charge that Rosenzweig's findings failed to pass muster *logically* as confirmations. On the contrary, he did refer to them as "confirmations" (*Bestätigungen*). Rather what disenchanted Freud was that in his view, these results were *probatively superfluous* or *redundant*, albeit harmless as such. But *why* did Freud look upon them as superfluous? As he stated, he regarded psychoanalytic hypotheses as already abundantly well established clinically by "a wealth of reliable observations." Hence, he saw no need for further substantiation by experiments conducted outside the psychoanalytic situation.

Three years after Freud's dismissive reply, Rosenzweig (1937: 65) commented on it by writing: "many analysts today would not agree with Freud's view . . . and . . . possibly Freud himself has in the interim changed his mind." Some psychoanalysts did indeed dissent from Freud's appraisal of Rosenzweig's claim of experimental confirmation. But while doing so, these other analysts *indicted* rather than endorsed Rosenzweig's contention that his findings support Freud's theory of repression. For they objected vehemently that, far from yielding harmlessly superfluous confirmations, Rosenzweig's work was fundamentally unsound, because his experiment simply did not qualify logically as a test of the *psychoanalytic* notion of repression (MacKinnon and Dukes 1964: 703-709). I concur completely with these other analysts that whatever relevance Rosenzweig's findings may have to *non*psychoanalytic accounts of forgetting, they patently have no evidential bearing on Freudian repression as that notion is articulated in Freud's classic 1915 paper (S.E. 1915, 14: 146-158). Indeed, it is most puzzling that this fact was not evident to Rosenzweig before others pointed it out. For in the aforecited 1934 article, Rosenzweig himself states explicitly at the outset (p. 248) what he takes to be the pertinent construal of Freud's 1915 paper. And I submit that the probative *irrelevance* of Rosenzweig's laboratory findings is immediately perspicuous from that very formulation. For our purposes, however, the details of this logical malfeasance need not concern us.

Despite their strong differences, both of the parties to the above dispute about the probative value of *clinical* data for the empirical appraisal of psychoanalytic theory do agree that at least part of the

Freudian corpus is indeed cogently testable by empirical findings of *some* sort: the Freudians have the support of Glymour, for example, in contending that *actually realizable* observations made within the confines of the treatment setting do afford epistemically sound testability, and such anti-Freudian protagonists as Eysenck make the contrary claim that epistemically well-conceived tests are actually realizable, at least in principle, but *only* in the controlled environment of the laboratory or in other *extra*clinical contexts. And clearly, the assumption of actual empirical testability shared by the disputants is likewise affirmed by someone who maintains that *both* clinical and extraclinical findings are suitable, at least in principle, for testing psychoanalysis.

Yet this shared assumption of actual testability has again been denied simplicity by Popper, who has even denied the *logical* possibility of testing psychoanalysis empirically. As recently as when he replied to his critics in 1974 (Popper 1974, 2: 984-985), he reiterated his earlier claim that Freud's theory, as well as Adler's, are "simply nontestable, irrefutable. There was no conceivable human behaviour which would contradict them" (Popper 1962: 37). It is then a mere corollary of this thesis of nontestability that *clinical* data, in particular, likewise cannot serve as a basis for genuine empirical tests. But when Popper claims that his falsifiability criterion of demarcation between science and nonscience bars psychoanalysis from the pantheon of the bona fide empirical sciences, his *principal* concern is not with Freudian theory as such, important though it is. Thus in 1974 he stressed the quite general role of his demarcation criterion within his overall philosophy, when he wrote:

my criterion of demarcation. . . is more than sharp enough to make a distinction between many physical theories on the one hand, and metaphysical theories, such as psychoanalysis, or Marxism (in its present [as distinct from its original] form), on the other. This is, of course, one of my main theses; and nobody who has not understood it can be said to have understood my theory. [1974: 984]

But our concern is with why Popper is so emphatic to be understood as claiming that, *unlike* Marxism, "psychoanalysis was immune [to falsification by any logically possible empirical findings] to start with, and remained so" (1974: 985). In the footnote that he appends to this very sentence, he steers us to his *Conjectures and Refutations* (1962). On turning to this earlier work (chap. 1, sections 1 and 2; pp. 156-157, 255-258), we find that not so much psychoanalysis itself (or present-day Marxism) is the prime target of his charge of nonfalsifiability, but rather its role as a *centerpiece* of his castigation of *inductivism* qua method of scientific theory-validation and/or criterion of demarcation. For, as I read it, we are told (pp. 33-38) that inductivism does countenance the claims of ubiquitous empirical confirmation of Freud's theory that are made by its adherents. And similarly, inductivism gives sanction, we learn, to the purported validations of Adler's revisionist version of psychoanalysis and of contemporary Marxism. Thus by 1919, Popper had convinced himself both that inductivism does not have the methodological resources to challenge the scientific credentials of psychoanalysis *and* that Freud's theory—as well as Adlerian revisionism and Marxism—is in fact empirically irrefutable. On this basis, Popper argued that the inductivist method of confirmation and its criterion of demarcation are *unacceptably permissive.*

Hence, the real philosophical villain of his story was inductivism rather than psychoanalysis or Marxism as such, although he deplored them in their own right. Having found to his dismay in 1919 that inductivism still held sway as a criterion of demarcation, Popper adduced psychoanalysis—Freudian and Adlerian—as the *pièce de résistance* of his case against it. He therefore concluded, "Thus there clearly was a need for a different criterion of demarcation" (1962: 256). In short, psychoanalysis was and—at least as of 1974—has remained Popper's prime illustration of the greater stringency that he claims for the falsifiability criterion he enunciated. But, clearly, if he were right that Freud's theory is simply untestable altogether, then it would be pointless to inquire whether this theory can be cogently tested *clinically.* Hence, it now behooves us to address Popper's stated challenge.

CAN POPPER'S INDICTMENT OF FREUDIAN THEORY BE SUSTAINED?

In earlier publications, I have argued that neither the Freudian theory of personality nor the therapeutic tenets of psychoanalysis are untestable in Popper's sense (Grünbaum 1976, 1977, 1979a). Furthermore, there I contended in detail that Popper's portrayal of psychoanalysis as a theory entitled to claim good *inductivist* credentials is predicated on a caricature of the requirements for theory validation laid down by such arch-inductivists as Bacon and Mill. Thus, I pointed out that Freud's theory is replete with *causal* hypotheses and that the evidential conditions that must be met to furnish genuine inductive support for *such* hypotheses are very demanding. But I emphasized that precisely these exacting inductivist conditions were pathetically *unfulfilled* by those

Freudians who claimed ubiquitous confirmation of the psychoanalytic corpus, to Popper's fully justified consternation.

My epistemological scrutiny of psychoanalysis as a scientific theory in some of these earlier articles elicited a very encouraging laudatory response from John Watkins (1978: 351-352; but see also p. 140 for the *context* of Watkins's response that is provided by the editors). He did not challenge my conclusion that psychoanalysis is actually falsifiable. Yet he questioned the *bearing* of this claim on Popper's demarcation criterion itself. As he put it, "suppose (with Grünbaum) that psychoanalytic theory is testable; then Popper was wrong about Freudian theory: it is better than he thought." Why, asks Watkins (1978: 351), would one presume that Popper's "demarcation-criterion was in trouble because it actually included something which Popper himself had mistakenly excluded"? And he objects that "Grünbaum seems to take the unscientific status of Freudian theory as a datum against which that demarcation-criterion should be judged, rather than the other way around" (p. 352). David Miller demurred in a similar vein (private communication).

But their objection overlooks the cardinal point I was concerned to make when I discussed Freud's theory in the context of Popper's philosophy of science. For the title of the relevant section of the earliest essay in which I dealt with this topic was "Popper's Historiography of Inductivism and the Test Case of Freudian Psychoanalytic Theory" (Grünbaum 1976: 215). Neither there nor elsewhere thereafter did I offer the refutability of psychoanalysis as a counterexample to Popper's falsificationist demarcation criterion as such. Instead, I adduced the falsifiability of Freudian theory against Popper's contention that this influential theory provides a centerpiece illustration of the following major thesis espoused by him: the falsifiability criterion of demarcation is *more restrictive* than the inductivist one, and hence ought to supersede it! There is no basis in my writings, I submit, for the depiction of my views given by Watkins (1978: 351) when he wrote: "Grünbaum claims that Popper's demarcation criterion is...too weak because, contrary to Popper's intention, it fails to exclude Freud's psychoanalytical theory." Rather, on the pertinent page (Grünbaum 1976: 227), I explicitly addressed what I called "Popper's demarcation *asymmetry*" (p. 214), which is the *contrast* drawn by Popper between his criterion of scientificality and the inductivist one. What I did maintain concerning this contrast was that it is "unsound" to ascribe *greater stringency* to Popper's falsifiability criterion, at least "with respect to psychoanalysis."

That my focus was on the *comparative* stringency of the two demarcation criteria when I discussed Freud vis-à-vis Popper—and *not* on the adequacy of Popper's criterion *as such!*—is further apparent in that I went on to assess the strictness of the inductivist criterion in the very next sentence. Speaking there of advocates of eliminative inductivism as distinct from the enumerative inductivism that Bacon disparaged as "puerile," I declared: "the mere fact that...inductivists try to use supportive instances to 'probabilify' or credibilify hypotheses does NOT commit them to granting credible scientific status to a hypothesis *solely* on the strength of existing positive instances, however numerous" (1976: 227-228). When I then gave "the upshot of my comparison of inductivist conceptions of scientificality with Popper's," I wrote that

the moral I draw is the following: Popper was seriously mistaken in claiming that IN THE ABSENCE OF NEGATIVE INSTANCES, all forms of inductivism are necessarily committed to the (probabilified) scientific credibility of a theory, merely because that theory can adduce numerous positive instances.

Finally, upon applying this import to "psychoanalysis in particular," I concluded:

Thus, the inductivist's willingness to either probabilify or somehow credibilify theories which *can* marshal genuinely supportive positive instances does *not* render the inductivist helpless to dismiss the positive instances adduced by psychoanalysts as non-probative. [1976: 229]

Hence, I think that Watkins's complaint against taking the unscientific status of Freudian theory "as a datum" by which to judge the falsifiability criterion of demarcation should not have been laid at my door at all. Indeed, I wonder whether Popper's own account of the logical role played by Freudian theory when he evolved his demarcation criterion (1962: chap. 1) would not justify directing Watkins's complaint against the reasoning then employed by Popper himself. Thus, as I read the first four pages of this chapter, Popper started out from the following premise: psychoanalysis, like astrology and the Marxist theory of history, "does not come up to scientific standards," but it *is* countenanced as such by the *"inductive"* empirical method of theory validation. He then saw his task, he tells us, as one of devising a criterion of demarcation more stringent than inductivism, at least to the extent of *excluding* psychoanalysis (besides Marxism) as being nonscientific: "My problem perhaps first took the simple form, 'What is wrong with Marxism, psychoanalysis, and individual [Adlerian] psychology? Why are they so different from physical theories, from Newton's theory, and especially from the theory of relativity?'" (1962: 34).

To Peter Urbach's mind, I have misread Popper's epistemic rejection of the ubiquitous confirmations claimed by the Freudians he encountered. For on Urbach's reading, Popper pointed to these alleged validations *not* as an indictment of the permissiveness of the confirmation criteria countenanced by inductivism; instead, as Urbach would have it, Popper was concerned to expose the *delusion* of the Freudians that the purported confirmations satisfy inductivist canons. But I submit that, besides straining charity, Urbach's reading boomerangs, for it completely undercuts Popper's avowed purpose to adduce psychoanalysis as a prime illustration of his thesis that the inductivist criterion of demarcation is unacceptably permissive, and that his falsificationist alternative is more stringent (Popper 1962: 33-36; 1974: 984).

Thus, when speaking of psychoanalysis, Adlerian psychology, and Marxism, Popper (1962: 36) declared: "it was practically impossible to describe any human behaviour that might not be claimed to be a verification of these theories," an assertion immediately followed by his falsificationist manifesto whose first contention states: "It is easy to obtain confirmations, or verifications, for nearly every theory—if we look for confirmations" (p. 36). Evidently Popper's complaint is not that the abundant confirmations claimed by Freudians are actually devoid of inductivist warrant; instead, his charge is precisely that inductivist criteria are helpless to disavow the credentials that Freudians had claimed for their theory!

In earlier articles, I have devoted attention to Popper's views on psychoanalysis. But there are further philosophical reproaches that he lodged against Freud (and Adler) that I have not examined heretofore. These additional strictures comprise both emphatic arguments for the untestability of psychoanalytic theory, and a censorious utilization of some purported textual exegesis of Freud's 1923 paper on the theory and practice of dream interpretation. I believe that Popper's further complaints call for critical scrutiny. But since my overall concern in the present essay is with the *clinical* credentials of psychoanalysis, I shall consider Popper's additional objections to Freud in a different subdivision as follows: (1) those that do *not* focus on *clinical* observations in particular, and (2) those offered to deny the probative relevance of *clinical* findings as such.

Let me now deal with the first of these two sets of additional Popperian indictments of psychoanalysis. I shall then defer the scrutiny of the second group until after I have argued in much detail that by *inductivist* standards, the clinical validation of Freudian theory is very largely spurious, despite the *heuristic* value of clinical data.

In his replies to critics, Popper (1974: 985) wrote:

Marxism was once a science, but one which was refuted by some of the facts which happened to clash with its predictions.

However, Marxism is no longer a science; for it broke the methodological rule that we must accept falsification, and it immunized itself against the most blatant refutations of its predictions.

Psychoanalysis is a very different case. It is an interesting psychological metaphysics (and no doubt there is some truth in it, as there is so often in metaphysical ideas), but it never was a science. There may be lots of people who are Freudian or Adlerian cases: Freud himself was clearly a Freudian case, and Adler an Adlerian case. But what prevents their theories from being scientific in the sense here described is, very simply, that they do not exclude any physically possible human behaviour. Whatever anybody may do is, in principle, explicable in Freudian or Adlerian terms. (Adler's break with Freud was more Adlerian than Freudian, but Freud never looked on it as a refutation of his theory.)

The point is very clear. Neither Freud nor Adler excludes any particular person's acting in any particular way, whatever the outward circumstances. Whether a man sacrificed his life to rescue a drowning child (a case of sublimation) or whether he murdered the child by drowning him (a case of repression) could not possibly be predicted or excluded by Freud's theory; *the theory was compatible with everything that could happen — even without any special immunization treatment.*

Thus while Marxism became nonscientific by its adoption of an immunizing strategy, psychoanalysis was immune to start with, and remained so.

This important passage prompts me to make the following series of critical comments:

1. Even a casual perusal of the mere *titles* of Freud's papers and lectures in the *Standard Edition* yields two examples of falsifiability. The second is a case of acknowledged falsification, to boot. The first is the paper "A Case of Paranoia Running Counter to the Psychoanalytic Theory of the Disease" (S.E. 1915, 14: 263-272); the second is the lecture "Revision of the Theory of Dreams" (S.E. 1933, 22: 7-30, especially pp. 28-30). Let us consider the first.

The "psychoanalytic theory of paranoia," which is at issue in the paper, is the hypothesis that *repressed* homosexual love is *causally necessary* for affliction by paranoid delusions (S.E. 1915, 14: 265-266). The patient was a young woman who had sought out a lawyer for protection from the molestations of a man with whom she had been having an affair. The lawyer suspected paranoia when she charged that her lover had gotten unseen witnesses to photograph them while making love, and that he was now in a position to use the photographs to disgrace her publicly and compel her to resign her job. Moreover, letters from her lover that she had turned over to the lawyer deplored that their beautiful and tender relationship was being destroyed by her unfortunate morbid idea. Nonetheless, aware that truth is sometimes stranger than fiction, the lawyer asked Freud for his psychiatric judgment as to whether the young woman was actually paranoid.

The lover's letters made "a very favorable impression" on Freud, thereby lending some credence to the delusional character of the young woman's complaints. But, assuming that she was indeed paranoid, Freud's initial session with her led to a theoretically disconcerting conclusion: "The girl seemed to be defending herself against love for a man by directly transforming the lover into a persecutor: there was no sign of the influence of a woman, no trace of a struggle against a homosexual attachment" (S.E. 1915, 14: 265). If she was indeed delusional, then this seeming total absence of repressed homosexuality "emphatically contradicted" Freud's prior hypothesis of a homosexual etiology for paranoia. Thus, he reasoned: "Either the theory must be given up or else, in view of this departure from our [theoretical] expectations, we must side with the lawyer and assume that this was no paranoic combination but an actual experience which had been correctly interpreted" (S.E. 1915, 14: 266). Furthermore: "In these circumstances the simplest thing would have been to abandon the theory that the delusion of persecution invariably depends on homosexuality" (p. 266). In short, Freud explicitly allowed that if the young woman *was* paranoid, then her case was a *refuting* instance of the etiology he had postulated for that disorder. Alternatively, he reckoned with the possibility that she was not paranoid.

As it turned out, during a second session the patient's report on episodes at her place of employment not only greatly enhanced the likelihood of her being afflicted by delusions but also accorded with the postulated etiology by revealing a conflict-ridden homosexual attachment to an elderly woman there. But the point is that the psychoanalytic etiology of paranoia is empirically falsifiable (disconfirmable) *and* that Freud explicitly recognized it. For, as we saw, this hypothesis states that a homosexual psychic conflict is causally necessary for the affliction. Empirical indicators can bespeak the absence of homosexual conflict as well as the presence of paranoid delusions so as to discredit the stated etiology.

Hence, this example has an important general moral: whenever empirical indicators can warrant the *absence* of a certain theoretical pathogen P as well as a differential diagnosis of the *presence* of a certain theoretical neurosis N, then an etiologic hypothesis of the strong form "P is causally necessary for N" is clearly empirically falsifiable. It will be falsified by any victim of N who had not been subjected to P. For the hypothesis *predicts* that anyone not so subjected will be spared the miseries of N, a prediction having significant prophylactic import.

Equivalently, the hypothesis *retrodicts* that any instance of N was also a case of P. Hence, if there are empirical indicators as well for the *presence* of P, then this retrodiction can be empirically instantiated by a person who instantiates both N and P.

Being a strict determinist, Freud's etiological quest was for *universal* hypotheses (S.E. 1915, 14: 265). But he believed he had empirical grounds for holding that the development of a disorder N after an individual I suffers a pathogenic experience P depended on I's hereditary vulnerability. Hence, his universal etiologic hypotheses typically asserted that exposure to P is *causally necessary* for the development of N, *not* that it is causally sufficient.

Indeed, by claiming that P is the "*specific*" pathogen of N, he was asserting not only that P is causally necessary for N but also that P is never, or hardly ever, an etiologic factor in the pathogenesis of any other nosologically distinct syndrome (S.E. 1895, 3: 135-139). Robert Koch's specific etiology of tuberculosis, i.e., the pathogenic tubercle bacillus, served as a model (S.E. 1895, 3: 137). By the same token, Freud pointed to the tubercle bacillus to illustrate that a pathogen can be quite explanatory, although its mere presence does not guarantee the occurrence of the illness (S.E. 1896, 3: 209). And Freud was wont to conjecture *specific* etiologies for the various psychoneuroses until late in his career (S.E. 1925, 20: 55). Hence, as illustrated by the above example of paranoia, these etiologies evidently have a high degree of empirical falsifiability whenever empirical indicators can attest a differential diagnosis of N, as well as the absence of P. For the hypothesis that P is the specific pathogen of N entails the universal prediction that every case of non-P will remain a non-N, and equivalently, the universal retrodiction that any N suffered P, although it does not predict whether a given exposure to P will issue in N. Thus, Glymour's account (1974) of Freud's case history of the Rat Man makes clear how Freud's specific etiology of the Rat Man's obsession was falsified by means of disconfirming the retrodiction that Freud had based on it.

Let us return to our paranoia example. As I pointed out in an earlier article (Grünbaum 1979a: 138-139), the etiology of paranoia postulated by psychoanalysis likewise makes an important "statistical" prediction that qualifies as "risky" with respect to any rival "background" theory that denies the etiologic relevance of repressed homosexuality for paranoia. By Popper's standards, the failure of this prediction would count against Freud's etiology, and its success would corroborate it.

To be specific, originally Freud (S.E. 1911, 12: 63) hypothesized the etiology of male paranoia (Schreber case) along the following lines. Given the social taboo on male homosexuality, the failure to repress homosexual impulses may well issue in feelings of severe anxiety and guilt. The latter anxiety could then be eliminated by converting the love emotion "I love him" into its opposite "I hate him," a type of transformation that Freud labeled "reaction formation." Thus, the pattern of reaction formation is that once a dangerous impulse has been largely repressed, it surfaces in the guise of a far more acceptable *contrary* feeling, a conversion that therefore serves as a *defense* against the *anxiety* associated with the underlying dangerous impulse. When the defense of reaction formation proves insufficient to alleviate the anxiety, however, the afflicted party may resort to the further defensive maneuver of "projection," in which "I hate him" is converted into "He hates me." This final stage of the employment of defenses is then the full-blown paranoia. Thus, this rather epigrammatic formulation depicts reaction formation and projection as the repressed defense mechanisms that are actuated by the postulated *specific* pathogen of paranoia. But if repressed homosexuality is indeed the specific etiologic factor in paranoia, then the decline of the taboo on homosexuality in our society should be accompanied by a decreased incidence of male paranoia. And, by the same token, there ought to have been relatively less paranoia in those ancient societies in which male homosexuality was condoned or even sanctioned, for the reduction of massive anxiety and repression with respect to homosexual feelings would contribute to the removal of Freud's *conditio sine qua non* for this syndrome.

Incidentally, as Freud explains (S.E. 1915, 14: 265), before he enunciated universally that homosexuality is the specific pathogen of paranoia, he had declared more cautiously in his earlier publication that it is "perhaps an invariable" etiologic factor (S.E. 1911, 12: 59-60, 62-63, especially p. 59). When I first drew the above "statistical" prediction from Freud's etiology (Grünbaum 1979a: 139), I allowed for Freud's more cautious early formulation. There I predicated the forecast of decreased incidence as a concomitant of taboo decline on the *ceteris paribus* clause that no other potential causes of paranoia become operative. But, by making repressed homosexuality the *conditio sine qua non* of the syndrome, Freud's specific etiology clearly enables the prediction to go through *without* any such proviso.

But even assertions of pathogenic causal relevance that are logically *weaker* than the specific etiologies can be empirically disconfirmable. They can have testable (disconfirmable) predictive import, although they fall short of declaring P to be causally necessary for N. Thus, when pertinent empirical data fail to bear out the prediction that P positively affects the incidence of N, they bespeak the causal *irrelevance* of P to N. Consequently, the currently hypothesized causal relevance of heavy cigarette smoking to lung cancer and cardiovascular disease is disconfirmable, as is the alleged causal relevance of laetrile to cancer remission, which was reportedly discredited by recent findings in the United States.

The etiology that Freud conjectured for one of his female homosexual patients furnishes a useful case in point. He states its substance as follows:

> It was just when the girl was experiencing the revival of her infantile Oedipus complex at puberty that she suffered her great disappointment. She became keenly conscious of the wish to have a child, and a male one; that what she desired was her *father's* child and an image of *him*, her consciousness was not allowed to know. And what happened next? It was not *she* who bore the child, but her unconsciously hated rival, her mother. Furiously resentful and embittered, she turned away from her father and from men altogether. After this first great reverse she forswore her womanhood and sought another goal for her libido. [S.E. 1920, 18: 157]

But later on, he cautions:

> We do not, therefore, mean to maintain that every girl who experiences a disappointment such as this of the longing for love that springs from the Oedipus attitude at puberty will necessarily on that account fall a victim to homosexuality. On the contrary, other kinds of reaction to this trauma are undoubtedly commoner. [S.E. 1920, 18: 168]

Thus, he is disclaiming the predictability of lesbianism from the stated pubescent disappointment *in any one given case*. Yet the frustration does have disconfirmable predictive import, although its causal relevance is not claimed to be that of a specific pathogen. For by designating the stated sort of disappointment as *an* etiologic factor for lesbianism, Freud is claiming that occurrences of such disappointment *positively affect* the incidence of lesbianism.

This predictive consequence should be borne in mind, since Freud's case history of his lesbian patient occasioned his general observation that the etiologic explanation of an already existing instance of a disorder is usually not matched by the predictability of the syndrome *in any one given case* (S.E. 1920, 18: 167-168). An apologist for Popper was thereby led to conclude that the limitation on predictability in psychoanalysis thus avowed by Freud is tantamount to generic nonpredictability and hence to nondisconfirmability. But oddly enough this apologist is not inclined to regard the causal relevance of heavy smoking to cardiovascular disease as wholly nonpredictive or nondisconfirmable, although chain smoking is not even held to be a specific pathogen for this disease, let alone a universal predictor of it.

The comments I have made so far in response to Popper's aforecited 1974 statement have focused largely on Freud's 1915 paper on paranoia, whose very title announces an instance of empirical falsifiability. Besides, Freud's 1933 "Revision of the Theory of Dreams" presents an acknowledged falsification by the recurrent dreams of war neurotics. But we shall have occasion to discuss the clinical credentials of the psychoanalytic dream theory in a later section. Hence, it will suffice to have merely mentioned Freud's 1933 revision here before proceeding to the second set of comments that are prompted by Popper's 1974 declaration.

2. At the 1980 Popper Symposium, I asked what *proof* Popper has offered that *none* of the *consequences* of the theoretical Freudian postulates are empirically testable, as claimed by his thesis of nonfalsifiability. One of Popper's disciples in effect volunteered the reply that this untestability is known by direct inspection of the postulates, as it were. To this I say that the failure of some philosophers of science to identify testable consequences by such inspection may have been grounds for suspecting untestability, but is hardly adequate to furnish the required proof of nonfalsifiability.

Indeed, the examples of falsifiability that I have already adduced have a quite different moral: the inability of certain philosophers of science to have discerned *any* testable consequences of Freud's theory betokens their insufficient command or scrutiny of its logical content rather than a scientific liability of psychoanalysis. It is as if those with only a rather cursory exposure to physics concluded by inspection that its high level hypotheses are not falsifiable, just because *they* cannot think of a way to test them. For instance, both expertise and ingenuity made it possible recently to devise tests capable of falsifying the hypothesis that neutrinos have a zero rest mass (Robinson 1980). By the same token, I reject the hubristic expectation that if high-level psychoanalytic hypotheses are testable at all, then almost any intellectually gifted academic ought to be able to devise potentially falsifying test designs for them. Failing that, some Popperians rashly suggest that the presumption of inherent nontestability is strong.

Hence, let me return to my stated question: what proof, if any, did Popper actually offer for his aforecited emphatic reiteration that the Freudian theoretical corpus is wholly devoid of empirically testable consequences? To furnish such a proof, it would be necessary to establish the *falsity* of the claim that there exists at least one empirical statement about human behavior among the logical consequences of the psychoanalytic theoretical postulates. But as Popper has admonished elsewhere, an existential statement asserting that an *infinite* class

A has at least one member that possesses a certain property *P* cannot be deductively falsified by any finite set of "basic" evidence sentences, each of which *denies* that some individual in *A* has *P*. Yet Popper has committed himself *tout court* to the *falsity* of the following *existential* statement: the infinite Tarskian consequence class of the psychoanalytic theoretical corpus does contain at least one member that qualifies as an empirical statement about human behavior.

Hence, I must ask: what *argument* has Popper given to sustain his denial of this existential statement? How did he manage to convince himself that the infinite consequence class of Freud's theory contains no testable members at all? Indeed, what would it be like to give a *proof* of this denial that is consonant with the requirements of a deductivist? Would one first try to axiomatize all of Freud's theory, perhaps with a view to availing oneself of Craig's method of reaxiomatization for the purpose of trying to eliminate all of the prima facie theoretical terms, and to determining whether all of the remaining theorems must somehow still be *generically "non*observational"? I do not profess to know the answer, but the problem is Popper's, not mine.

What he does offer in lieu of anything like such a *general* argument is a procedure that has at least the appearance of reliance on his methodological bête noire: induction by enumeration. For in the above citation and elsewhere, he invokes mere examples. Thus, he points to the quite different behavior of two men toward a child, one of whom would try to rescue it from drowning, the other who would attempt to kill it by drowning. Popper had also adduced this supposed illustration with a little more detail in his earlier writings (1962: 35). He gives no indication whatever whether he drew this example from any actual case history or publication of Freud's (or Adler's). Yet if Freud and Adler did play fast and loose with the ascription of dispositions to people in the manner of Popper's example, then their case histories surely ought to be rich in actual illustrations of such malfeasance. As the example stands, however, it appears grossly contrived. And I contend that, in any case, it is unavailing.

But here we can forego a detailed statement of my reasons for this judgment, for I have previously set them forth elsewhere (1979a: 134-135). There I did so by reference to Popper's more detailed original statement of his example.

Let me say here, however, that if Popper's case of the drowning child is to have any cogency at all, he would need to show that Freud's theory grants unrestricted *license* to postulate *at will* whatever potentially explanatory initial conditions we may fancy as to the motivations or dispositions of a given person in particular external circumstances.

One looks in vain for Popper's documentation of such utter license in psychoanalysis. Yet in the aforecited passage, he again implicitly assumes it by simply telling us that "whatever anybody may do is, in principle, explicable in Freudian or Adlerian terms." This, in the face of the fact that Freud scorned the attribution of such universal explanatory power to his theory as a vulgar misunderstanding, when he referred to psychoanalysis and wrote: "It has never dreamt of trying to explain 'everything'" (S.E. 1923, 18: 252).

Hence, in an earlier article (1979a: 135) I asked concerning psychoanalysis: "Is it clear that the postulation of initial conditions *ad libitum* without any *independent* evidence of their fulfillment is quite generally countenanced by that theory to a far greater extent than in, say, physics, which Popper deems to be a bona fide science?" I claim that Freud's writings warrant a negative answer to this question. Moreover, William Goosens has made my evaluation of the case of the drowning child succinct by pointing out that Popper's use of this example to support his charge of nonfalsifiability boomerangs. For by gratuitously assuming unbridled freedom to postulate initial conditions in the manner of the example, it could be adapted, *mutatis mutandis*, to do the following: one would simply say that Newton's physics "does not exclude any particular particle's acting in any particular way," after having made just such gratuitous use of the failure of Newton's *laws* of motion themselves to restrict the direction in which a particle may move through a given point.

On the heels of saying that Freud's and Adler's theories do not exclude any physically possible human behavior, Popper told us that "whatever anybody may do is, in principle, explicable in Freudian or Adlerian terms." But if a theory *does not exclude* any behavior at all, no matter what the initial conditions, how then can it deductively *explain* any *particular* behavior? To explain deductively is to exclude: as Spinoza emphasized, to assert *p* is to deny every proposition incompatible with it. I can use two notions introduced by Michael Martin (1978: 10-16) to refine the statement of the relevant connection between the falsifiability of psychoanalysis, on the one hand, and its ability to explain facets of human thought or conduct, on the other. As Martin noted, the consequences of a theory may be empirically vague, and/or it may be unclear just what empirical statements the theory entails. Thus, he speaks respectively of "consequence vagueness" and of "deductive indeterminacy," and he points out that either of these two properties adversely affects the testability of a theory. Using these locutions, I maintain that insofar as consequence vagueness and/or deductive indeterminacy do militate against the empirical falsifiability of Freud's theory, they undercut its *explanatory capability* as well as its *inductive confirmability*, and vice versa.

3. In the 1974 passage cited above, Popper seems to have made a parenthetical gesture in the direction of documentation from Freud by trying to *illustrate* the nonfalsifiability of psychoanalysis and/or Freud's inhospitality to falsifications as follows: "Adler's break with Freud was more Adlerian than Freudian, but Freud never looked on it as a refutation of his theory." I submit that qua illustration of Freud's purported inhospitality to refutation, Popper's aside about the rift between Freud and Adler is unavailing and rather frivolous.

When Adler was still a Freudian, he reportedly told Freud that it was hardly gratifying for him to spend his entire life being intellectually overshadowed by Freud (Colby 1951: 230). Hence, it has been conjectured that Adler's doctrinal break with Freud was at least partly motivated by the desire to be a recognized innovative thinker in his own right. In his own psychological theory, Adler then went on to subordinate the sexual drive to the drive to assert oneself and to overcome a sense of inferiority even in sexual encounters. Perhaps Popper was referring to Adler's declared desire *not* to be Freud's understudy, when Popper said that "Adler's break with Freud was more Adlerian than Freudian." I myself do *not* see that the phenomenon of Adler's dissent does qualify as a *disconfirming* instance for Freud's theory. But *if* it does so qualify — as Popper seems to suggest here — then why does Popper feel entitled to claim that its falsifying force is lessened just because "Freud never looked on it as a refutation of his theory"?

In contrast, if Freud's theory is indeed as empirically *empty* as claimed by Popper by reference to his example of the drowning child, then how can Popper claim to *know* — as he does in the citation — that "Freud himself was clearly a Freudian case, and Adler an Adlerian case"? For, if psychoanalysis and Adlerian psychology are each thus devoid of empirical import, as alleged by Popper, how can even Freud's self-analysis and Adler's "masculine protest" defiance of Freud sustain Popper's assertion here that their respective personalities instantiated their respective theories?

More fundamentally, if Freud's theory is a mere "psychological metaphysics" or "myth," which only the future might see transformed into a testable theory — much as Empedocles' theory of evolution was a mere myth for a long time (Popper 1962: 38) — how, then, could Popper claim to know in 1974, by his own standards of factual empirical knowledge, that "there is some [nontautological] truth in it"? Unfortunately, he gives us no details. Far from being *unable*, like a myth, to make falsifiable predictions, psychoanalytic theory even makes predictions that qualify as "risky" by Popper's standards. Our discussion of "symptom substitution" in a later section will furnish another illustration of such a prediction. My earlier example featured the expected decline in the incidence of paranoia as homosexuality becomes more accepted.

4. Freud made a major retraction in regard to the *distinctive* therapeutic merits he had claimed emphatically for his own modality of psychiatric treatment. Thus, in his fullest account of the dynamics he postulated for his version of analytic therapy (S.E. 1917, 16: 448-463), he had contended that, unlike other therapies—which substitute cosmetics for the extirpation of the pathogens that keep neuroses alive—analysis acts "like surgery" (p. 450) by overcoming resistances to the patient's educative insight into the role of these pathogens (see also S.E. 1925, 20: 43). And on this basis, he maintained in that 1917 account, as well as a few pages earlier (pp. 444-445), that psychoanalytic treatment has the uniquely *prophylactic* power of not only averting the patient's relapse into his prior affliction but also preventing his becoming ill with a different, fresh neurosis. Yet in his famous paper "Analysis Terminable and Interminable" (S.E. 1937, 23: 216-254), Freud repudiated both of these prophylactic capabilities. (The editors of the *Standard Edition* point out (23: 214-215), however, that Freud *seems* to have reinstated the durability of the therapeutic conquest of a *prior* neurosis in a paper that he wrote only a year later, but which was published posthumously [S.E. 1940, 23: 179].) Incidentally, throughout this essay, the term "analytic therapy" will be used to refer to *Freud's* own pioneering conception and/or practice of Breuer's therapeutic legacy, unless explicitly indicated otherwise.

F. J. Sulloway (1979), in a lengthy historical account of the evolution of Freud's theories under the influence of their initial biological moorings, and R. E. Fancher (1973), in an earlier depiction of the development of psychoanalytic psychology, give ample evidence that Freud's successive modifications of many of his hypotheses throughout most of his life were hardly empirically unmotivated, capricious, or idiosyncratic. What reconstruction, I ask, would or could Popper give us of Freud's rationale for these repeated theory changes, and still cling to his charge of nonfalsifiability and/or to his charge that Freud was inhospitable to adverse evidence? I see no escape from the conclusion that this charge ought never to have been leveled in the first place, or at least should not have been repeated by Popper as late as 1974. To have reached this conclusion, one need only to have read Freud's letters to Wilhelm Fliess, which were available in print two decades earlier than

Popper's last statement on this matter (Freud 1954). Thus, to take a dramatic example, we learn from a letter that Freud wrote in 1897 how adverse evidence that he himself had uncovered drove him to repudiate his previously cherished seduction etiology of hysteria (Freud 1954, letter #69: 215-218). And even his at least occasional *intellectual hospitality* to refutation by others is apparent from the concluding sentence of a letter to Fliess in which he privately outlined the substance of his first 1895 paper on anxiety neurosis (Freud 1954, draft E: 88-94). The last sentence of this letter reads: "Suggestions, amplifications, *indeed refutations* and explanations, will be received with extreme gratitude [emphasis added]." In fact, as we shall now see, that 1895 paper offered a falsifiable etiology.

5. In his instructive 1895 "Reply to Criticisms of My Paper on Anxiety Neurosis" (S.E. 1895, 3: 123-139), Freud stated explicitly what sort of finding he would acknowledge to be a *refuting* instance for his hypothesized etiology of anxiety neurosis. Indeed, this reply, as well as the original paper defended in it, throw a great deal of light on Freud's understanding of the standards that need to be met when validating causal hypotheses. An account of his argument in these two 1895 papers on anxiety neurosis will illuminate just how the early Freud functioned as a *methodologist*, even though his theory of anxiety neurosis is not part of *psychoanalytic* theory proper.

And why is Freud's theory of anxiety neurosis not part of psychoanalytic theory proper? He hypothesized that no repressed ideas are the pathogens of anxiety neurosis, a syndrome that he detached as a distinct nosologic entity from neurasthenia, after the American neurologist Beard had singled out the latter as a clinical object. Since unconscious ideation is thus not implicated in the etiology of anxiety neurosis, the *psychoanalytic* method is not able, let alone necessary, to uncover its pathogenesis. By the same token, analytic *therapy* is not only unavailing for it but inapplicable to it. Indeed, the very etiology Freud conjectured for it entailed that only an alteration in the patient's current sexual life—not the probing of the unconscious legacy of his childhood—can remove its presumed *somatic* pathogen.

As Freud tells us, he had detached anxiety neurosis from Beard's neurasthenia as a distinct clinical entity because the symptoms of the former "are clinically much more closely related to one another" than to the typical symptoms of neurasthenia: "they frequently appear together and they replace one another in the course of the illness." And he labeled the underlying theoretical syndrome "anxiety neurosis," because all of its manifestations can be grouped around its chief nuclear symptom of anxiety (S.E. 1895, 3: 91). Thus, having enumerated the members of this *cluster* of symptoms and their incidence in specified life situations, Freud saw himself able to make fallible differential diagnoses of the presence of this cluster.

When proceeding to offer, in quite theoretical terms, his hypothesis as to the underlying etiology of this syndrome, he exempts two sorts of cases from its purview: (1) patients who give evidence that their affliction is a matter of "a grave hereditary taint," and (2) avowedly *very rare* and hence *negligible* cases in which "the etiology is doubtful or different" (S.E. 1895, 3: 99, 127). As for the first case type, he emphasizes that if "no heredity is to be discovered" in a given instance of the syndrome, he will "hold the case to be an acquired one," and will claim that his hypothesized etiology does apply to it (S.E. 1895, 3: 135). But what did Freud count as evidence for the presence of "a grave hereditary taint"?

Although he does not tell us in this particular paper, Breuer and he gave some indication of his answer in the same year on the opening page of the foundational case history of Anna O. Increased incidence of the disorder among "more distant relatives" is the criterion they give there for a neuropathic heredity (S.E. 1895, 2: 21). Yet as Freud noted in his "Heredity and Aetiology of the Neuroses," "a retrospective diagnosis of the illnesses of ancestors or absent members of a family can only very rarely be successfully made" (S.E. 1896, 3: 144). The importance he presumably attached to the stated requirement that the relatives showing higher-than-average incidence of the symptoms be "more distant" can be gauged from his admonition not to infer hereditariness carelessly from mere increased incidence among siblings or cousins who lived together. As he emphasizes, the latter increased incidence could well be a matter of "pseudo-heredity" (S.E. 1896, 3: 209, 156).

Nowadays, when determining whether heredity enhances vulnerability to an affective disorder, investigators would seek such information as the comparative incidence of the disorder among separated monozygotic and dizygotic twins, as well as the incidence in the general population (Winokur 1975). *A fortiori* quite stringent probative demands would be made, if those suffering from a given disorder were to be subdivided into hereditary and acquired cases, as proposed by Freud. But even during his own time, Freud surely was all too aware that his decision to count a case of anxiety neurosis as "acquired" on the mere strength of not being *demonstrably* hereditary was fraught with the risk of misclassifying a bona fide hereditary case as "acquired" from sheer lack of information. By not fulfilling the antecedent pathogenic conditions required by Freud's specific etiology, such a *pseudo*acquired case can then *spuriously falsify* that etiologic hypothesis, which is restricted to *acquired* cases. Though Freud presumably appreciated this risk of spurious falsification no less than we do, the fact remains that he was willing to run it. And apparently, he was likewise willing to chance that the test cases he would face when being challenged by his critics would not happen to be the very rare etiologically anomalous ones, whose existence he had acknowledged at the outset. For as we shall see, he explicitly called on his critic Löwenfeld to confront him with cases of the syndrome in which the antecedent required by his specific etiology was *missing*. Thus, he was committing himself to accept such a finding as falsifying.

He had postulated that the psychically unassimilated neurophysiological effect of unrelieved or aborted, purely somatic sexual excitation is the specific pathogen of anxiety neurosis. For example, the forfeiture of the relief of sexual tension by either partner in coitus interruptus or reservatus often issues in the creation of the very condition he had thus hypothesized to be etiological. Freud explains how he tested his hypothesis in these cases by a procedure akin to J. S. Mill's joint method of agreement and difference, and found that it stood up well under such testing. But, as Benjamin Rubinstein has remarked, we do not know what sampling method Freud used, nor whether his findings were statistically significant.

What matters for us now is just how Freud dealt, in his second 1895 paper on anxiety neurosis (S.E. 1895, 3: 123-139), with the critique of his postulated etiology offered by the psychiatrist Leopold Löwenfeld, who claimed to have refuted it by clinical findings.

To recapitulate, Freud had made the strong quasi-*universal* claim that unless the etiology of the anxiety syndrome is easily seen to be *purely* hereditary in a given patient, the stated impairment of sexual life is the "specific cause" of this syndrome in the following twofold sense: this sexual impairment is well-nigh causally *necessary* for the occurrence of the syndrome, and furthermore, this sexual deficit is never (or hardly ever) an etiologic factor in any *other* distinct syndrome (S.E. 1895, 3: 99, 127, 134-139). Thus, Freud was claiming, among other things, that the stated abnormality of the sexual life had to have been present in practically *every* person who suffers from *acquired* (rather than purely hereditary) anxiety neurosis. Accordingly, he pointedly declared (S.E. 1895, 3: 128) that if Löwenfeld were to refute this claim, Löwenfeld would have to confront him with cases of the acquired syndrome in which Freud's postulated specific pathogen is missing. Freud makes clear that he regards an observably normal sex life to be an *empirically sufficient* indicator for the *absence* of this hypothesized pathogen, for he challenged Löwenfeld to confront him "with cases in which anxiety neurosis has arisen after a psychical shock although the subject has (on the whole) led a *normal vita sexualis.*" Furthermore, he noted that Löwenfeld had not fulfilled this condition when adducing the case of a woman patient whose anxiety neurosis Löwenfeld had attributed to a single frightening experience (S.E. 1895, 3: 129). Hence, speaking of anxiety neurosis also as "phobia," Freud provided a summary statement that would do any falsificationist proud.

The main thing about . . . phobias seems to me to be that *when the vita sexualis is normal* — when the specific condition, a disturbance of sexual life in the sense of a deflection of the somatic from the psychical, is not fulfilled — *phobias do not appear at all*. However much else may be obscure about the mechanism of phobias, my theory can only be refuted when I have been shown phobias where sexual life is normal. [S.E. 1895, 3: 134]

It has been objected that Freud's challenge to Löwenfeld was empty after all. For suppose that, in a given patient, they both agree that the differential diagnosis is anxiety neurosis. And assume further that, by all accounts, the patient's sex life is normal. Then the complaint is that everyone's sex life can be held to be abnormal in *some* respect, so that Freud could always escape refutation by pleading some such abnormality. But I should point out that, in a later paper, Freud explicitly disavowed such an evasive maneuver: "Since minor deviations from a normal *vita sexualis* are much too common for us to attach any value to their discovery, we shall only allow a serious and long-continued abnormality in the sexual life of a neurotic patient to carry weight as an explanation" (S.E. 1898, 3: 269). Besides, even in the above citation from his 1895 paper, he had barred such an escape by allowing parenthetically that a refuting instance would be present, even if the anxiety neurotic's sex life is normal only "on the whole."

But what of repudiating the differential diagnosis to evade falsification when the phobic patient's sex life is blissful? At *first* sight, one can get the quite mistaken impression that the retraction of a differential diagnosis for the sake of upholding an etiology *must* be illicit, and that Freud was guilty of just that. True, he did preserve the etiology of neurasthenia, though not of anxiety neurosis, by repudiating initial differential diagnoses. As he reports:

So far as the theory of the sexual aetiology of neurasthenia is concerned, there are no negative cases. In my mind, at least, the conviction has become so certain that where an interrogation has shown a negative result, I have turned this to account too for diagnostic purposes. I have told myself, that is, that such a case cannot be one of neurasthenia. [S.E. 1898. 3: 269]

It is immaterial that this report pertains to neurasthenia rather than anxiety neurosis, for it is safe to assume that Freud was not loath to follow the same procedure with respect to the etiology of anxiety neurosis. And since our concern is with the latter, I shall make this assumption, at least for expository purposes. But then I must point out that on the heels of reporting his retraction of a differential diagnosis to preserve his etiology, Freud hastened to emphasize the following: his retractions soon turned out to be supported by *independent* evidence for an *alternative* diagnosis (S.E. 1898, 3: 269-270). To provide perspective for gauging the merits of Freud's detailed handling of this independent confirmation, let us first see how non-Freudians deal with similar problems today.

Nowadays, just as in Freud's day, the differential diagnosis of anxiety neurosis presents at least two sorts of problems: (1) to differentiate it as a primary syndrome from organic diseases that often *mimic* many of the same symptoms, (2) to discriminate between anxiety neurosis and other psychiatric afflictions, notably depression. As for the first problem, even if the patient presents a typical cluster of anxiety-related symptoms, it is essential to rule out such physical disorders as ischemia (e.g., coronary insufficiency), hyperthyroidism, caffeinism, paroxysmal atrial tachycardia, psychomotor epilepsy, hypoglycemia, drug abuse, and drug withdrawal syndrome, among others. And in regard to the second problem, note that the symptoms of the two psychiatric disorders always overlap, at least in regard to disturbances of sleep, appetite, and sexuality. It is generally recognized that unless a symptom cluster is pathognostic for one particular disease, it is typically very difficult indeed to make a unique diagnosis by exclusion of potential diagnostic pitfalls (Slater and Roth 1977: 96-97).

Now suppose that an initial differential diagnosis classified some patients as belonging to a certain nosologic category *C*. But assume further that, thus classified, their prior histories are incompatible with a previously hypothesized etiology of *C* that had been accepted. Or that, when the patients classified as *C* underwent a treatment *t* previously deemed effective for *C*, they responded poorly, thereby impugning the therapy *t*. Then the very fallibility of differential diagnoses may make it reasonable to retract the initial differential diagnosis and preserve previously accepted etiologic or therapeutic hypotheses, provided that independent evidence for an alternative diagnosis is then forthcoming. Just such a procedure is illustrated in a standard textbook of psychiatry whose authors are anything but Freudians (Slater and Roth 1977).

As they point out in effect (p. 97), when patients who are prima facie depressives react by acute exacerbation of their symptoms to treatments that are deemed effective for depression, the latter claim of therapeutic effectiveness is not rejected; instead, the treatment fiasco is taken to be good grounds for then making a new differential diagnosis of anxiety neurosis. Thus, when particular patients initially classified as depressives get worse after treatment by presumably antidepressant tricyclic compounds or by electroshock, the therapeuticity of these treatments for bona fide depressives is not impugned; rather, it is then inferred that the given patients ought to be reclassified as suffering from anxiety neurosis. Independent evidence to sustain the reclassification is not easily procured: modern statistical methods were needed to achieve a satisfactory degree of differentiation between depression and anxiety neurosis (Slater and Roth 1977: 226).

With this perspective, let us ask: when Freud preserved his etiologies by the retraction of initial differential diagnoses, did he make his continued adherence to this inference contingent on the production of *independent* evidence for the unsoundness of the initial diagnoses? As he reports, when a number of prima facie neurasthenics turned out to have personal histories incompatible with his postulated sexual etiology of neurasthenia, he was driven to reclassify them as victims of progressive paralysis. And, Freud maintains, "The further course of those cases later confirmed my view" (S.E. 1898, 3: 269). In another case, the alternative diagnosis that a physical ailment is aping the symptoms of neurasthenia received independent confirmation (pp. 269-270).

But the procurement of independent evidence for an alternative differential diagnosis became more murky when it just called for reliance on the psychoanalytic method. The etiologies Freud had enunciated for both anxiety neurosis and neurasthenia *excluded* repressed ideation from their pathogenesis. Hence, the diagnostic identification of patients suffering from these so-called "actual" neuroses provided no scope for the use of the psychoanalytic method of clinical investigation, whose hallmark was the exposure of repressions. Breuer's work on hysterics, however, had led Freud to postulate repression etiologies for the "psychoneuroses" of hysteria and obsessional disorder. Hence, when there was a need to *confirm* that a patient's presenting symptoms ought to be rediagnosed as betokening one of the psychoneuroses rather than one of the "actual" neuroses, reliance on the psychoanalytic method became essential in order to find etiologic corroboration.

Just this need for independent confirmation by the psychoanalytic method arose when Freud resorted to an alternative diagnosis of psychoneurosis to prevent the refutation of the etiologies he had enunciated for the actual neuroses.

Sometimes an interrogation discloses the presence of a normal sexual life in a patient whose neurosis, on a superficial view, does in fact closely resemble neurasthenia or anxiety neurosis. But a more deep-going investigation regularly reveals the true state of affairs. Behind such cases, which have been taken for neurasthenia, there lies a psychoneurosis—hysteria or obsessional neurosis. . . . Falling back on psychoneurosis when a case of neurasthenia shows a negative sexual result, is, however, no cheap way out of the difficulty; the proof that we are right is to be obtained by the method which alone unmasks hysteria with certainty—the method of psycho-analysis. [S.E. 1898, 3: 270]

In short, Freud's procedure was to invoke the etiologies of the psychoneuroses—which he had evolved by means of the psychoanalytic method—as a basis for independently confirming alternative diagnoses required to preserve his etiologies of the actual neuroses. For when prima facie cases of anxiety neurosis or neurasthenia did not fulfill the antecedents demanded by Freud's etiologies, he then *rediagnosed* them as cases of psychoneurosis. Unless the psychoanalytic method is fundamentally flawed and/or there is reason to doubt the etiologies predicated upon it, Freud is entitled to claim that this procedure is indeed not a "cheap way out of the difficulty."

It is the central thesis of this essay that the clinical psychoanalytic method and the causal (etiologic) inferences based upon it are fundamentally flawed epistemically, but for reasons *other than* nonfalsifiability. What is now relevant, instead, to the appraisal of Freud's reliance on *psychoanalytic* rediagnoses of prima facie neurasthenics is a matter of personal scientific integrity raised by Glymour (private communication): we know from Freud's private 1897 letter (number 69) to Fliess that, by the time he *denied* having used a "cheap way out," he had good reason to be quite diffident about *such* rediagnoses, because his seduction etiology of hysteria lay in shambles. Indeed, we know from one of his 1898 letters to Fliess that Freud was fairly cynical about the entire 1898 article in which he espoused rediagnoses: "You must promise me to expect nothing from the chit-chat article. It really is nothing but tittle-tattle, good enough for the public, but not worth mentioning between ourselves" (Freud 1954, letter #81: 243). Yet, having started his self-analysis in the summer of 1897 (see S.E., 3: 262), and having thereby been led to postulate the Oedipus complex by October 1897 (Freud 1954, letter #71: 223), perhaps Freud entertained hopes by early 1898 of vindicating the psychoanalytic method after all.

In any case, a proper appraisal of Freud's methodology even during the formative years of psychoanalysis defies Popper's crude categories. But deplorably, the simplistic verdicts Popper was able to generate by his obliviousness to Freud's actual writings have not only gained wide currency but are still in vogue. One need only turn to such very recent books as those by Stannard (1980: chaps. 3, 4) and Clark (1980). Yet I trust it will become clear from the scrutiny of clinical validation I shall offer in this essay just why Popper's application of his falsifiability criterion is too insensitive to exhibit the most *egregious* of the epistemic defects bedeviling the Freudian etiologies, interpretation of dreams, theory of parapraxes, etc. Indeed, as I shall argue, time-honored inductivist canons for the validation of causal claims have precisely that capability.

6. In 1937, two years before his death, Freud published his "Constructions in Analysis" (S.E. 1937, 23: 257-269). This methodologically crucial paper is devoted to the logic of clinical disconfirmation and confirmation of psychoanalytic interpretations and reconstructions of the patient's past, which are the epistemic lifeblood of Freud's entire theory. In a later section, I shall argue for the spuriousness of the *consilience* of clinical inductions espoused by Freud in that 1937 paper. But this spuriousness does not make it any less odd that anyone should have pen in hand and charge Freud with total insensitivity to falsifiability without even allowing for the following opening paragraph of that key paper:

A certain well-known man of science . . . gave expression to an opinion upon analytic technique which was at once derogatory and unjust. He said that in giving interpretations to a patient we treat him upon the famous principle of "Heads I win, tails you lose." That is to say, if the patient agrees with us, then the interpretation is right; but if he contradicts us, that is only a sign of his resistance, which again shows that we are right. In this way we are always in the right against the poor helpless wretch whom we are analysing, no matter how he may respond to what we put forward. Now . . . it is in fact true that a "No" from one of our patients is not as a rule enough to make us abandon an interpretation as incorrect. . . . It is therefore worth while to give a detailed account of how we are accustomed to arrive at an assessment of the "Yes" or "No" of our patients during analytic treatment—of their expression of agreement or of denial. [S.E. 1937, 23: 257]

7. Although Popper did not mention ambivalence in the 1974 statement quoted earlier, let me comment here on his rhetorical question of whether the psychoanalytic concept of ambivalence is not typical of a whole family of Freudian notions, "which would make it difficult, if not impossible, to agree" (Popper 1962: 38, n.3) on criteria for falsifying the explanatory relevance of such concepts. Incidentally, Popper combines this rhetorical question with the tantalizing parenthetical caveat that he does not deny the existence of ambivalence. But I submit that insofar as there is actual agreement on definite *criteria* for falsification in those theories that Popper does deem "scientific," I do not see why such agreement should be, in principle, more elusive in the case of ambiva-

lence, *modulo* Duhemian excursions into the quite elastic Lakatosian protective belts. For let us turn to Freud's ascription of ambivalence to Little Hans or more generally, say, to children (Laplanche and Pontalis 1973: 26-28), where there is testability, I suggest, for the following reason: to predicate ambivalence of children toward their parents is to say that there will be *some* behavioral manifestations of hostility as well as some overt expressions of affection, and *one* of these two contrary affects may be largely unconscious or covert at any one time. If there were no such mixed behavioral orientation at all, the ascription of ambivalence would be disconfirmed. Of course, Freud's theory of child ambivalence does not predict which one of the two polar affects a child will display on a given occasion. But *such* nonpredictability is not tantamount to untestability.

So much for my scrutiny of those Popperian objections to Freud that were *not specifically* aimed at impugning the probative relevance of the *clinical* data from analytic treatment sessions.

DOES NEO-BACONIAN INDUCTIVISM SANCTION THE VALIDATION OF PSYCHOANALYTIC THEORY BY CLINICAL DATA?

I should remind the reader that "clinical data" are here construed as findings coming from *within* the psychoanalytic treatment sessions. When I am concerned with contrasting these data from the couch with observational results secured from *outside* the psychoanalytic interview, I shall speak of the former as "*intra*clinical" for emphasis.

Let me now outline the theses for which I shall argue:

1. Freud gave a cardinal epistemological defense of the psychoanalytic method of clinical investigation that seems to have hitherto gone entirely unnoticed. I have dubbed this pivotal defense 'The Tally Argument" in earlier publications (Grünbaum 1979b, 1980). It was *this* defense—or its bold lawlike premise—I maintain, that was all at once his basis for five claims, each of which is of the first importance for the legitimation of the central parts of his theory. These five claims are the following:

(i) Denial of an irremediable epistemic contamination of clinical data by suggestion

(ii) Affirmation of a crucial difference, in regard to the *dynamics* of therapy, between psychoanalytic treatment and all rival therapies that actually operate entirely by suggestion

(iii) Assertion that the psychoanalytic method is able to validate its major causal claims — such as its specific sexual etiologies of the various psychoneuroses — by essentially *retrospective* methods without vitiation by *post hoc ergo propter hoc*, and without the burdens of prospective studies employing the controls of experimental inquiries

(iv) Contention that favorable therapeutic outcome can be warrantedly attributed to psychoanalytic intervention *without* statistical comparisons pertaining to the results from untreated control groups

(v) Avowal that, once the patient's motivations are no longer distorted or hidden by repressed conflicts, credence can rightly be given to his or her introspective self-observations, because these data then do supply probatively significant information (cf. Kohut 1959; Waelder 1962: 628-629)

2. The epistemological considerations that prompted Freud to enunciate his Tally Argument make him a sophisticated scientific methodologist, far superior than is allowed by the appraisals of friendly critics like Fisher and Greenberg (1977) or Glymour (1980), let alone by very severe critics like Eysenck.

Yet evidence accumulating in the most recent decades makes the principal premise of the Tally Argument well-nigh empirically untenable, and thus devastatingly undermines the conclusions that Freud drew from it. Indeed, no empirically plausible alternative to that crucial discredited premise capable of yielding Freud's desired conclusions seems to be in sight.

3. Without a viable replacement for Freud's Tally Argument, however, there is woefully insufficient ground to vindicate the intraclinical testability of the cardinal tenets of psychoanalysis (especially its ubiquitous causal claims) — a testability espoused traditionally by analysts, and more recently by Glymour on the strength of the pincer-and-bootstrap strategy. This unfavorable conclusion is reached by the application of neo-Baconian inductivist standards, whose demands for the validation of causal claims can clearly not be met intraclinically unless the psychoanalytic method is buttressed by a powerful substitute for the defunct Tally Argument. Moreover, in the absence of such a substitute, the epistemic decontamination of the bulk of the patient's productions on the couch from the suggestive effects of the analyst's communications appears to be quite utopian.

4. Insofar as the credentials of psychoanalytic theory are currently held to rest on clinical findings, as most of its official spokesmen would have us believe, the dearth of acceptable and probatively cogent clinical data renders these credentials quite weak. Thus, lacking a viable alternative to the aborted Tally Argument with comparable scope and ambition, the future validation of Freudian theory, if any, will have to come very largely from *extra*clinical findings.

5. Two years before his death, Freud invoked the *consilience* of clinical inductions (in the sense of William Whewell) to determine the probative cogency of the patient's assent or dissent in response to the interpretations presented by the analyst (S.E. 1937, 23: 257-269). But such a reliance on consilience is unavailing until and unless there emerges an as yet unimagined trustworthy method for epistemically decontaminating each of the *seemingly* independent consilient pieces of clinical evidence. For, as I shall argue, the methodological defects of Freud's "fundamental rule" of free association (S.E. 1923, 18: 238; 1925, 20: 41; 1940, 23: 174) ingress *alike* into the interpretation of several of these prima facie independent pieces of evidence (e.g., manifest dream content, parapraxes, waking fantasies). This multiple ingression renders the seeming consilience probatively spurious. But even if the consilient emergence of a repression were genuine, this would still not show that repressions *engender* neuroses, dreams or "slips."

6. Given the aforementioned dismal inductivist verdict on clinical testability, that traditional inductivist methodology of theory appraisal no more countenances the *clinical* validation of psychoanalysis than Popper does (1962: 38, n.3). Hence, the specifically clinical confirmations claimed by many Freudians but abjured as spurious by inductivist canons are unavailable as a basis for Popper's charge of undue permissiveness against an inductivist criterion of demarcation. And, as I have already argued, the actual falsifiability of psychoanalysis undercuts Popper's reliance on Freud's theory as a basis for claiming greater stringency for his criterion of demarcation.

Finally, Popper's astonishing omission of Freud's explicit reference to the Tally Argument from a passage that Popper adduced against him renders Popper's exegesis of Freud highly unfair and misleading. It was only by simply ignoring and omitting mention of Freud's reference to the Tally Argument when citing the passage in question that Popper was able to indict Freud for being incredibly oblivious to the contaminating effects of suggestion. Indeed, Freud's concern with these effects was always unflagging.

I shall now offer justifications for this series of theses, starting with my account of Freud's rationale for putting clinical confirmation on an epistemic throne.

FREUD'S TALLY ARGUMENT

Despite Freud's fundamental epistemic reliance on clinical testing, he did indeed acknowledge the challenge that data from the couch ought to be discounted as being inadmissibly contaminated. Even friendly critics like Wilhelm Fliess charged that analysts induce their docile patients by suggestion to furnish the very clinical responses needed to validate the psychoanalytic theory of personality (Freud 1954: pp. 334-337). Freud himself deemed it necessary to counter decisively this ominous charge of *spurious* clinical confirmation. For he was keenly aware that unless the methodologically damaging import of the patient's compliance with his doctor's expectations can somehow be neutralized, the doctor is on thin ice when purporting to mediate veridical insights to his client rather than only fanciful *pseudo*insights persuasively endowed with the ring of verisimilitude. Indeed, if the probative value of the analysand's responses is thus negated by brainwashing, then Freudian therapy might reasonably be held to function as an emotional corrective *not* because it enables the analysand to acquire bona fide self-knowledge, but instead because he or she succumbs to proselytizing *suggestion*, which operates the more insidiously under the pretense that analysis is *non*directive.

After Freud had practiced analysis for some time by communicating his interpretations of the patient's unconscious motivations, he felt himself driven to modify the dynamics of his therapy by according the role of a catalyst, vehicle, or ice-breaker to the patient's positive feelings for the analyst. For Freud had to mobilize these positive feelings to overcome the analysand's resistances with a view to eliciting confirmation from the latter's memory, whenever possible (S.E. 1920, 18: 18). And depending on whether the analysand's feelings toward his doctor were positive or negative, Freud spoke of the emotional relationship as a positive or negative "transference" (S.E. 1912, 12: 105). When thus acknowledging the vehicular therapeutic role of the positive transference relationship and attributing it to the doctor's authority qua parent surrogate, Freud knew all too well (S.E. 1917, 16: 446-447) that he was playing right into the hands of those critics who made the following complaints: clinical data have no probative value for the confirmation of the psychoanalytic theory of personality, and any therapeutic gains from analysis are *not* wrought by true insightful self-discovery but rather are the placebo effects induced by the analyst's suggestive influence. Thus, Freud gave ammunition to just these critics when he acknowledged the following: in order to overcome the patient's fierce resistances to the analyst's interpretations of his unconscious conflicts, the analyst cannot rely on the patient's intellectual insight but must decisively enlist the patient's need for his doctor's approval qua parental surrogate (S.E. 1917, 16: 445; 1919, 17: 159). In fact, Freud himself points out that precisely this affectionate help-seeking subservience on the part of the analysand "clothes the doctor with authority and is transformed into belief in his communications and explanations" (S.E. 1917, 16: 445). In this vein, Freud asks the patient to believe in the analyst's theoretical retrodictions of significant happenings in the client's early life when the patient himself is *unable to recall* these hypothesized remote events (S.E. 1920, 18: 18-19). For, as Freud tells us: "The patient cannot remember the whole of what is repressed in him, and what he cannot remember may be precisely the essential part of it. Thus he acquires no sense of conviction of the correctness of the construction that has been communicated to him" (S.E. 1920, 18: 18).

Thus, despite his best efforts, the analyst may well be stymied when seeking confirmation of his reconstructions of the patient's childhood by retrieving the latter's repressed memories. In such situations, Freud justifies his demand for the patient's faith in his retrodictions by the assumption that the analysand has a "compulsion to repeat" or reenact prototypic conflictual childhood themes with the doctor: "He [the patient] is obliged to *repeat* the repressed material as a contemporary experience instead of, as the physician would prefer to see, *remembering* it as something belonging to the past" (S.E. 1920, 18: 18). The repeated themes are held to derive from infantile sexual yearnings once entertained by the patient toward his parents (S.E. 1925, 20: 43). Now the main evidence that Freud adduces for his repetition-compulsion postulate is that the adult realities at the time of the analytic transaction show the patient's positive feelings toward his analyst to be extravagant in degree as well as grotesque in character (S.E. 1914, 12: 150; 1917, 16: 439-444). Yet this very state of mind clearly heightens the patient's suggestibility via intellectual and psychological subordination to his doctor. And this suggestibility is not lessened, especially in regard to genetic transference interpretations, in an analysis employing the technique recommended by Merton Gill (1980:287), who accords a role to genetic transference interpretations but urges that "the bulk of the analytic work should take place in the transference in the here and now" (p. 286).

Moreover, ever since Freud had studied with Charcot in 1885 and had then used prohibitory suggestion to order hypnotized patients to

shed their symptoms, he had appreciated the power of pure suggestion to effect impressive even if only temporary remissions (S.E. 1905,
7: 301-302). Thus, in 1893, when Breuer and he published their joint
Preliminary Communication on Breuer's cathartic method for treating
hysteria (S.E. 1893, 2: 3-17), they pointedly *argued* that *not* suggestion
but rather the cathartic release of strangulated affect associated with a
traumatic memory is responsible for the therapeutic gains of hysterics
who had been treated by that method (S.E. 1893, 2: 7). Freud was wont
to repeat this disavowal of prohibitory suggestion in later years when
speaking of Breuer's original hypnotic version of the cathartic method
(e.g., in S.E. 1904, 7: 250). And once Freud had modified Breuer's
method so as to transform it into full-fledged psychoanalysis, he was at
pains again and again — even before his 1917 landmark paper "Analytic
Therapy" — to *dissociate* the dynamics of his therapy from the prohibitory suggestion devices of other treatment modalities, just as Breuer
and he had thus dissociated the cathartic method itself (S.E. 1895,
2: 99, 305; 1904, 7: 250, 260-261, 301; 1910, 11: 146-147; 1912, 12: 105-106;
1913, 12: 125-126; 1913, 12: 143-144; 1914, 12: 155-156).

Indeed, Breuer and Freud *predicated* their *etiologic* identification of
repressed traumatic memories as being *pathogens* on precisely their
"observation" that the therapeutic successes of the cathartic method
are wrought by the hypnotized patient's abreactive recall of the forgotten traumatic experience, and not by prohibitory suggestion. Thus,
therapeutic recall of a repressed memory emerged as a kind of proto
insight into the pathogen of the patient's psychoneurosis. Once Freud
had replaced hypnosis by free association in the psychoanalytic
method of treatment and investigation, the moral he drew from the
cathartic method was that any genuine therapeutic gain attained by his
patients *requires* insight into the actual pathogens of their affliction.
Hence, the durable achievement of substantial therapeutic progress
could be held to betoken the correctness of the etiology inferred by
means of the psychoanalytic method of inquiry.

No wonder, therefore, that Freud saw the clinical confirmations of
his *etiologic* hypotheses placed in some jeopardy when critics seized on
the avowed *catalytic* remedial role of the patient's transference relationship to his analyst. Critics adduced the role of transference to *deny* that
veridical insight into the pathogens of the analysand's neurosis is the
therapeutically effective ingredient of an analysis. Thus, at the end of
his 1917 lecture "Transference," which beautifully set the stage for the
crucial next one, "Analytic Therapy," Freud squarely addressed the
portentous challenge of suggestibility as follows:

It must dawn on us that in our technique we have abandoned hypnosis only to rediscover suggestion in the shape of transference.

But here I will pause, and let you have a word; for I see an objection boiling up in you so fiercely that it would make you incapable of listening if it were not put into words: "Ah! so you've admitted it at last! You work with the help of suggestion, just like the hypnotists! That is what we've thought for a long time. But, if so, why the roundabout road by way of memories of the past, discovering the unconscious, interpreting and translating back distortions — this immense expenditure of labour, time and money — when the one effective thing is after all only suggestion? Why do you not make direct suggestions against the symptoms, as the others do — the honest hypnotists? Moreover, if you try to excuse yourself for your long detour on the ground that you have made a number of important psychological discoveries which are hidden by direct suggestion — what about the certainty of these discoveries now? Are not they a result of suggestion too, of unintentional suggestion? Is it not possible that you are forcing on the patient what you want and what seems to you correct in this field as well?"

What you are throwing up at me in this is uncommonly interesting and must be answered. [S.E. 1917, 16: 446-447]

This thoroughgoing recognition of the double bombshell of suggestibility *and* the careful 1917 argument Freud then offered in an attempt to defuse it stands in refreshing contrast to the manner in which typical contemporary analysts insouciantly ignore the heart of the matter or make light of it.

Thus, Linn A. Campbell (1978: 1, 8-9, 20-21) maintains that the *deliberate* use of suggestion with a view to obtaining an *uncritical* or unreflective response from the patient is antithetical to the *exploratory aims* of analytic therapy. But Campbell does not even consider how the therapist's good intention to let the patient be critical can be expected to provide prophylaxis against compliant yet reflective patient responses that issue in spurious clinical confirmations. The closest Campbell comes to entertaining that the elicitation of such patient responses might actually be unavoidable is as follows: he acknowledges the risk of *inadvertent* covert suggestion by the analyst when the latter has an unconscious neurotic need for a shortcut to the patient's gratitude (pp. 19-20). Yet Campbell soothingly assures us that, in any such case, truth will out: any symptom relief ensuing from such an unconscious misalliance between patient and therapist will be transient, since the patient will be left vulnerable to later stresses. Thus, by the end of Campbell's article the central issue has been successfully sidetracked.

In another recent article on psychoanalysis and suggestion, the German analyst Helmut Thomä (1977: 51) claims that the patient's scepticism counteracts the analyst's suggestive influences, especially when the analysand has hostile feelings toward his doctor, But it is a commonplace among analysts that even patients who have angrily abandoned their initial therapist and enter reanalysis with another, turn out to retain notions they acquired from their first analyst. Yet on the strength of patient scepticism, Thomä manages to remain unruffled by the problem to which his entire article is presumably addressed.

As a last illustration of the epistemic laxity of respected present-day analysts, I quote from the senior Chicago analyst Michael Basch (1980: 70-71), who wrote:

Only the hope of fulfilling infantile wishes can mobilize a patient for the therapeutic task. In adulthood, as in childhood, only the hope for love and the fear that love will be withdrawn can overcome the resistance to examining defensive patterns that have, after all, been established to avoid anxiety.

A patient who has a positive transference to the therapist wants to please him and will talk about what she thinks will interest him. . . . A patient lets himself be known, even though he fears exposing himself to humiliation and punishment, because he wants the therapist's affection and approval, not simply because he wants to get well. To know this about a patient is to be alert to the dangers of the transference relationship. The patient in a positive transference will, unconsciously, do his best to conform to the therapist's wishes as he, the patient, understands them. If the therapist wants to talk in terms of the Oedipus complex and incestuous sexuality, the patient will do his utmost to bring out material in such a way that it will fit that set; if another therapist approaches the same patient in a different framework, the latter will oblige that therapist in turn.

But when Basch points to the latter compliance as an illustration of the dangers inherent in the patient's eagerness to please his analyst, he cheerfully disregards the *epistemic* ravages of that compliance; for he tells us that "all is well" so long as the therapy sessions do not stagnate or become boring, and the patient's behavior changes. If such stagnation is avoided, we are told, the patient may safely be presumed to be acquiring bona fide insights. Only the stated kind of stagnation is held to bespeak that "the therapist's focus was not accurate and that he must lead the patient's introspection in a different direction" (p. 71). But this ignores that the patient may be undergoing brainwashing and may embrace mythological analytic interpretations even as his symptoms improve and as he finds the sessions interesting.

I shall be concerned to discuss just how Freud himself brilliantly, albeit unsuccessfully, came to grips with the full dimensions of the mortal challenge of suggestibility, which he himself stated so eloquently. When he picked up this gauntlet in his 1917 lecture, "Analytic Therapy," he gave us his cardinal epistemological rationale for the psychoanalytic method of clinical investigation and testing, a pivotal rationale whose import had gone completely unnoticed in the literature, as far as I know, until I called attention to its significance in two recent papers (Grünbaum 1979b, 1980). There I dubbed Freud's fundamental 1917 defense of his clinical epistemology "The Tally Argument."

Freud begins his 1917 "Analytic Therapy" lecture by recalling the question that he is about to address. As he puts it:

> You asked me why we do not make use of direct suggestion in psycho-analytic therapy, when we admit that our influence rests essentially on transference [which amounts to the utilization of the patient's personal relationship to the analyst] — that is, on suggestion; and you added a doubt whether, in view of this predominance of suggestion, we are still able to claim that our psychological discoveries are objective [rather than self-fulfilling products of *unintentional* suggestion]. I promised I would give you a detailed reply. [S.E. 1917, 16:448]

The careful reply he then proceeds to give falls into two parts.

First, he tries to explain meticulously that in *hypnosis*, suggestion serves the *pivotal* role of simply ceremonially *forbidding* the symptoms to exist, whereas in the dynamics of psychoanalytic therapy, the function of suggestion is that of being a *catalyst* or "vehicle" in the *educative* excavation of the repressed underlying etiology of the symptoms. And as he stressed nearly a decade later, "it would be a mistake to believe that this factor [of suggestion] is the vehicle and promoter of the treatment throughout its length. At the beginning, no doubt" (S.E. 1926, 20: 190). Secondly, far from begging the question by just *asserting* this epistemically wholesome role for suggestion in analysis, he justifies his assertion by enunciating the following premise: the veridical disclosure of the patient's hidden conflicts, which are the pathogens of his or her neurosis, is causally necessary for the durable and thoroughgoing conquest of his or her illness. But the disclosure thus requisite for therapeutic success will occur, in turn, *only* if incorrect analytic interpretations spuriously confirmed by *contaminated* responses from the patient have been discarded in favor of correct constructions derived from clinical data *not* distorted by the patient's compliance with the analyst's communicated expectations. In short, in the second part of his reply to the stated charge of contamination, Freud gives an *argument* for deeming the therapeutically favorable outcome of an analysis to be adequate reason for attributing the following probative merit to such a successful analysis: "Whatever in the doctor's conjectures is inaccurate drops out in the course of the analysis" (S.E. 1917, 16:452).

Let us now look at Freud's more detailed statement of his twofold reply to the basic question posed by him at the start of his 1917 lecture. As he points out (S.E. 1917, 16: 449-450), the elimination of symptoms by hypnosis is usually only temporary and hence requires a quasi-addictive repetition of the treatment. In the course of thus forbidding the symptoms, the doctor learns nothing as to their "sense and meaning." Thus, he tells us:

In the light of the knowledge we have gained from psycho-analysis we can describe the difference between hypnotic and psycho-analytic suggestion as follows. Hypnotic treatment seeks to cover up and gloss over something in mental life; analytic treatment seeks to expose and get rid of something [footnote omitted]. The former acts like a cosmetic, the latter like surgery. The former makes use of suggestion in order to forbid the symptoms; it strengthens the repressions, but, apart from that, leaves all the processes that have led to the formation of the symptoms unaltered. Analytic treatment makes its impact further back towards the roots, where the conflicts are which gave rise to the symptoms, and uses suggestion in order to alter the outcome of those conflicts. Hypnotic treatment leaves the patient inert and unchanged, and for that reason, too, equally unable to resist any fresh occasion for falling ill. An analytic treatment demands from both doctor and patient the accomplishment of serious work, which is employed in lifting internal resistances. Through the overcoming of these resistances the patient's mental life is permanently changed, is raised to a high level of development and remains protected against fresh possibilities of falling ill [footnote omitted]. This work of overcoming resistances is the essential function of analytic treatment; the patient has to accomplish it and the doctor makes this possible for him with the help of suggestion operating in an *educative* sense. For that reason psycho-analytic treatment has justly been described as a kind of *after-education* [footnote omitted]. [S.E. 1917, 16: 450-451]

After a theoretical interlude to which we shall turn shortly, Freud completes his account of the difference between the *therapeutic* employment of suggestion in hypnosis, on the one hand, and in analysis, on the other. Thus, he explains further:

We endeavour by a careful technique to avoid the occurrence of premature successes due to suggestion; but no harm is done even if they do occur, for we are not satisfied by a first success. We do not regard an analysis as at an end until all the obscurities of the case are cleared up, the gaps in the patient's memory filled in, the precipitating causes of the repression discovered. We look upon successes that set in too soon as obstacles rather than as a help to the work of analysis; and we put an end to such successes by constantly resolving the transference on which they are based [which is to analyze the patient's emotional attachment to the analyst *and* to wean him from the dependence engendered by it]. It is this last characteristic which is the fundamental distinction between analytic and purely suggestive therapy, and which frees the results of analysis from the suspicion of being successes due to suggestion. In every other kind of suggestive treatment the transference is carefully preserved and left untouched; in analysis it is itself subjected to treatment and is dissected in all the shapes in which it appears. At the end of an analytic treatment the transference must itself be cleared away; and if success is then obtained or continues, it rests, not on suggestion, but on the achievement by its means of an overcoming of internal resistances, on the internal change that has been brought about in the patient.

The acceptance of suggestions on individual points is no doubt discouraged by the fact that during the treatment we are struggling unceasingly against resistances which are able to transform themselves into negative (hostile) transferences. [S.E. 1917, 16: 452-453]

But note that, as Freud himself emphasizes, the doctor makes it possible for the patient to overcome resistances "with the help of suggestion operating in the *educative* sense" (S.E. 1917, 16: 451). And, as we recall, he had acknowledged that the patient's transference attachment to the analyst "clothes the doctor with authority and is transformed into belief in his communications" (S.E. 1917, 16: 445). Hence, it can readily be objected that precisely because the doctor is thus leading the patient—much as a lawyer may be leading a witness in the courtroom—the asserted *therapeutic* differences between hyp- nosis and analysis boomerang, since an avowedly *educative* use of suggestion provides even more scope for indoctrinating the patient to become an ideological disciple than the prohibitory kind of suggestion, which is essentially confined to the symptoms.

Characteristically, Freud is alert to the legitimacy of this challenge, and he addresses it head-on in what I regard as epistemologically perhaps the most pregnant single passage in his writings:

But you will now tell me that, no matter whether we call the motive force of our analysis transference or suggestion, there is a risk that the influencing of our patient may make the objective certainty of our findings doubtful. What is advantageous to our therapy is damaging to our researches. This is the objection that is most often raised against psycho-analysis, and it must be admitted that, though it is groundless, it cannot be rejected as unreasonable. If it were justified, psycho-analysis would be nothing more than a particularly well-disguised and particularly effective form of suggestive treatment and we should have to attach little weight to all that it tells us about what influences our lives, the dynamics of the mind or the unconscious. That is what our opponents believe; and in especial they think that we have "talked" the patients into everything relating to the importance of sexual experiences — or even into those experiences themselves — after such notions have grown up in our own depraved imagination. These accusations are contradicted more easily by an appeal to experience than by the help of theory. Anyone who has himself carried out psycho-analyses will have been able to convince himself on countless occasions that it is impossible to make suggestions to a patient in that way. The doctor has no difficulty, of course, in making him a supporter of some particular theory and in thus making him share some possible error of his own. In this respect the patient is behaving like anyone else — like a pupil — but this only affects his intelligence, not his illness. After all, his conflicts will only be successfully solved and his resistances overcome if the anticipatory ideas he is given tally with what is real in him. Whatever in the doctor's conjectures is inaccurate drops out in the course of the analysis [footnote omitted]; it has to be withdrawn and replaced by something more correct. [S.E. 1917, 16: 452]

Note at once that Freud acknowledges the patient's *intellectual* docility. But he emphasizes that while the doctor therefore "has no difficulty, of course, in making him . . . share some possible error of his own . . . this only affects his intelligence, not his illness." Thus, Freud is clearly relying on the alleged refractoriness of the neurosis to dislodgment by the mere pseudoinsights generated by incorrect conjectures on the part of the analyst. And he depends on that purported refractoriness to serve as nothing less than the epistemic underwriter of the clinical validation of his entire theory. For Freud allows that the objection most often raised against psychoanalysis is as follows: epistemologically, therapeutic success is *non*probative, because it is achieved *not* by imparting veridical insight but rather by the persuasive suggestion of fanciful pseudoinsights that merely ring verisimilar to the docile patient. He leaves no doubt as to the utter devastation that would be wrought by this objection if it could not be overcome. As he explains, "If it were justified, psycho-analysis would be nothing more than a particularly well-disguised and particularly effective form of suggestive treatment and we should have to attach little weight to all that it tells us about what influences our lives, the dynamics of the mind or the unconscious" (S.E. 1917, 16: 452].

Let us now articulate systematically the *argument* he uses to counter the charge of epistemic contamination of clinical data by suggestion, and his attempt to avert the ominous import of that charge. His counterargument does invoke *therapeutic* success. Hence, let us be mindful that the successful therapeutic conquest of the analysand's neurosis is held to consist in an adaptive restructuring of the intrapsychic personality dispositions such that there is concomitant lasting overt symptom relief without symptom substitution. The intrapsychic restructuring is deemed crucial to safeguard the quality and durability of overt symptomatic improvement.

Immediately after asserting that the doctor's theoretical stance, *if erroneous*, can persuasively affect the patient's intelligence but *cannot* dislodge his illness, Freud gives us the fundamental premise on which he rests this imperviousness of the patient's neurosis: "After all, his conflicts will only be successfully solved and his resistances overcome if the anticipatory ideas [i.e., interpretative depictions of analytic meaning] he is given tally [both objectively and subjectively] with what is real in him" (S.E. 1917, 16: 452). This bold assertion of the *causal indispensability* of psychoanalytic insight for the conquest of the patient's psychoneurosis is a terse enunciation of the thesis that Freud had previously formulated more explicitly in his 1909 case history of Little Hans, where he wrote:

In a psycho-analysis the physician always gives his patient (sometimes to a greater and sometimes to a less extent) the conscious anticipatory ideas by the help of which he is put in a position to recognize and to grasp the unconscious material. For there are some patients who need more of such assistance and some who need less; but there are none who get through without some of it. Slight disorders may perhaps be brought to an end by the subject's unaided efforts, but never a neurosis—a thing which has set itself up against the ego as an element alien to it. To get the better of such an element another person must be brought in, and in so far as that other person can be of assistance the neurosis will be curable. [S.E. 1909, 10: 104]

The assumptions that Freud actually invokes in this context can be stated as a conjunction of two causally necessary conditions as follows: (1) only the psychoanalytic method of interpretation and treatment can yield or mediate to the patient correct insight into the unconscious pathogens of his psychoneurosis, and (2) the analysand's correct insight into the etiology of his affliction and into the unconscious dynamics of his character is, in turn, *causally necessary* for the therapeutic conquest of this neurosis. I shall refer to the *conjunction* of these two Freudian claims as his "Necessary Condition Thesis" or, for brevity, "NCT." I have been careful to formulate this thesis with respect to the "psychoneuroses," as distinct from the so-called "actual" neuroses. For, as we shall see further on, Freud denied that NCT holds for the *actual* neuroses, and I ask that this important restriction be borne in mind even when I omit the qualification for brevity. Clearly, NCT entails not only that there is no spontaneous remission of psychoneuroses but also that, if there are any cures at all, psychoanalysis is *uniquely* therapeutic for such disorders as compared to any *rival* therapies.

Armed with his daring NCT, Freud promptly uses it to legitimate probatively the clinical data furnished by psychoneurotic patients whose analyses presumably had been successful. Nay, upon asserting the existence of such therapeutically successful patients P, as well as Freud's NCT, *two* conclusions follow in regard to any and all patients P who emerged cured from their analyses:

Conclusion 1. The psychoanalytic interpretations of the hidden causes of P's behavior given to him by his analyst are indeed correct, and thus—as Freud put it—these interpretations "tally with what is real" in P.

Conclusion 2. Only analytic treatment could have wrought the conquest of *P*'s psychoneurosis.

In view of Freud's use of the appealing phrase "tally with what is real," I have used the label "Tally Argument" for the argument whose two premises and two conclusions I have just stated.

It is of capital importance to appreciate that Freud is at pains to employ the Tally Argument in order to justify the following epistemo-logical claim: actual *durable* therapeutic success guarantees *not only* that the pertinent analytic interpretations *ring* true or credible to the analysand *but also* that they *are* indeed veridical, or at least quite close to the mark. Freud then relies on this bold intermediate contention to conclude nothing less than the following: collectively, the successful outcomes of analyses do constitute *cogent* evidence for all that general psychoanalytic theory tells us about the influences of the unconscious dynamics of the mind on our lives. In short, psychoanalytic treatment successes as a whole vouch for the truth of the Freudian theory of personality, including its specific etiologies of the psychoneuroses and even its general theory of psychosexual development.

Thus, Freud thought his theory of personality ought to command the assent of the scientific public. After all, the first conclusion of the Tally Argument had, in effect, absolved the psychoanalytic method of investigation from cognitive vitiation by the fact that the imperious analyst subjects the hapless patient to *educative* suggestion. And as we saw in his "Analytic Therapy" lecture, which is number 28 of his 1917 Introductory Lectures, he had predicated this vindication on the exis-tence of genuinely successful treatment outcomes from analysis by claiming that the analyst *can* indoctrinate the patient erroneously but cannot thereby dislodge his illness.

Yet in his earlier lecture (number 16) of the same series, he simply ignored the pivotal role that therapeutic success was to play in his Tally Argument. For in the earlier lecture he declared:

Even if psycho-analysis showed itself as unsuccessful in every other form of nervous and psychical disease as it does in delusions, it would still remain completely justified as an irreplaceable instrument of scientific research. [S.E. 1917, 16: 255]

But in the face of the suggestibility challenge, this statement is a gratuitous piece of salesmanship, unworthy of the Freud who gave us the Tally Argument. In fact, Freud emphasizes (S.E. 1917, 16: 438-439, 445-446) that within the class of psychoneuroses, the subclass of so-called "narcissistic neuroses"—as distinct from the "transference neuroses" (Laplanche and Pontalis 1973: 258, 462)—are simply *refractory* to his therapy. Hence, in the case of the former subclass of disorders, the Tally Argument is, of course, unavailable to authenticate his clinically inferred etiologies by means of therapeutic success. Yet, in another lecture (number 27), he explicitly gave the same epistemic sanction to the clinical etiologies of the two subclasses of psychoneuroses (S.E. 1917, 16: 438-439). And presumably he did so by *extrapolating* the therapeutic vindication of the psychoanalytic method of etiologic investigation from the transference neuroses to the narcissistic ones.

I have called attention to *two* conclusions that follow from the premises of Freud's Tally Argument. One of them asserts the truth of the psychoanalytic theory of personality; the other claims unique efficacy for analytic therapy. But Freud himself explicitly deduced only the first of these two conclusions, and stated the second quite separately in the same 1917 paper, as if it needed to stand on its own feet epistemically.

Thus, well after having inferred the first claim, he tells us (S.E. 1917, 16: 458) that the therapeutic successes of analysis are not only "second to none of the finest in the field of internal medicine" but also that psychoanalytic treatment gains "could not have been achieved by any other procedure," let alone spontaneously. The latter assertion of unique therapeutic potency is a reiteration of the equally sanguine claim he had made in 1895 when evaluating his therapeutic results from the cathartic precursor of analysis. For at that much earlier time, he had declared, "I . . . have accomplished some things which no other therapeutic procedure could have achieved" (S.E. 1895, 2: 266). Small wonder, therefore, that Freud concluded his 1917 "Analytic Therapy" paper by blithely dismissing doubts as to the therapeutic efficacy of analysis, after merely alluding to the difficulties of statistical comparisons of treatment outcome with results from untreated control groups, let alone with the results from rival therapies. The very same complacent position is taken, for example, by Erich Fromm (1970: 15), who does not hesitate to tell us that "many patients have experienced a new sense of vitality and capacity for joy, and no other method than psychoanalysis could have produced these changes."

Note that *if* Freud is warranted in postulating his NCT, and if psychoanalytic treatment outcome does bespeak its therapeutic efficacy, then he is surely entitled to *dissociate* the remedial insight dynamics of his treatment process from the mechanisms of the purely suggestive therapies. In thus setting his therapy apart from mere or prohibitory suggestion, he can then be undaunted by the catalytic,

vehicular role he had been led to accord to the transference relationship. Indeed, he focuses on the role of the transference in the patient's
achievement of insight when he explicitly sets forth the fundamental
characteristic that, in his view, "frees the results of analysis from the
suspicion of being successes due to suggestion" (S.E. 1917, 16: 453).
Freud does acknowledge, of course, that "the special personal influence of the analyst. . . exists and plays a large part in analysis" (S.E.
1926, 20: 190), but as he points out at once, "it would be a mistake to
believe that this factor is the vehicle and promoter of the treatment
throughout its length. At the beginning no doubt" (S.E. 1926, 20: 190);
for it is a cardinal therapeutic aim of an analysis to afford the patient
insight into his unconscious conflicts. Yet ironically the patient's transference of his infantile conflicts onto the analyst is activated and
functions *obstructively* as a diversion just when the most sensitive
repressed material is threatened by exposure: "in analysis [positive and
negative] transference emerges as *the most powerful resistance* to the
treatment" (S.E. 1912, 12: 101).

Hence, if the patient is to "work through" and overcome the resistances that obfuscate his access to the desired insight, his transference
attachment must be dissected and *resolved*, whereas it is left untouched
and *preserved* in the suggestive therapies (S.E. 1917, 16: 453). An
analysis is intended to issue in the patient's emotional *independence*
from the doctor; merely suggestive treatment, however, preserves the
dependence on the therapist. Freud deems just this difference in
dealing with the transference to be "the fundamental distinction
between analytic and purely suggestive therapy" (S.E. 1917, 16: 453;
see also 1914, 12: 155-156). As he put it:

it is perfectly true that psycho-analysis, like other psycho-therapeutic
methods, employs the instrument of suggestion (or transference). But the
difference is this: that in analysis it is not allowed to play the decisive part in
determining the therapeutic results. It is used instead to induce the patient to
perform a piece of psychical work—the overcoming of his transference-
resistances—which involves a permanent alteration in his mental economy.
The transference is made conscious to the patient by the analyst, and it is
resolved by convincing him that in his transference-attitude he is *re-experiencing* emotional relations which had their origin in his earliest object-attachments
during the repressed period of his childhood. In this way the transference is
changed from the strongest weapon of the resistance into the best instrument
of the analytic treatment. Nevertheless its handling remains the most difficult
as well as the most important part of the technique of analysis. [S.E. 1925,
20: 42-43]

By the same token, he differentiates between transference remissions
and analytic cures:

Often enough the transference is able to remove the symptoms of the disease by itself, but only for a while—only for as long as it itself lasts. In this case the treatment is a treatment by suggestion, and not a psycho-analysis at all. It only deserves the latter name if the intensity of the transference has been utilized for the overcoming of resistances. Only then has being ill become impossible, even when the transference has once more been dissolved, which is its destined end. [S.E. 1913, 12: 143]

Astonishingly, the *analysis* and resolution of the patient's transference subordination to his analyst has itself been invoked to *discredit* the following reproach: because of the epistemically confounding effects of the patient's doctrinal acquiescence to the analyst's quasi-parental authority, the ensuing clinical data are liable to furnish only *spurious* confirmations of psychoanalytic hypotheses. But what is the basis for the alleged capability of the analysis of the transference to purge psychoanalytic investigation of self-fulfilling bogus findings? It is that the patient's childlike doctrinal compliance with his therapist is *itself* formally part and parcel of the targets of the resolution of his "transference neurosis." Yet I cannot emphasize strongly enough that such an invocation of the analysis of the transference to rebut the charge of self-validation is logically a viciously circular bootstrap operation.

For clearly, the psychoanalytic dissection of the patient's deferential submission to his doctor already presupposes the empirical validity of the very hypotheses whose spurious confirmation by the analysand's clinical responses was at issue from the outset! As Freud told us explicitly, "The transference is made conscious to the patient by the analyst, and it is resolved by convincing him that in his transference-attitude he is *re-experiencing* emotional relations which had their origin in his earliest object-attachments during the repressed period of his childhood" (S.E. 1925, 20: 43). But the etiologic hypotheses employed to furnish just these purported insights and convictions to the patient are themselves avowedly predicated on clinical data, and all of these data have been admittedly suspect all along as being confounded by indoctrination.

Hence, it is plainly altogether question begging and self-validating to maintain by way of rebuttal that the analysis of the transference precludes spurious confirmation by guaranteeing the patient's emancipation from compliance with the analyst's communicated expectations. This specious disposition of the stated complaint of spurious clinical confirmation is hardly remedied upon heeding a recent injunction from Merton Gill (1980: 286), who declares: "the bulk of the analytic work should take place in the transference in the here and now." For obviously, analytic work having the latter focus rests on hypotheses whose validation is no less in question than the credentials of the *genetic* transference interpretations whose role Gill wishes to reduce.

But let us return to Freud's own account of the analysis of the transference. Toward achieving its resolution, he remarks "it is the analyst's task constantly to tear the patient out of his menacing illusion [of loving the analyst] and to show him again and again that what he takes to be new real life [i.e., realistic affection] is a reflection of the past" (S.E. 1940, 23: 177). Quite naturally, therefore, it is a recurring theme in Freud's writings that his therapy extirpates the pathogens of the patient's symptoms in surgical fashion, whereas the basic pathology is left intact by the suggestive treatments, which are thus merely cosmetic (S.E. 1917, 16: 450, 459; 1910, 11: 52, 146; 1905, 7: 260-261). Incidentally, this contrast between psychoanalytic treatment and mere suggestion is not retracted at all by Freud's 1921 reiteration that suggestibility is a "riddle." He then professed anew his lifelong agnosticism regarding the causal mechanism of individual suggestibility whereby group suggestion effects illogical psychological dominance over individuals and results in a change of their behavior (S.E. 1921, 18: 88-90).

A caveat recently issued by a contemporary analyst exemplifies the continuing allegiance, in at least some quarters, to Freud's distinction between (1) transference-induced symptom remissions, which are deemed ephemeral or fragile under new stresses, and (2) the analytic eradication of the underlying pathogens. In an article on transference, Brian Bird (1972: 285-286) writes:

One of the most serious problems of analysis is the very substantial help which the patient receives directly from the analyst and the analytic situation. For many a patient, the analyst in the analytic situation is in fact the most stable, reasonable, wise, and understanding person he has ever met, and the setting in which they meet may actually be the most honest, open, direct, and regular relationship he has ever experienced. . . . Taken altogether, the total *real* value to the patient of the analytic situation can easily be immense. The trouble with this kind of help is that if it goes on and on, it may have such a real, direct, and continuing impact upon the patient that he can never get deeply enough involved in transference situations to allow him to resolve, or even to become acquainted with, his most crippling internal difficulties. The trouble, in a sense, is that the direct nonanalytical helpfulness of the analytic situation is far too good! The trouble also is that we as analysts apparently cannot resist the seductiveness of being directly helpful.

Despite Freud's theoretical disavowal of mere suggestion as a remedial tool, he was not above making therapeutic promises to patients that, by his own account, were at best just hopes at the time. Thus, in 1910 he tells us that even "when I alone represented psycho-analysis...I assured my patients that I knew how to relieve them permanently of their sufferings" (S.E. 1910, 11: 146). Yet on the next page, he allows that these assurances may well be unjustified. For after pointing out that even rival therapies deriving suggestive force from being fashionable are unable "to get the better of neuroses," he says, "time will show whether psycho-analytic treatment can accomplish more."

As long as Freud saw himself entitled to adduce his NCT, he felt able — with a *single* stroke — to rebuff the twin suggestibility attacks on the dynamics of his therapy as well as on the cognitive reliability of the clinical data gathered by psychoanalytic investigation. Precisely because the crucial NCT premise of his Tally Argument declared correct *etiologic* insight to be therapeutically indispensable, this argument legitimated Freud's confidence in the following proposition: his *retrospective* clinical ascertainment of the etiologies of the psychoneuroses and of the causes of normal personality development *by the psychoanalytic method* was not vitiated by pitfalls of causal inference such as *post hoc ergo propter hoc*, but rather was methodologically sound. No wonder he felt justified in saying, "In psycho-analysis there has existed from the very first [i.e., even in the original cathartic method] an inseparable bond between cure and research. . . . Our analytic procedure is the only one in which this precious conjunction is assured" (S.E. 1926, 20: 256). Indeed, as Freud had told us as early as 1893, "Breuer learnt from his first patient that the attempt at discovering the determining cause of a symptom was at the same time a therapeutic manoeuvre" (S.E. 1893, 3: 35). Thus, he maintained that in psycho-analysis, "scientific research and therapeutic effort coincide" (S.E. 1923, 18: 236). One is therefore dumbfounded by the statement of analyst Judd Marmor (1968: 6): "I suspect that it was largely the historical accident that Freud was attempting to earn a living as a psychiatric practitioner that drove him to utilize his investigative tool simultaneously as a therapeutic instrument."

The explicit conclusion that Freud drew from his Tally Argument has essentially been reiterated in recent decades by prominent analysts. One of the more articulate endorsements is given by the Freudian Robert Waelder. In his review article on Sidney Hook's well-known symposium (1959), Waelder (1962: 629-630) writes:

Whenever a psychoanalyst is satisfied that he has untied the Gordian knot of a neurosis and has correctly understood its dynamics and its psychogenesis, his confidence is based on two kinds of data, one of outside observation of events, the other of the patient's self-observation. The first is the experience, repeated countless times during the working-through period of the analysis and again countless times during the person's later life, that this particular interpretation, or set of interpretations, and no other, can dispel the symptoms when they reappear, that they alone are the key that opens the lock; because particularly in the more serious neurosis of long standing, successful analytic therapy often does not bring about an ideal "cure" in the sense of our utopian desires, a traceless disappearance of disturbances without any price to be paid for it, but rather the ability to conquer them and to maintain a good, though contrived rather than stable, balance by vigilance and effort.

Then . . . there is an inner experience; what had been unconscious can now be consciously felt.

Waelder contrasts psychoanalysis with "a purely physicalistic discipline" by characterizing it epistemically as "largely, though by no means entirely, a matter of introspection and empathy" (pp. 628-629). Hence, he *also* invokes confirmation of the analyst's interpretations by the patient's *introspections* to espouse Freud's Tally Argument claim that "whatever in the doctor's conjectures is inaccurate drops out in the course of the analysis" (S.E. 1917, 16: 452). Thus, Waelder (1962: 629) elaborates on the contribution made by "the patient's self-observation" to the analyst's confidence in having "correctly understood" the psychogenesis and dynamics of his client's neurosis:

The interpretations offered by the psychoanalyst to his patient point out inner connections that can be fully experienced. Of course, any individual interpretation that is suggested in the course of an analysis may or may not be correct; the patient may or may not accept it, and his acceptance or rejection may be caused by realistic estimates or by emotional prejudices. But as analysis proceeds, mistaken interpretations will gradually wither away, inaccurate or incomplete interpretations will gradually be amended or completed, and emotional prejudices of the patient will gradually be overcome. In a successful analysis, the patient eventually becomes aware of the previously unconscious elements in his neurosis: he can fully feel and experience how his neurotic symptoms grew out of the conflicts of which he is now conscious; and he can fully feel and experience how facing up to these conflicts dispels the symptoms and, as Freud put it, "transforms neurotic suffering into everyday misery"; and how flinching will bring the symptoms back again.

Incidentally, as I have shown elsewhere in detail (Grünbaum 1980: pp. 354-367), just this accolade to the epistemic reliability of the analysand's introspections when validating etiologic and therapeutic claims is gainsaid by the recent conclusions of the cognitive psychologists Nisbett and Wilson.

Very recently, the analyst Michael Basch (1980: 171) echoed Freud's NCT:

"Insight," "psychoanalytically oriented" or "depth" psychotherapy . . . is based on Freud's recognition that psychological problems are developmental, and that only by obtaining [veridical] insight into the process that gives rise to them can a resolution based on cause [as distinct from a shallow and fragile symptom remission] be reached.

Like Waelder, Basch (p. 83) points to the "repeated experience" of failing to achieve the desired change in the patient's behavior in response to some entirely plausible interpretation, but then scoring a therapeutic breakthrough after offering some *particular* interpretation. And, just like Waelder, Basch takes this finding to be *evidence* for the correctness and insightfulness — rather than the mere *persuasiveness* for the patient — of the *one* interpretation that issued in significant therapeutic gain. But can any such therapeutic episode actually count in favor of Freud's NCT? Surely not until and unless there are good grounds for claiming that the "repeated experience" adduced by Basch may indeed be taken to bespeak the truth — *not* just the *congeniality!* — of the therapeutically distinguished interpretation, as well as the falsity of the therapeutically barren analytic conjectures. Yet neither Basch nor Waelder have supplied such grounds.

What clues does Freud himself give us as to the evidence that led him to champion his NCT until at least 1917? Clearly, this question is imperative, because the *empirical tenability* of this cardinal premise of his Tally Argument is the pivot on which he rested his generic tribute to the probative value of the clinical data obtainable by the psychoanalytic method of inquiry. It would seem that until at least 1917, Freud regarded NCT as supported by the *dynamics* he avowedly felt driven to postulate in order to make intelligible the *patterns* of therapeutic success *and* failure resulting from the use of the following two treatment modalities: (1) Josef Breuer's cathartic method of abreaction, which still employed hypnosis on hysterics, and (2) Freud's own innovative psychoanalytic version of Breuer's method, which replaced hypnosis by the technique of free association to treat psychoneurotics. Indeed, the pioneering reasoning by which Freud responded to his therapeutic successes and failures countenanced the sort of inferences that we already encountered in the aforecited writings by the analysts Waelder and Basch. Let us see how Freud was led to that reasoning.

Breuer's findings seemed to betoken the therapeuticity of the patient's abreactive and articulate recall of the repressed traumatic experience during which a particular hysterical symptom presumably first appeared. The positive therapeutic results that Breuer and Freud first obtained by means of such catharsis then served as their *evidence* for identifying the traumatic experience in question etiologically as the specific cause, or *pathogen*, of the given symptoms (S.E. 1893, 2: 6-7;

1893, 3: 29-30; 1896, 3: 193). In this way, Breuer had concluded, for example, that his patient Anna O's strong aversion to drinking water had been caused by strangulated and repressed disgust at the sight of seeing a companion's dog drink water from a glass (S.E. 1895, 2: 34-35). Once the etiology of the patient's hydrophobic behavior has been thus inferred, it can serve to explain that behavior.

But quite *apart* from therapeutic success, Freud lays down two generic necessary conditions of adequacy that must be met by any traumatic experience, *if* that trauma is to furnish a *satisfactory etiologic explanation* of the given symptom by qualifying as its "specific cause." Freud gives the following example to motivate these conditions of adequacy:

> Let us suppose that the symptom under consideration is hysterical vomiting; in that case we shall feel that we have been able to understand its causation (except for a certain [hereditary] residue) if the analysis traces the symptom back to an experience which *justifiably produced a high amount of disgust* — for instance, the sight of a decomposing dead body. But if, instead of this, the analysis shows us that the vomiting arose from a great fright, e.g., from a railway accident, we shall feel dissatisfied and will have to ask ourselves how it is that the fright has led to the particular symptoms of vomiting. This derivation lacks *suitability as a determinant*. We shall have another instance of an insufficient explanation if the vomiting is supposed to have arisen from, let us say, eating a fruit which had partly gone bad. Here, it is true, the vomiting *is* determined by disgust, but we cannot understand how, in this instance, the disgust could have become so powerful as to be perpetuated in a hysterical symptom; the experience lacks *traumatic force*. [S.E. 1896, 3: 193-194]

Accordingly, he enunciates his generic requirements:

> Tracing a hysterical symptom back to a traumatic scene assists our understanding only if the scene satisfies two conditions; if it possesses the relevant *suitability to serve as a determinant* and if it recognizably possesses the necessary *traumatic force*. [S.E. 1896, 3: 193]

Yet, in fact, any and *every* repressed traumatic experience satisfying these two conditions of explanatory adequacy might well be *etiologically irrelevant* to hysteria, if only because Breuer's and Freud's fundamental hypothesis of a *repression etiology* may be generically false! And, *if* so, then Breuer was surely mistaken in attributing crucial pathogenic significance to the *particular* traumatic experience that occasioned the *onset* of a given hysterical symptom, an experience I shall hereafter denote "occasioning trauma" for brevity. But for quite different reasons, Freud was persuaded to downgrade the etiologic role of the occasioning trauma from a "specific" cause to a mere precipitating (releasing) cause (S.E. 1895, 3: 135-136).

As Freud explains (S.E. 1896, 3: 193-197), his reasons were the following: (1) with overwhelming frequency, the occasioning trauma violated at least one of Freud's two stated requirements for etiologic adequacy, and (2) whenever his psychoanalytic procedure uncovered a repressed occasioning trauma that violated both of these adequacy conditions, the undoing of *this* repression was altogether useless therapeutically. In all such cases, "we also fail to secure any therapeutic gain; the patient retains his symptoms unaltered" (S.E. 1896, 3: 195)!

We must appreciate why Freud took this therapeutic fiasco to cast additional doubt on the pathogenic potency of the occasioning trauma. It was because he expected therapeutic success once the patient was no longer repressing an *etiologically essential* memory. This expectation was based on the general moral of Breuer's cathartic method, which Freud still took seriously and which he had rendered concisely as follows: "Breuer learnt from his first patient that the [successful] attempt at discovering the [psychically sequestered] determining cause of a symptom was at the same time a therapeutic manoeuvre" (S.E. 1893, 3: 35).

Though Freud therefore demoted the *occasioning* trauma etiologically, he insisted that the *generic* postulation of a repression etiology for hysteria was empirically warranted. This warrant came from the psychoanalytic disclosure of a much *earlier* sexual trauma which, in his view, did have impressive pathogenic earmarks (S.E. 1896, 3: 193). As he put it:

> We finally make our way from the hysterical symptom to the scene which is really operative traumatically and which is satisfactory in every respect, both therapeutically and analytically. . . . If the first-discovered scene is unsatisfactory, we tell our patient that this experience explains nothing, but that behind it there must be hidden a more significant, earlier, experience; and we direct his attention by the same technique to the associative thread which connects the two memories—the one that has been discovered and the one that has still to be discovered [footnote omitted]. A continuation of the analysis then leads in every instance to the reproduction of new scenes of the character we expect. [S.E. 1896, 3: 195-196]

> The most important finding that is arrived at if an analysis is thus consistently pursued is this. Whatever case and whatever symptom we take as our point of departure, *in the end we infallibly come to the field of sexual experience*. So here for the first time we seem to have discovered an aetiological precondition for hysterical symptoms. [S.E. 1896, 3: 199]

In short, Freud had inferred a substantial difference in pathogenic significance between the occasioning trauma, on the one hand, and the presumed earlier sexual trauma, on the other. And he related that difference to his own emendation of the etiologic assumption governing Breuer's cathartic therapy: "Thus a sexual trauma [during child-hood] stepped into the place of an ordinary [occasioning] trauma [from later life] and the latter was seen to owe its aetiological significance to an associative or symbolic connection with the former, which had preceded it" (S.E. 1923, 18: 243).

Thus, in the 1896 paper from which we have been citing, Freud reported therapeutic failures and successes, respectively, as follows: (1) psychoanalytic treatment issued in a therapeutic fiasco whenever the patient was clearly left without any insight into the actual specific etiology of his neurosis, which had remained sequestered in his uncon-scious while the shallow analysis was uncovering only a *precipitating* cause of his affliction; and (2) cases in which the psychoanalytic undoing of the patient's repression of a trauma was "satisfactory in every respect both therapeutically and analytically," these therapeuti-cally successful cases being instances in which the patient achieved bona fide etiological insight, since the pertinent trauma had all the earmarks of being "really operative" pathogenically (S.E. 1896, 3: 195). Note that Freud's two conditions for etiologic adequacy are avowedly only necessary rather than sufficient conditions for identifying a trauma as being etiologically essential for hysteria. Yet he seems to take it for granted here that the concrete features of a repressed trauma can collectively vouch for its pathogenic potency, *independently* of any *therapeutic benefit* engendered by its mnemic restoration to the patient's consciousness (S.E. 1896, 3: 202-203). As Edward Erwin has remarked to me, if such direct etiologic identifiability were indeed granted, then Freud could have spared himself the circuitous detour of trying to vindicate it via NCT.

But perhaps Freud thought that such *direct* identifiability is feasible in *some* cases and not possible in others. If so, then the etiologic inferences in the *latter* cases would first be vindicated via NCT, once its bold second conjunct can claim evidential support. This conjunct asserts that correct insight into the essential etiology of the patient's neurosis is causally necessary for his therapeutic conquest of it. Evi-dential support for this assertion would be provided, in turn, once the purported cases of direct etiologic identifiability are invoked to buttress the stated two correlations as to therapeutic outcome; for the afore-mentioned concomitances bespeak the kind of causal relevance of insight to therapeutic outcome that is avowed by NCT. In any case, it would seem that, even in the remainder of the same 1896 paper, Freud did not hesitate to adduce just this daring NCT claim, as I shall now show.

When reporting that the vast majority of *occasioning* traumatic scenes *violated* at least one of his two conditions for etiologic adequacy, Freud recorded some rare exceptions: "The traumatic scene in which the symptom originated [i.e., the occasioning trauma] does in fact occasionally possess both the qualities—suitability as a determinant and traumatic force—which we require for an understanding of the symptom" (S.E. 1896, 3: 194). Then he declared emphatically that the pathogenesis of hysteria can *never* be effected by the occasioning trauma without the etiologic contribution of *earlier* painful experiences, no matter what other qualities that later trauma possesses. Immediately after enunciating this proposition, he reverts to those avowedly *rare* occasioning traumata that *do* satisfy his two etiologic adequacy conditions:

> You might suppose that the rare instances in which analysis is able to trace the symptom back direct [*sic*] to a traumatic scene [i.e., occasioning trauma] that is thoroughly suitable as a determinant and possesses traumatic force, and is able, by thus tracing it back, at the same time to remove it (in the way described in Breuer's case history of Anna O.)—you might suppose that such instances must, after all, constitute powerful objections to the general validity of the proposition [of the etiologic *parasitism* of the occasioning traumata] I have just put forward. It certainly looks so. But I must assure you that I have the best grounds for assuming that even in such instances there exists a chain of [etiologically] operative memories which stretches far back behind the first [occasioning] traumatic scene, *even though* the reproduction of the latter alone may have the result of removing the symptom. [S.E. 1896, 3: 197]

Here Freud is acknowledging that prima facie his proposition of etiologic parasitism faces "powerful objections" from those rare occasioning traumata that satisfy his two *necessary* conditions for etiologic adequacy *and* whose restoration to the patient's consciousness issues in symptom removal. He then uses the italicized words *even though* to single out this *therapeutic* outcome as a special challenge to the proposition that he had enunciated just before.

But why should he suppose at all that symptom removal, engendered by the patient's recall of occasioning traumata that satisfy his two necessary conditions, would prima facie gainsay the etiologic parasitism that his proposition attributed to every occasioning trauma? I submit that *his rationale* for this supposition *is furnished by none other than his NCT*, which declared insight into the *essential* etiology of a neurosis to be causally necessary for a cure. For clearly the fulfillment of the two *necessary* conditions of etiologic adequacy by some occasioning traumata is entirely compatible with the etiologic parasitism of *all* such traumata, since these necessary conditions are not also jointly sufficient. Instead, as is patent from Freud's use of the words *even though*, the etiologic parasitism of occasioning traumata *seems* to run counter to the symptom removal that did ensue in some cases when the analysis retrieved *only* an *occasioning* trauma!

Hence, I ask anew: even prima facie, why should this positive therapeutic outcome not be achieved in the wake of insight into an etiologically *marginal* trauma? And I answer: because — if the resulting symptom removal *were* tantamount to the conquest of the underlying neurosis — then the remission would violate NCT's demand for insight into the *essential* etiology of the neurosis as a condition requisite for its conquest.

Fortunately, after having presented the tantalizing challenge posed by the symptom remissions, Freud does not leave us wondering indefinitely whether and how he does reconcile his NCT with this positive treatment outcome from etiologically marginal insight. Later in his paper (S.E. 1896, 3: 206), he cautions that the patient's symptom removal need not be tantamount to his "radical cure," if only because the analysand may be prone to relapses. Aware that a *symptom* cure may actually *not* betoken the conquest of the *underlying* neurosis, he explicitly deems fragile any symptom cure occurring in the wake of the *failure*, on the part of the patient's etiologic insight, to penetrate beyond the occasioning trauma to the "specific aetiology" (S.E. 1896, 3: 209-210) of his affliction. Hence, he has preserved compatibility with NCT. As he explains:

In a number of cases therapeutic evidence of the genuineness of the [traumatic] infantile scenes can also be brought forward. There are cases in which a complete or partial cure can be obtained without our having to go as deep as the infantile experiences. And there are others in which no success at all is obtained until the analysis has come to its natural end with the uncovering of the earliest traumas. In the former cases we are not, I believe, secure against relapses, and my expectation is that a complete psycho-analysis implies a radical cure of the hysteria. [S.E. 1896, 3: 206]

But Freud leaves unclear here *on what grounds* he takes the stated therapeutic results to be "evidence" for his seduction etiology. Could he be invoking NCT, no less than he surely seems to have done earlier in the same paper? The same exegetical question as to the role of NCT is posed by his reliance on therapeutic success to "confirm" his analytically inferred sexual etiology of hysteria, when avowedly submitting the credentials of that etiology "to the strictest examination":

If you submit my assertion that the aetiology of hysteria lies in sexual life to the strictest examination, you will find that it is supported by the fact that in some eighteen cases of hysteria I have been able to discover this connection in every single symptom, and, where the circumstances allowed, to confirm it by therapeutic success. [S.E. 1896, 3: 199]

When reading these passages, we must be mindful of his etiological ranking of the earliest traumata vis-à-vis the later ones.

All the events subsequent to puberty to which an influence must be attributed upon the development of the hysterical neurosis and upon the formation of its symptoms are in fact only concurrent causes — *"agents provocateurs."* . . . These accessory agents are not subject to the strict conditions imposed on the specific causes; analysis demonstrates in an irrefutable fashion that they enjoy a pathogenic influence for hysteria only owing to their faculty for awakening the unconscious psychical trace of the childhood event. [S.E. 1896, 3: 154-155]

While thus stressing the causal ranking among the etiological factors, Freud called attention to their cumulativity (S.E. 1896, 3: 214, 216). Moreover, in one of his 1895 case histories (Fräulein Elisabeth von R.), Freud had not only downgraded the occasioning trauma etiologically but had asserted the bold second conjunct of NCT even with respect to *symptom removal*:

Indeed, in the great majority of instances we find that a first trauma has left no symptom behind, while a later trauma of the same kind produces a symptom, and yet that the latter could not have come into existence without the co-operation of the earlier provoking cause; nor can it be cleared up without taking all the provoking causes into account. [S.E. 1896, 2: 173]

In another 1895 case history, Freud had adumbrated the role he attributed to the patient's inherited constitution in the auxiliary etiology of hysteria:

Frau von N. was undoubtedly a personality with a severe neuropathic hered-ity. It seems likely that there can be no hysteria apart from a disposition of this kind. But on the other hand disposition alone does not make hysteria. There must be reasons that bring it about, and, in my opinion, these reasons must be appropriate: the aetiology is of a specific character. [S.E. 1895, 2:102]

In this way, he gave a partial answer to the question about the *causally sufficient* condition for this disorder, a question he put as follows: "What can the other factors be which the 'specific aetiology' of hysteria still needs in order actually to produce the neurosis?" [S.E. 1896, 3: 210]

Incidentally, in recent years there have been allegations that cases of classical hysteria of the sort seen by Freud have since disappeared. Clearly, if there is no temporal stability in the diagnostic criteria used to identify patients as hysterics, then the *reported* secular decline in the prevalence of this disorder hardly bespeaks an actual decrease in its incidence. As the analyst Kaplan (1981: 15) explains illuminatingly:

The diagnosis of hysteria, however, was applied to a diverse group of patients with not only conversion, but with phobic and other symptoms paralleling the development of our psychoanalytic theories and new preformed conceptions about hysteria.

There is also evidence that the classically described hysteria is still commonly seen today, more often in less sophisticated patients, but in all social classes, not necessarily by psychoanalysts, but by psychiatrists and other physicians [footnote omitted]. Now as we look back, many of the patients previously seen as suffering from hysteria would no longer be so diagnosed.

Cognizant of Freud's distinction between a symptom cure and a radical one, analysts have perennially prided themselves on treating the causes of neuroses, rather than the mere symptoms, by means of undoing repressions psychoanalytically. But in his 1917 lecture "Transference," Freud qualified the sense in which analysis can claim to be a "causal therapy." For there he pointed out that much as lifting repressions is a more thoroughgoing attack on a neurosis than mere symptom removal, it is not an attack on those *earlier* roots of the etiological series in the patient's constitution, which first make the patient at all *vulnerable* to pathogenic experiences (S.E. 1917, 16: 435-436). The latter kind of assault on the pathogenic dispositions—perhaps "by some chemical means," he tells us—"would be a causal therapy in the true sense of the word" (p. 436). But until and unless Freud's etiologies do have adequate credentials, his therapy has no claim to being any kind of "causal therapy."

As we have seen, his distinction between a symptom cure, perhaps induced by the transference relationship, and a cure of the underlying neurosis serves to obviate a spurious counterexample to his NCT, which is generated by failure to allow for this distinction. That this caveat is salutary is further illustrated by its relevance to the proper construal of a cryptic statement in his 1917 "Analytic Therapy" lecture. There (S.E. 1917, 16: 449), only a few pages before making use of NCT in the Tally Argument, he recalls his disappointments when he practiced both Bernheim's and Breuer's versions of hypnotic therapy. The procedure could be used with some patients but not with others, was unaccountably quite helpful with some while achieving little with others, and even when successful, the resulting improvement was not durable. This lack of permanence necessitated an addictive repetition of the treatment, which deprived the patient of his self-reliance (see also S.E. 1905, 7: 301). Having registered these complaints, Freud nonetheless punctuated them by the following cryptic demurrer: "Admittedly sometimes things went entirely as one would wish: after a few efforts, success was complete and permanent. But the conditions determining such a favourable outcome remained unknown" (S.E. 1917, 16: 449). A footnote appended to the term "permanent" by the editors of the *Standard Edition* steers the reader to an instance of this kind in Freud's paper "A Case of Successful Treatment by Hypnotism" (S.E. 1892 1: 117-28), which appeared in two parts in December 1892 and January 1893.

But when we turn to this paper, it becomes clear that Freud expressed himself misleadingly by describing the success of the hypnotic treatment reported there as "permanent," and that this success consisted of symptom removals which do *not* gainsay NCT. The patient was a woman whose various hysterical symptoms prevented her from breast-feeding her first child. Two sessions of prohibitory hypnotic suggestion à la Bernheim did suffice to remove all of her symptoms. But this removal was "permanent" only until she had a second child a year later, when her symptoms returned and had to be removed hypnotically once again. That Freud regarded such hypnotic symptom removals as shallow, ephemeral transference cures is evident from the following 1904 statement by him, which is must less cryptic than the aforecited 1917 demurrer:

I gave up the suggestive technique, and with it hypnosis, so early in my practice because I despaired of making suggestion powerful and enduring enough to effect permanent cures. In every severe case I saw the suggestions which had been applied crumble away again; after which the disease or some substitute for it was back once more. [S.E. 1905, 7: 261]

He reiterated his distinction between a psychoanalytic "radical cure" of a full-fledged neurosis and a shallow one by "more convenient methods of treatment" (S.E. 1905, 7: 262-263), and allowed for "slighter, episodic cases which we see recovering under all kinds of influences and even spontaneously." And, as we recall, as part of his 1909 enunciation of NCT, he again allowed that "slight disorders may perhaps be brought to an end by the subject's unaided efforts, but never a neurosis" (S.E. 1909, 10: 104).

It will be recalled that in 1896, Freud had marshaled both therapeutic and other clinical findings that he regarded as evidence for the pathogenic role of the inferred infantile seduction scenes (S.E. 1896, 3: 199, 206). But in the same 1896 paper, he took special pains to address doubts as to whether these episodes had occurred at all, not merely whether—if genuine—they were also the specific pathogens of hysteria. Though Freud privately repudiated even the very occurrence of the seductions only a year and a half later (Freud 1954, letter #69 to Wilhelm Fliess: 215-217), it is instructive to see just what doubts he canvassed, and how he rebuffed them in 1896.

Ever mindful of the challenge of suggestibility, he asked rhetorically:

Is it not very possible either that the physician forces such scenes upon his docile patients, alleging that they are memories, or else that the patients tell the physician things which they have deliberately invented or have imagined and that he accepts those things as true? [S.E. 1896, 3: 204]

And he replies to the first doubt:

I have never yet succeeded in forcing on a patient a scene I was expecting to find, in such a way that he seemed to be living through it with all the appropriate feelings. [S.E. 1896, 3: 205]

Here Freud is undaunted, although he himself had mentioned earlier in the paper that if the occasioning trauma is etiologically unsatisfactory, "we tell our patient that his experience explains nothing, but that behind it there must be hidden a more significant, earlier, experience" (S.E. 1896, 3: 195-196). Even twenty-eight years after his repudiation of the seduction etiology, he is unrelenting on this point: "I do not believe even now that I forced the seduction phantasies on my patients, that I 'suggested' them" (S.E. 1925, 20: 34). Yet, at that later time, he did retract his 1896 reply to the charge that his patients had manufactured the seduction scenes and had duped the analyst. His confident reply in 1896 had been that there is "conclusive proof" to the contrary:

The behaviour of patients while they are reproducing these infantile experiences is in every respect incompatible with the assumption that the scenes are anything else than a reality which is being felt with distress and reproduced with the greatest reluctance. . . .

Why should patients assure me so emphatically of their unbelief, if what they want to discredit is something which — from whatever motive — they themselves have invented? [S.E. 1896, 3: 204]

But as he explains in 1925:

When, however, I was at last obliged to recognize that these scenes of seduction had never taken place, and that they were only phantasies which my patients had made up or which I myself had perhaps forced on them, I was for some time completely at a loss. My confidence alike in my technique and it its results suffered a severe blow; it could not be disputed that I had arrived at these scenes by a technical method which I considered correct, and their subject-matter was unquestionably related to the symptoms from which my investigation had started. [S.E. 1925, 20: 34]

And in an earlier historical account, he reports that the mistaken etiology "might have been almost fatal to the young science" of psychoanalysis:

When this aetiology broke down under the weight of its own improbability and contradiction in definitely ascertainable circumstances. . . I would gladly have given up the whole work, just as my esteemed predecessor, Breuer, had done when he made his unwelcome discovery. Perhaps I persevered only because I no longer had any choice and could not then begin again at anything else. [S.E. 1914, 14: 17]

Though the seduction etiology debacle thus jeopardized the psychoanalytic enterprise in general, it did *not* refute the bold second conjunct of NCT in particular. Clearly, NCT would have been strongly disconfirmed *if* there had been cases of patients who had been genuinely cured after being given *pseudo*insight by their analysis into episodes of sexual abuse that had presumably never occurred in *their* childhood, though probably in others. But the very first of the three reasons that Freud gave Fliess in 1897 for abandoning the seduction theory was precisely that no such therapeutic conquests of the underlying neurosis materialized. Indeed, as he pointed out, such remedial gains as he did achieve were of the sort that could readily have been wrought by suggestion:

The first group of factors were the continual disappointment of my attempts to bring my analyses to a real conclusion, the running away of people who for a time had seemed my most favourably inclined patients, the lack of the complete success on which I had counted, and the possibility of explaining my partial successes in other, familiar, ways [i.e., suggestion]. [Freud 1954: 215]

But these therapeutic disclaimers are second thoughts, since he had twice adduced therapeutic results in support of his seduction etiology only the year before, as we saw. If Freud's more considered, unfavorable therapeutic inventory is assumed, then his replacement of actual by fancied seductions as the pathogens of hysteria did not serve to gainsay his NCT. Thus, the compatibility of NCT, including its first conjunct, with the collapse of the seduction etiology shows that this debacle, at any rate, provides no basis for judging Freud to have been intellectually dishonest when he explicitly enunciated NCT in 1909 and 1917. Nonetheless, his scientific candor does appear questionable in the light of the nine years he permitted to elapse before even *publicly intimating* his change of view (S.E. 1906, 7: 274-275).

Is the Tally Argument Viable?

The capacity of Freud's 1917 Tally Argument to *warrant* the actual truth of its conclusions depends, of course, on the empirical tenability of its two premises. As noted before, NCT is the pivot that gave any therapeutic triumphs achieved by analysis the leverage to vouch for the authenticity of its clinical data. Hence, to the extent that Freud disavowed one or both of these premises in later years, he forfeited his erstwhile reliance on this argument to vindicate the psychoanalytic method of inquiry and/or the conclusions he had reached by means of it. Again, to the extent that analytic treatment nowadays continues not to effect real cures of neuroses, and NCT is rendered dubious by currently available empirical information, Freudian theory is now devoid of this vindication in the face of the remaining twin challenge from suggestibility.

For a number of decades, Freud did claim empirical sanction for both of the premises in his Tally Argument. But ironically, in his later years he himself undermined this argument by gradually renouncing or significantly weakening each premise. Thus, in an important 1937 paper (S.E. 1937, 23: 216-254), his disparagement of the quality and durability of actual psychoanalytic treatment outcome bordered on a repudiation of treatment success. But even when Freud was not quite that pessimistic about the caliber of therapeutic outcome (S.E. 1926, 20: 265), he gainsaid his erstwhile NCT in 1926 by conceding the existence of spontaneous remission as follows: "As a rule our therapy must be content with bringing about more quickly, more reliably and with less expenditure of energy than would otherwise be the case the good result which in favourable circumstances would have occurred of itself" (S.E. 1926, 20: 154). Of course, the label "spontaneous remission" is to convey that gains made by an afflicted person were caused entirely by extraclinical life events rather than by professional therapists, not that these benefits were uncaused. Notably, Freud grants that neuroses yielding to analytic therapy would, in due course, remit spontaneously anyway. Hence, even Freud's own evidence placed his NCT premise in serious jeopardy.

Other analysts have likewise made concessions to spontaneous remission and have acknowledged that "all pervading" psychic improvements or cures can be effected without psychoanalytic insight by theoretically rival treatment modalities such as behavior therapy (Malan 1976: 172-173, 269, 147). It is to be understood that various treatment modalities are held to be "rivals" of one another in the sense that there is a divergence between their *theories* of the rationale, dynamics, methods, or techniques of the therapeutic process. Notably in psychoanalysis and behavior therapy, but perhaps also in some of the other modalities, the underlying theoretical rationale also comprises hypotheses pertaining to personality development, etiology, and the current dynamics of pathological behavior. Thus, the divergences between the rival therapies naturally extend to *these* causal hypotheses as well. Notoriously, there is a plethora of such rival therapeutic modalities, at least well over 125.

Ironically, in the case of some psychoanalytic theoreticians, the willingness to countenance the existence of spontaneous remission of full-fledged neuroses in *contravention* of NCT was prompted by the need to cope with a difficulty posed by behavior therapy for the *received* Freudian theory of the origin *and* maintenance of neurotic symptoms. To articulate the pertinent difficulty, note what would be expected to happen, according to this received account of symptom formation, when a symptom is extinguished by a direct attack on it, while its underlying neurosis is left intact. A neurotic symptom is held to be a compromise, *formed* in response to an unresolved conflict between a forbidden unconscious impulse and the ego's defense against it. The symptom is held to be *sustained* at any given time by a *coexisting*, ongoing unconscious conflict, which—as claimed by NCT—does not resolve itself without psychoanalytic intervention. Hence, if the repression of the unconscious wish is not lifted psychoanalytically, the underlying neurosis will persist, even if behavior therapy or hypnosis, for example, extinguishes the particular symptom that only *manifests* the neurosis at the time. As long as the neurotic conflict does persist, the patient's psyche will call for the defensive service previously rendered by the banished symptom. Hence, typically and especially in severe cases, the unresolved conflict ought to engender a *new* symptom. And incidentally, this expectation qualifies as a "risky" prediction in Popper's sense.

Thus, when Freud explained his disappointments with hypnotic therapy, he claimed, as we saw, that in every severe case he had treated suggestively, the patient either relapsed or developed *"some substitute"* for the original symptoms (emphasis added; S.E. 1905, 7: 261). But is such so-called "symptom substitution," which is the *replacement* of an extinguished symptom by a new one, in fact a normal occurrence? Fisher and Greenberg (1977: 370) have summarized empirical studies of the incidence of *new* symptoms, construed as "behaviors judged socially or personally maladaptive":

The evidence is consistent and solid that in many types of cases, symptoms can be removed by behavioral treatments with no indication that the patient suffers any negative consequences. . . . In fact, many of the investigations find signs of generalized improvement in functioning after the removal of an incapacitating symptom.

More recently, in a long-term follow-up of agoraphobic patients who had received behavior therapy, these patients were not only "much better at follow-up than they had been before treatment" but there was also no evidence of any symptom substitution (Munby and Johnston 1980: 418). This, then, is the difficulty posed for the analytic dynamics of symptom maintenance by behavioristic symptom extinction without relapse.

As Edward Erwin (1978: 161) has noted, some pro-Freudian writers have proposed to accommodate this dearth of symptom substitution, and they have done so by postulating that there are indeed remissions of neuroses *without* benefit of psychoanalytically mediated insight as follows: though all symptoms are *initially* generated defensively, in a good many cases their underlying conflicts are resolved by spontaneous ego maturation, and in such instances the sheer inertia of an acquired habit may well preserve the symptoms as "ghosts" of the erstwhile neurosis. Hence, when a symptom is only a relic of a spontaneously conquered neurosis, the behavioristic extinction of the latter's "ghost" ought *not* to issue in any substitute for it. Such replacement by a new symptom ought to occur only when the vanished one was a manifestation of an *ongoing* conflict, rather than a ghost. Rhoads and Feather (1974: 17) claim to be able to tell whether a given symptom is a ghost symptom or not. Furthermore, they report having "found that classical [behavioristic] desensitization proceeds quickly and rapidly when used to treat 'ghost' symptoms," whereas such therapy does not have this effect in the case of *non*–ghost symptoms.

But clearly, this proposed division of existing symptoms into "ghosts" and "nonghosts" invokes the spontaneous remission of neuroses. Thus, the postulate of vestige symptoms repudiates NCT—a veritable pillar of Freudian therapeutic doctrine—as well as the received psychoanalytic dynamics of symptom maintenance (S.E. 1893, 2: 6), for the sake of accommodating the sparsity of symptom substitution. And, as I shall now show, by rejecting the received analytic view that *present* symptoms are manifestations of coexisting and ongoing repressed conflicts, the ghost-symptom theorists unwittingly effect an *epistemic subversion* of the Freudian etiology of *initial* symptom *origination*, which they are anxious to retain. This epistemic undercutting results because the hypothesis of symptom maintenance repudiated by the ghost-symptom theorists has been the major avenue for the purported clinical inferability of etiology ever since Breuer and Freud had enunciated it (S.E. 1893, 2: 6).

In order to *justify* their etiologic identification of an original act of repression as the specific pathogen responsible, at the outset, for the initial formation of the symptom, the founders of psychoanalysis extrapolated backward from the maintenance dynamics they postulated for the continuing existence of the symptom. The evidence they marshaled, in turn, to justify this dynamics was that therapeutic symptom removal ensued from the abreactive lifting of a *coexisting* repression. In this way, they inferred etiologies via symptom maintenance from cathartic treatment success. The importance of the role they assigned to this ongoing repression as the cause of the current existence of a symptom is betokened by the pains they take to *reject* the notion that the symptom "leads an independent existence" as a mere vestige, once it has been engendered by an initial and subsequently forgotten trauma. Thus, they declare: "We must presume rather that the psychical trauma—or more precisely the [repressed] memory of the trauma—acts like a foreign body which long after its entry must continue to be regarded as an agent that is still at work" (S.E. 1893, 2: 6).

Clearly then, in order to certify the etiologic identification of the original repression as the prime pathogen on the basis of the therapeutic results they adduce, Breuer and Freud rely on their causal account of symptom maintenance. Even long after Freud had introduced free association as the key to fathoming repressions—as, for example, in the interpretation of manifest dream content—that venerable account of symptom maintenance remained the principal epistemic avenue for the inferability of etiology by means of the clinical data obtained from psychoanalytic investigation! Yet precisely that time-honored explanation of why symptoms persist when they do is incompatible with the "ghost thesis" that while they persist, there is frequent spontaneous dissipation of the initial repression, which purportedly engendered the symptoms to begin with.

It emerges, therefore, that Freudians who espouse the ghost-symptom hypothesis (e.g., Weitzman 1967: 307) do so on pain of severing a vital inferential link that has been paradigmatic for the clinical validation of Freud's etiologies. Hence, the resort to ghost symptoms for the sake of accommodating the sparsity of symptom substitution boomerangs: the cost of this accommodation is the epistemic subversion of the psychoanalytic etiology of original symptom formation, an etiology that the Freudian ghost theoreticians avowedly wish to preserve. This cost must then be added to the epistemic sacrifice incurred by the disavowal of NCT, which we have already tallied.

Furthermore, note that the ghost-symptom hypothesis explains the low incidence of symptom substitution by the high prevalence of ghost symptoms. For just this reason, the hypothesis ironically provides theoretical grounds for deeming psychoanalytic therapy very largely superfluous, at least for all those nosologic categories of patients which featured the sparsity of symptom substitution. Indeed, on that hypothesis, the presenting symptoms of the typical patient who is accepted for analysis are likely to be ghost symptoms, since people of high ego-strength presumably have a good chance of spontaneous ego-maturation. Hence, the permanent removal of these presenting symptoms without risk of being replaced by others hardly requires the pain, time, and expense exacted by psychoanalysis. If such symptoms yield to treatment at all, their short-term nonanalytic extinction will do. Analysis is then reduced to being the treatment of choice for only that small minority of psychoneurotics who are now presumed to be afflicted by *non*–ghost symptoms. In the great majority of cases, psychoanalysis must then be deemed a *placebo* therapy (Grünbaum 1980: 325-350; 1981). Yet Freud had insisted that the working through of the patient's conflicts is the crucial therapeutic factor in treatment, and indeed the ingredient "which distinguishes analytic treatment from any kind of treatment by suggestion" (S.E. 1914, 12: 155-156).

In short, opting for ghost symptoms gainsays NCT, undermines the received clinical epistemology of Freud's etiologies of the psychoneuroses, and makes analytic therapy largely superfluous to boot. This is a high price to pay.

Did Freud himself ever countenance the possibility of spontaneous erosion of the pathological repressions, while the symptoms persist as mere vestiges of the repressions? Late in his career, in a footnote to his disappointingly fuzzy 1926 essay on anxiety, Freud entertained, even if he did not espouse, this ghost-symptom hypothesis (S.E. 1926, 20: 142, n. 1). There he explained that the 1923 advent of his *second* topographic model of the mind—which featured the id, ego, and superego as agencies—prompted him to question his erstwhile view of symptom maintenance. At least in the case of psychoanalytically untreated victims of neurotic symptoms, he had believed in the continuing unconscious survival of initially repressed instinctual impulses. It seems "ready to hand and certain," he tells us, "that the old, repressed wishes must still be present in the unconscious since we still find their derivatives, the symptoms, in operation." Yet by 1926, "we begin to suspect that it is not self-evident, perhaps not even usual, that those impulses should remain unaltered and unalterable in this way." Hence, by that time, he had come to deem his entrenched view unduly restrictive: "It does not enable us to decide between two possibilities: either that the old wish is now operating only through its derivatives, having transferred the whole of its cathectic energy to them, or that it is itself still in existence too." This is Freud's plea for entertaining, if not embracing, the ghost-symptom hypothesis.

Weitzman (1967: 307) calls attention to this plea in order to make two points: (1) "successful symptomatic treatment may be taken as evidence" for the ghost-symptom hypothesis, and (2) this hypothesis "might be extended and elaborated in ways entirely compatible with analytic theory." Evidently Weitzman is quite unaware that, for the reasons I have given, the incorporation of the ghost postulate in analytic theory devastatingly undermines it epistemically. Besides, it largely negates such relevance as analysts have been wont to claim for Freud's therapy.

The difficulties besetting NCT and/or the Tally Argument that I have set forth augment the already massive ones I had recently developed elsewhere *in detail* (Grünbaum 1980: 319-354; pp. 326-342 of this reference are amplified in Grünbaum 1981). And since the Tally Argument is thus gravely undercut, any therapeutic successes scored by analysts, even if spectacular, have become *probatively* unavailing to the validation of psychoanalytic theory via that argument. Indeed, as I took pains to show (Grünbaum 1980: 343-352), not only is NCT discredited but no empirically warranted *alternative* premise that could take its place and yield the desired sanguine conclusions seems to be in sight. Hence, currently no viable surrogate for the defunct Tally Argument appears on the horizon. But this leaves unanswered the gravamen of the reproach that the psychoanalytic method of inquiry issues in bogus confirmations; for Freud had placed cardinal reliance on the Tally Argument to counter the indictment that clinical data are inauthentic as a result of suggestibility.

The vital legitimating role that NCT would have played epistemically if it were viable points up a linkage between Freud's therapy and the attempted clinical validation of his general theory of unconscious motivations that was intrinsic to the psychoanalytic enterprise from the start. As he explained: "In psycho-analysis there has existed from the very first an inseparable bond between cure and research" (S.E. 1926, 20: 256). Indeed, we saw that in the cathartic method the epistemic dependence of the inferred etiology on therapeutic results was a crucial one: it was the therapy that enabled Breuer and Freud at all to propel the patients' various clinical responses under hypnosis into repression etiologies.

Thus, psychoanalytic hypotheses that do *not* themselves pertain at all to either the dynamics or the outcome of analytic therapy nonetheless have been *epistemically parasitic* on therapeutic results, partly to legitimate the probity of nontherapeutic clinical data, and partly to support the etiologies directly in the manner of the "Preliminary Communication" by Breuer and Freud. Yet Freud's essential reliance on positive therapeutic outcome to vindicate the probity of clinical data via NCT in the face of suggestibility is being widely overlooked. Those who have made it fashionable nowadays to dissociate the credentials of Freud's theory of personality—the "science"—from the credentials of his therapy ought to face that they are stepping on very thin ice indeed. But before I turn to taking the measure of this thinness, I need to juxtapose two major sets of prima facie divergent methodological injunctions to which Freud adhered; for this juxtaposition will permit a reappraisal of Freud as a methodologist.

The first of the two methodological directives is to use the psychoanalytic method for the clinical ascertainment of the specific etiologies of the *psycho*neuroses, and more generally to validate *causal* hypotheses pertaining to unconscious motivations intraclinically *without* experimental controls. Freud considered this injunction to be vindicated by his Tally Argument. The second injunction pertained to the etiologic investigation of disorders such as anxiety neurosis, to which the psychoanalytic method of inquiry *and* therapy is avowedly *inapplicable*, because repressed ideation is held to play no role in their pathogenesis. In regard to probing the etiology of such afflictions, Freud gave the explicit admonition against victimization by *post hoc ergo propter hoc* and other pitfalls of causal inference, a caveat that he issued and applied devastatingly in his 1895 reply to Löwenfeld. I shall now set forth Freud's handling of the second of these two injunctions in order to put into still bolder relief his reliance on his NCT to legitimate the psychoanalytic method of clinical investigation as a means of validating hypotheses pertaining to unconscious motivations. As a corollary, I shall then challenge the unduly disparaging verdicts that even friendly critics have reached on him as a methodologist.

Freud's explicit warning against victimization by the pitfalls of causal inference in etiological inquiry is set forth in his searching 1895 "Reply to Löwenfeld" (S.E. 1895, 3: 123-139), which we had occasion to adduce against Popper earlier. Near the end of this reply, Freud articulates an admirably rich and lucid typology of the different senses in which diverse etiological factors may be causally relevant to a neurosis (pp. 135-136). It will be recalled that Löwenfeld had offered a critique of Freud's specific etiology of anxiety neurosis, a syndrome that Freud had been concerned to distinguish from neurasthenia, both clinically and etiologically. Löwenfeld claimed to have evidence that the psychical shock of a suddenly frightening experience—rather than any

sexual disturbance—was the pathogen of anxiety neurosis. But Freud
upheld his thesis that the specific etiology of this syndrome is sexual,
and he did so in a two-part argument as follows: (1) he chided Löwenfeld for having fallaciously inferred the rival *non*sexual etiology that
fright is the pathogen of anxiety neurosis by illicit causal reasoning
based on *post hoc ergo propter hoc*, and (2) he referred to the investigation
he himself had carried out in his first paper on anxiety neurosis (S.E.
1895, 3: 90-115) to validate the specific sexual etiology he had postulated for that syndrome. As for the first part of his argument, note
Freud's keen appreciation of methodological pitfalls that are commonly laid at his door by critics:

> About the facts themselves, which Löwenfeld uses against me, there is not the
> slightest doubt.
>   But there *is* doubt about their interpretation. Are we to accept the *post hoc
> ergo propter hoc* conclusion straight away and spare ourselves any critical
> consideration of the raw material? There are examples enough in which the
> final, releasing cause has not, in the face of critical analysis, maintained its
> position as the *causa efficiens*. One has only to think, for instance, of the
> relationship between trauma and gout. . . . It is clear to the meanest capacity
> that it is absurd to suppose that the trauma has "caused" the gout instead of
> having merely provoked it [i.e., provoked its *onset*]. It is bound to make us
> thoughtful when we come across aetiological factors of this sort—"stock"
> factors, as I should like to call them [footnote omitted]—in the aetiology of the
> most varied forms of illness. Emotion, fright, is also a stock factor of this
> kind. . . . I am justified in drawing the following conclusion: if the same specific
> cause can be shown to exist in the aetiology of all, or the great majority, of cases
> of anxiety neurosis, our view of the matter need not be shaken by the fact that
> the illness does not break out until one or other stock factor, such as emotion,
> has come into operation.
>   So it was with my cases of anxiety neurosis. [S.E. 1895, 3: 127]

But what *positive* reasons had Freud adduced in support of the
specific sexual etiology he had inferred for anxiety neurosis? He
reasoned essentially in the fashion of J. S. Mill's joint method of
agreement and difference, using the particular case in which the
inferred specific etiologic factor was realized by the practice of coitus
interruptus. But note that Freud was careful (S.E. 1895, 3: 114) to
distinguish between the underlying factor in the nervous system,
which he had hypothesized to be specifically etiologic for a given
syndrome, on the one hand, and the kinds of overt activities (or
inactivities) that often—though not always!—*realize* this factor, on the
other.[2]

Two major points in Freud's argument for his specific sexual etiology
of anxiety neurosis deserve notice: (1) he was careful to guard against

the inferential pitfall of *post hoc ergo propter hoc* by producing a variety of instances in which the *absence* of the presumed cause issued in the *absence* of the anxiety attacks; and (2) the "*therapeutic* proof" of his hypothesized etiology is furnished, as he tells us, by the results produced upon the patient's alteration of his or her sexual practices (S.E. 1895, 3: 104); for his cases of anxiety neurosis *cured themselves* when coitus interruptus was suspended in favor of normal inter-course. Thus, far from claiming that *only* psychoanalysis can cure anxiety neurosis, Freud drew on the specific etiology he had inferred for it from *non*psychoanalytic clinical data to provide theoretical grounds for concluding that anxiety neurosis is *not even amenable* to psychoanalytic treatment. As he explains, "Anxiety neurosis...is the product of all those factors which prevent the somatic sexual excitation from being worked over psychically" (S.E. 1895, 3: 109), an assertion he reaffirmed as late as 1926 (S.E. 1926, 20: 141). Hence, in anxiety neurosis, "the affect does not originate in a repressed idea but turns out to be *not further reducible by psychological analysis, nor amenable to psycho-therapy* [emphasis in original]" (S.E. 1895, 3: 97). Clearly, anxiety neu-rosis, and any other neurosis in whose pathogenesis repression is held to play no role, is excluded from the purview of NCT.

As Freud emphasizes here, no repressed idea and no "psychic working over" play any etiological role in anxiety neurosis, which results from the *direct* transformation of *somatic* sexual excitation into the symptoms (S.E. 1895, 3: 81, 124). Therefore, analytic treatment cannot remove its specific cause by means of psychoanalytic insight into the significance of its symptoms. It follows that the very etiology of anxiety neurosis that Freud had inferred by causal inquiry à la J. S. Mill provided theoretical reasons for concluding that this specific etiology could never have been disclosed, let alone validated, by the *intra*clini-cal devices of psychoanalytic investigation. Moreover, the pathogenic events specific to anxiety neurosis occur during the patient's adult life rather than during infancy or childhood and are therefore essentially contemporary or "actual."

This array of etiological and therapeutic results pertaining to this neurosis—and also to neurasthenia—contrasts sharply with the corresponding ones that Freud believed to have established for hyste-ria, obsessional neurosis, and paranoia by means of the *psychoanalytic* method of investigation and therapy. He therefore separately classified anxiety neurosis and neurasthenia as "actual neuroses," and dis-tinguished them from the psychoanalytically tractable "psychoneu-roses" (S.E. 1898, 3: 278-279; but see also the 1896 statement in 3: 167-168). It is now clear why I was concerned to formulate Freud's NCT initially as pertaining to the *psycho*neuroses and to exclude the actual neuroses from its purview.

As shown by his 1895 debate with Löwenfeld on anxiety neurosis, Freud obviously had a keen appreciation of the methodological safeguards afforded by controlled prospective causal inquiry, no less than of the pitfalls of *post hoc ergo propter hoc* inferences in the validation of the specific *contemporary* etiologies of the actual neuroses. But in 1895, Freud published not only his two papers on anxiety neurosis but also the *Studies on Hysteria*, which he had coauthored with Breuer. How, then, could that same Freud have forsaken the methodological safeguards of prospective causal inquiry, and have been content to employ the purely *intra*clinical psychoanalytic method to discover and validate the *infantile* etiologies of the psychoneuroses retrospectively? I trust I have shown why I claim that, at least as long as he was inclined to try to meet the challenge of suggestibility, Freud would very probably have given the following answer: *in the case of the psychoneuroses, the Tally Argument is the epistemic underwriter of clinical validation* by means of the psychoanalytic method of etiologic investigation, whereas no such underwriter is available to permit dispensing with the prospective methods of controlled causal inquiry in the case of the *actual* neuroses. Thus, as long as he felt able to rely on the Tally Argument, he felt quite justified when he expressed a sovereign patronizing serenity in the face of the following *dismissal* of his scientific credibility: the therapeutic successes of psychoanalysis as an emotional corrective are *not* achieved by imparting veridical self-knowledge, but rather by using suggestion to induce the compliant production of just those clinical data required to validate its theory, which therefore derives only *spurious* confirmation from these data.

The methodological vindication that Freud had put forward was apparently overlooked by his friendly critics Fisher and Greenberg, who judged him to be epistemologically uncritical on exactly this score as follows: "While therapist suggestion may lead to patient changes, therapist suggestion does not lead to data acceptable for validating hypotheses about personality. Freud never really came to terms with the differences involved in trying to learn about people as opposed to trying to change them" (Fisher and Greenberg 1977: 363). True, after the empirical demise of NCT, Freudians are no longer entitled to adduce therapeutic success as evidence for the veridicality of the analysts' interpretations. But since Freud did offer the Tally Argument, it would seem that, at one stage, he did come to terms, *albeit unsuccessfully,* "with the differences involved in trying to learn about people as opposed to trying to change them." For there, he addressed head-on the challenge: "What is advantageous to our therapy is damaging to our researches" (S.E. 1917, 16: 452).

A similar conditional exoneration of Freud applies, I believe, to Fisher and Greenberg's reaction to the admission made by Freud when he said: "Quite often we do not succeed in bringing the patient to recollect what has been repressed. Instead of that, if the analysis is carried out correctly, we produce in him an assured conviction of the truth of the construction which achieves the same therapeutic result as a recaptured memory" (S.E. 1937, 23: 265-266). After citing this passage, Fisher and Greenberg comment:

The retreat from confidence in the analyst's ability to establish "what really happened" in childhood to a method emphasizing "this is what must have happened to you" is an open acknowledgment of suggestion occurring in the treatment. It also, of course, raises some serious questions about how a theory of infantile sexuality could be validated solely on the basis of information obtained from psychoanalytic therapy. [Fisher and Greenberg 1977: 367]

Here again, these sympathetic critics seem to have overlooked that precisely in this context, Freud—at an earlier stage of his career, when he still espoused NCT—would have pointed to his Tally Argument, in which he at least tackled, though unsuccessfully, just the issue they raise.

To my knowledge, writers on Freud have simply failed to appreciate that he offered this argument and have even typically taken no cognizance of the pertinent part of his 1917 lecture (number 28). The psychologist N. S. Sutherland (1977: 114-115) is the one author known to me who did cite and criticize precisely this portion. It is therefore quite disappointing that the significance of Freud's enunciation of the NCT premise was completely lost on him. As will be recalled, the issue posed by Freud at the very start of the passage in question is whether it is true of analysts—as charged by their opponents—that "the influencing of our patient may make the objective certainty of our findings doubtful" (S.E. 1917, 16: 452). As I have argued, the question thus posed by Freud is *addressed* rather than begged when he responds by adducing NCT to claim that it is not damaging, though reasonable: "After all, his conflicts will only be successfully solved and his resistances overcome if the anticipatory ideas he is given tally with what is real in him" (p. 452). Yet Sutherland complains of question begging by commenting as follows:

Note the skill with which Freud makes concessions to his opponents—"the objection... cannot be rejected as unreasonable"—only to trounce them at the expense of taking for granted the very point he is trying to prove. "After all, his conflicts will only be successfully solved and his resistances overcome if the anticipatory ideas he is given tally with what is real in him." [Sutherland 1977: 115].

I have juxtaposed the causal reasoning that Freud displayed in his reply to Löwenfeld with his concern to *vindicate* psychoanalytic investigation as a probatively cogent method of inquiry by means of the Tally Argument. And I have argued that once cognizance is taken of this argument, his stature as a scientific methodologist appears in a rather more favorable light than even friendly critics like Fisher and Greenberg have been prepared to allow.

Yet once Freud gave up NCT, he seems to have simply disregarded his own 1917 avowal that the authenticity of clinical data is epistemically parasitic on therapeutic achievements. Thus, in the very year in which he acknowledged that neuroses do remit spontaneously in due course (S.E. 1926, 20: 154), he proclaimed himself "a supporter of the inherent [scientific] value of psychoanalysis and of its independence of its application to medicine" (S.E. 1926, 20: 254). Hence, he demanded: "I only want to feel assured that the therapy will not destroy the science." But by precisely the account he gave in his "Analytic Therapy" lecture, once intraclinical validation is bereft of the legitimation that he drew from therapeutic success via the Tally Argument, the menacing suggestibility problem, which he had held at bay by means of this argument, comes back to haunt data from the couch with a vengeance. Therefore, unless analytic treatment is the paragon of the therapies as claimed in the Tally Argument, Freud himself has acknowledged that he cannot be assured of the inherent scientific value of psychoanalysis, no matter how devoutly he desires it.

A host of epistemic liabilities other than suggestibility intermingle with it to bedevil clinical validation. An account of the range and depth of these further pitfalls will now serve to justify the third of my stated six main theses. Moreover, the major pillars of the theory of repression will turn out to be ill-founded, *even if clinical data could be taken at face value as being uncontaminated epistemically.*

THE CORNERSTONE OF THE PSYCHOANALYTIC EDIFICE: IS THE FREUDIAN THEORY OF REPRESSION WELL-FOUNDED?

Freud's method of free association has been hailed as the master key to unlocking all sorts of repressed ideation (S.E. Editor's Introduction, 2: xvi-xviii). Its products have been claimed to be uncontaminated excavations of buried mentation precisely because the flow of associations generated when the patient adheres to the governing "fundamental rule" is allegedly "free." As Freud maintains, it was "confirmed by wide experience" that the *contents* of all the associations that flow in the patient's mind from a given initial content do stand in an *internal causal connection* to that initial content (S.E. 1923, 18: 238). By avowedly being purely *internal*, this causal relatedness rules out the mediation of externally injected content in the strictly deterministic linkages that Freud postulates to exist between the initial mental content and the ensuing associations. And *if* there actually is no such external mediation, then the patient's flow of associations is indeed immune to contamination by distorting influences emanating from the analyst's suggestions! Thus, the analyst could then be held to function as a neutral catalyst or expeditor of the flow of his patient's free associations, even when he prompts the analysand to continue them after he suspects that they are being censored by internal resistances. In this way, the chain of the patient's associations is purported to serve as a pathway to the psychoanalytic unmasking of his repressions.

Freud recognized, it is true, that "free association is not really free," *to the extent* that "the patient remains under the influence of the analytic situation even though he is not directing his mental activities on to a particular subject. We shall be justified in assuming that nothing will occur to him that has not some reference to that situation" (S.E. 1925, 20: 40-41). But he makes it quite clear on the same page that this acknowledgment of a *global* influence by the analytic situation is *not* tantamount to admitting epistemic contamination of the products of free association by the analyst's influence: "it [free association] guarantees to a great extent that... nothing will be introduced into it by the expectations of the analyst" (p. 41). Thus, unencumbered by the stated qualifications, Freud deems free association to qualify as the "open sesame" for entry into the thoughts and feelings sequestered in the unconscious by repression.

For argument's sake, let us grant just for now that the patient's adherence to the fundamental rule of free association does safeguard the uncontaminated emergence of actually existing *repressed* wishes, anger, guilt, fear, or what have you. Why should the disclosure of these unconscious states be so very important? Clearly, it is because repressed ideation is held to have central dynamic significance in psychoanalytic theory. As Freud explains, "The theory of repression is the cornerstone on which the whole structure of psycho-analysis rests. It is the most essential part of it" (S.E. 1914, 14: 16). Hence, the cardinal epistemic value that is claimed for free association depends on the credentials of the theory of repression. It therefore behooves us now to examine the logical foundations of this theory in some detail. The upshot of that scrutiny will be that the reasoning by which Freud sought to justify the very foundation of his theory was grievously flawed. Thereupon we shall be able to appraise the probative value of free association.

Freud had emphasized that Breuer's "cathartic method [of therapy and clinical investigation] was the immediate precursor of psychoanalysis; and, in spite of every extension of experience and of every modification of theory, is still contained within it as its nucleus" (S.E. 1924, 19: 194). Josef Breuer used hypnosis to revive and articulate the patient's memory of a *repressed* traumatic experience that had presumably occasioned the first appearance of a particular hysterical symptom. Thereby Freud's mentor induced a purgative release of the pent-up emotional distress that had been originally bound to the trauma. Since such cathartic reliving of a repressed trauma seemed to yield relief from the particular hysterical symptom, Breuer and Freud hypothesized that repression is the sine qua non for the pathogenesis of the patient's psychoneurosis (S.E. 1893, 2: 6-7; 1893, 3: 29-30).

This *etiologic* role of repressed ideation then became prototypic for much of Freud's own theory of unconscious motivations. Repressed *wishes* were postulated to be the motives of *all* dreaming. Sundry repressed mentation was deemed to cause the *bungling* of actions at which the subject is normally successful ("parapraxes," such as slips of the tongue or pen, instances of mishearing or misreading, cases of forgetting words, intentions, or events, and the mislaying or losing of objects) (S.E. 1916, 15: 25, 67). Thus, even in the case of "normal" people, Freud saw manifest dream content and various sorts of "slips" as the telltale symptoms of (temporary) *mini*neuroses, engendered by repressions.

Freud arrived at the purported sexual repression-etiologies of the psychoneuroses, as well as at the supposed causes of dreams and parapraxes, by lifting presumed repressions via the patient's allegedly "free" associations. At the same time, excavation of the pertinent repressed ideation was to remove the pathogens of the patient's afflictions. Hence, scientifically, Freud deemed the psychoanalytic method of investigation to be both heuristic *and* probative, over and above being a method of therapy. By the same token, he declared that "the theory of repression is the cornerstone on which the whole structure of psychoanalysis rests. It is the most essential part of it" (S.E. 1914, 14: 16). And he claimed that clinical evidence furnishes compelling support for this theoretical cornerstone.

Therefore, we can scrutinize the logical foundations of psychoanalytic theory by examining Freud's clinical arguments for the repression etiology of the psychoneuroses and for the cardinal causal role of repressed ideation in committing "Freudian slips" and in dreaming. This portion of my essay is devoted to just such a scrutiny, and its upshot will be that the reasoning by which Freud sought to justify the very foundation of his theory was grievously flawed.

THE REPRESSION ETIOLOGY OF THE PSYCHONEUROSES

Breuer and Freud explicitly adduced the separate *therapeutic* removal of particular neurotic symptoms, by means of undoing repressions having a thematic and associative affinity to these very symptoms, as their *evidence* for attributing a cardinal *causal* role in symptom formation to the repression of traumatic events. Let us look at the intermediate reasoning on which the founders of psychoanalysis relied to claim therapeutic support for their etiologic identification of an original act of repression as the specific pathogen initially responsible for the formation of the neurotic symptom.

Breuer and Freud extrapolated this account of the origination of the symptom backward from the dynamics they had postulated for the subsequently continuing existence of the symptom. They had been led to attribute the *maintenance* of the symptom, in turn, to a *coexisting* ongoing repression of the traumatic *memory*, which "acts like a foreign body which long after its entry must continue to be regarded as an agent that is still at work." But what is their basis for this attribution? As they explain at once: "we find the evidence for this in a highly remarkable phenomenon," which they describe as follows: "*each individual hysterical symptom immediately and permanently disappeared when we had succeeded in bringing clearly to light the memory of the event by which it was provoked and in arousing its accompanying affect* [emphasis in original]" (S.E. 1893, 2: 6).

What, then, is the evidence they give for their etiologic identification of the repressed experience of a particular traumatic event E as the pathogen—avowedly *not* as the mere precipitator!—of a given symptom S that first appeared at the time of E? Plainly and emphatically, they predicate their identification of the repression of E as the pathogen of S on the fact that the abreactive lifting of that repression issued in the durable *removal* of S. And, as their wording shows, they appreciate all too well that *without* this symptom removal, neither the mere painfulness of the event E, nor its temporal coincidence with S's first appearance, nor yet the mere fact that the hysteric patient had *repressed* the trauma *E* could justify, even together, blaming the pathogenesis of *S* on the repression of *E*. Thus, the credibility of the repression etiology is crucially dependent on the reportedly durable separate removal of various particular symptoms, a therapeutic outcome deemed supportive because it appears to have been wrought by *separately* lifting particular repressions!

This epistemic dependence of the repression etiology on the presumed cathartic dynamics of effecting positive therapeutic outcome is further accentuated by the pains that Breuer and Freud take promptly to argue that their symptom removals are the result of the lifting of repressions rather than of suggestion: "It is plausible to suppose that . . . the patient expects to be relieved of his sufferings by this procedure, and it is this expectation . . . which is the [therapeutically] operative factor. This, however, is not so. . . . The symptoms, which sprang from separate causes were separately removed" (S.E. 1893, 2: 7). Thus, the separate symptom removals are made to carry the vital probative burden of discrediting the threatening rival hypothesis of placebo effect, wrought by mere suggestion (cf. Grünbaum, 1981).

Believing to have met this challenge, Breuer and Freud at once reiterate their epoch-making repression etiology. Let us now recapitulate the essential steps of the reasoning that prompted them to postulate this etiology. First, they attributed their positive therapeutic results to the lifting of repressions. Having assumed such a *therapeutic connection*, they wished to *explain* it. Then they saw that it would indeed be explained deductively by the following etiologic hypothesis: the particular repression whose undoing removed a given symptom *S* is *causally necessary* for the initial formation *and* maintenance of *S*. Thus, the nub of their inductive argument for inferring a repression etiology can be formulated as follows: the *removal* of a hysterical symptom *S* *by means of lifting* a repression *R* is *cogent evidence* that the repression *R* was *causally necessary* for the formation of the symptom *S* (S.E. 1893, 2: 7).

Clearly, the attribution of *therapeutic* success to the undoing of repressions—rather than to mere suggestion—was the foundation, both logically and historically, for the central dynamical significance that unconscious ideation acquired in psychoanalytic theory: without reliance on the presumed dynamics of their *therapeutic* results, Breuer and Freud could never have propelled clinical data into repression etiologies.

As we saw, they had argued pointedly that the therapeutic gains made by their cathartically treated patients were *not* wrought by suggestion. Instead, they attributed these remedial results to the abreactive recall of those *repressed* traumata during which the distressing symptoms had first appeared. Since these traumata occasioned the onset of the hysterical symptoms, I shall refer to them as "occasioning" traumata. Hence, we can say that Breuer and Freud had credited the patient's improvements to the *lifting* of the particular repression by which he had sequestered the memory of the *occasioning* trauma in his unconscious. Yet, when Freud himself treated additional patients by Breuer's cathartic method, this treatment failed to achieve *lasting* therapeutic gains. Indeed, the ensuing correlation of symptom relapses and intermittent removals, on the one hand, with the vicissitudes of his personal relations to the patient, on the other, led him to *repudiate* the *decisive* therapeutic role that Breuer and he had attributed to undoing the repression of the *occasioning* trauma!

The evidence and reasoning that had driven Freud to this repudiation by 1896 are poignantly recalled by him in his 1925 "Autobiographical Study":

Even the most brilliant [therapeutic] results were liable to be suddenly wiped away if my personal relation with the patient became disturbed. It was true that they would be reestablished if a reconciliation could be effected; but such an occurrence proved that the personal emotional relation between doctor and patient was after all stronger than the whole cathartic process. [S.E. 1925, 20: 27]

Freud's therapeutic repudiation of abreactively retrieving the memory of the *occasioning* trauma also had a momentous corollary: he likewise renounced the major *etiologic* significance that he and Breuer had originally attributed to the *repression* of *this* trauma (S.E. 1896, 3: 194-195). Yet he adhered undauntedly to the research program of seeking the pathogens of neuroses among *some* repressed traumata or *other* (S.E. 1896, 3: 195-199). And, though the disappointments of cathartic treatment outcome had undercut the very basis for giving decisive remedial credit to the lifting of repressions, he unflinchingly clung to the therapeutic view that the excavation of *some* repression or *other* would remove the pathogen of the patient's affliction. But, as I shall now argue, the empirical rationale that Breuer and Freud had used for postulating a *repression* etiology *at all* was altogether undermined by just the findings that induced Freud himself to repudiate the attribution of therapeutic gain to the undoing of the repression of the occasioning trauma.

The aforementioned symptom *relapses*, which ensued after Freud had lifted the patient's repression of the occasioning trauma, showed him that the undoing of this repression failed to uproot the *cause* of the neurotic symptoms. Moreover, the fragile, ephemeral symptom remissions achieved by patients who received Breuer's cathartic treatment could hardly be credited to the lifting of this repression. By Freud's own 1925 account, giving such therapeutic credit had very soon run afoul of a stubborn fact: "The personal emotional relation between doctor and patient was after all [therapeutically] stronger than the whole cathartic process" (S.E. 1925, 20: 27). For even *after* the patient's repression of the occasioning trauma had indeed been undone cathartically, the alternation between his remissions and relapses still depended *decisively* on the ups and downs of how well he got along emotionally with his doctor.

Yet, as we saw earlier, the 1893 postulation of a repression etiology of neurosis in Breuer and Freud's foundational communication had rested *crucially* on the premise that the patient's symptom removals had actually been wrought by lifting his repression of the memory of the occasioning trauma. Thus, Freud's own abandonment of just this therapeutic premise completely negated the very reason that Breuer and he had invoked for postulating the pathogenicity of repression at all. In short, I claim that *the moral of Freud's therapeutic disappointments in the use of the cathartic method after 1893 was nothing less than the collapse of the epoch-making 1893 argument for the repression etiology of neurosis*, which Breuer and he had propounded.

Why, I ask, did Freud adamantly retain the generic repression etiology instead of allowing that this etiology itself had simply become baseless? And why, in the face of this baselessness, was he content with his mere etiologic demotion of the repressed *occasioning* trauma, while clinging to the view that the pathogen is bound to be some other earlier repressed trauma of a sexual nature, to be excavated via free associations (S.E. 1896, 3: 195-199)? Whatever his reason, he seemingly did not appreciate that the etiologic fiasco suffered by Breuer's account in the wake of the disappointingly fragile therapeutic results had made a shambles of the very cornerstone of this psychoanalytic edifice; for such an appreciation would have been tantamount to his realization that the etiology of neurosis still posed the same fundamental challenge as it had *before* Anna O. enabled Breuer to stumble upon the alleged "talking cure." Instead, Freud avowedly committed himself to a "prolonged search for the traumatic experience from which hysterical symptoms appeared to be derived" (S.E. 1923, 18: 243), just when the initially plausible traumatic etiology had been found to be baseless after all.

I have stressed the collapse of the 1893 therapeutic argument on which Breuer and Freud rested their originally hypothesized repression etiology of neurosis. Yet I need to forestall a possible misunderstanding of my methodological complaint against Freud's tenacious search for evidence that might have warranted the *rehabilitation* of the repression etiology in a *new* version. Hence, let me emphasize that I do *not* fault the pursuit of this research program per se after the demise of the cathartic method. What I do find objectionable, however, is Freud's all too ready willingness—once he was no longer collaborating with Breuer—to claim pathogenicity for purported childhood repressions on evidence *far less cogent* than the *separate* symptom removals that Breuer and he had pointedly adduced in 1893. In short, having embarked on the program of retaining the repression etiology *somehow*, Freud was prepared to draw etiologic conclusions whose credentials just did not live up to Breuer's initial 1893 standard. Even that higher original standard, I contend, was still not high enough.

Indeed, I maintain that the repression etiology of neurosis would have lacked adequate empirical credentials, even if the therapeutic gains from cathartic treatment had turned out to be both durable and splendid. For, as I shall argue further on in detail, the retrospective validation of repression as the initial pathogen lacks the sort of controls that are needed to attest *causal relevance*, and there is doubt about the reliability of purported memories elicited under the suggestive conditions of hypnosis. Incidentally, despite the replacement of hypnosis by free association in psychoanalytic treatment, Freudian therapy has retained an important tenet of its cathartic predecessor: "Recollection without affect almost invariably produces no [therapeutic] result" (S.E. 1893, 2: 6).

As we saw above, Freud's own subsequent (1917) *therapeutic* defense of his sexual version of the repression etiology by means of the Tally Argument has fared no better empirically than the original reliance on cathartic treatment success as evidence for the pathogenicity of repression. Hence, whatever his own evidential or personal motivations for retaining the repression etiology, I claim that it should now be regarded as *generically* devoid of clinical evidential support, no less than Breuer's particular version of it, which Freud repudiated as clinically unfounded. By the same token, I maintain that the demise of the therapeutic justification for the repression etiology fundamentally impugns the *investigative* utility of lifting repressions via "free" associations in the conduct of etiologic inquiry. In short, the collapse of the therapeutic argument for the repression etiology seriously undermines the purported *clinical research* value of free associations, which are given pride of place as an epistemic avenue to the presumed pathogens.

Though the repression etiology of psychoneurotic disorders was thus itself in grave jeopardy from lack of cogent clinical support, Freud extrapolated it by postulating that repressions engender "slips" (parapraxes) and dreams no less than they spawn full-blown neuroses. For example, he assimilated a slip of the tongue to the status of a mini-neurotic symptom by viewing the slip as a *compromise* between a repressed motive that crops out in the form of a disturbance, on the one hand, and the conscious intention to make a certain utterance, on the other. But as against this generalized explanatory reliance on repressed mentation, I shall argue for the following thesis: even if the original *therapeutic* defense of the repression etiology of neuroses had actually turned out to be empirically viable, Freud's compromise models of parapraxes and of manifest dream content would be *misextrapolations* of that etiology, precisely because they lacked any corresponding therapeutic base at the outset. For in 1900 Freud defended the heuristic and probative use of free association in *interpreting dreams* by pointing to its primary use in *etiologic* inquiry. And he explicitly adduced *therapeutic* results, in turn, to legitimate free association as a reliable means of identifying the pathogens etiologically. As he put it: "We might also point out in our defense that our procedure in interpreting dreams [by means of free association] is identical with the procedure by which we resolve hysterical symptoms; and there the correctness of our method is warranted by the coincident emergence and disappearance of the symptoms" (S.E. 1900, 5: 528).

PARAPRAXES AS MINI-NEUROTIC SYMPTOMS

One of Freud's paradigm cases of a slip of the tongue will now serve to exhibit the poverty of the empirical credentials of his compromise model of parapraxes. The example involves the forgetting of a pronoun in a Latin quotation.

On one of his trips, Freud became reacquainted with an academically trained young man who was familiar with some of his psychoanalytic writings. The young man, an Austrian Jew whom we shall call "AJ," conveys to Freud that he resented the social and career handicaps resulting from religious discrimination. To vent this frustration, he *tries* to quote the line from Virgil's *Aeneid* in which the despairing and abandoned Dido exclaims: *Exoriare aliquis nostris ex ossibus ultor*

("Would that someone arise from our bones as an avenger!"). But AJ's memory is defective, and he not only inverts the word order of *nostris ex* but altogether *omits* the indefinite pronoun *aliquis* ("someone"). Aware that something was missing in the line, AJ asks for help, whereupon Freud quotes the line correctly (S.E. 1901, 6: 9).

The young man then asks Freud to explain the memory lapse. Being glad to oblige, Freud then enjoins him to associate freely, whereupon AJ begins by decomposing *aliquis* into *a* and *liquis*. After a series of intermediate associations, the young man comes up with the thought of St. Januarius, the Christian martyr who became the patron saint of Naples, and brings up the purported miracle of this saint's clotted blood. Freud points out that St. Januarius and St. Augustine, whom AJ had mentioned earlier, "both have to do with the calendar." Then Freud asks: "But won't you remind me about the miracle of his blood?" After responding that this relic is kept in a vial stored in a Neapolitan church and liquefies at regular intervals, AJ pauses. Thereupon Freud says, "Well, go on. Why do you pause?" After AJ responds "Well, something *has* come into my mind... but it's too intimate to pass on. ... Besides, I don't see any connection, or any necessity for saying it [ellipsis points in original]," Freud assures him in a schoolmasterly manner, "You can leave the connection to me" (S.E. 1901, 6: 10-11).

When AJ then volunteers that his intimate sudden thought was "of a lady from whom I might easily hear a piece of news that would be very awkward for both of us," Freud asks rhetorically, "That her periods have stopped?" He explains reasonably enough that he had interpreted the young man's prior association to the miracle of St. Januarius' blood as an allusion to a woman's period.

AJ did actually have good reason to fear that his paramour was pregnant by him. The anxiety he had felt because of this ominous possibility had indeed emerged, however tortuously, from the process of association in which he had engaged. Moreover, AJ himself was well aware of these facts, yet he was prompted to query the alleged *causal bearing* of his genuine worry on his *aliquis* lapse: "And you really mean to say that it was this anxious expectation that made me unable to produce an unimportant word like *aliquis*?" With sovereign confidence, Freud retorted, "It seems to me undeniable."

Judging by Freud's account, it is unclear whether AJ had actually *repressed* his fear of pregnancy rather than merely relegated it to his own so-called preconscious by diverting his attention to other stimuli. But let us assume that this thought had been in a repressed state, at least prior to the time t_1 when AJ committed the parapraxis of forgetting *aliquis*. Soon after Freud restored this forgotten word to AJ's awareness, the young man used the restored word as the point of departure for associations, which he began to generate at time t_2. Then the anxiety-laden thought of a confirmed unwanted pregnancy emerged at time t_3. For brevity, I shall say that there was a "memory lapse" at time t_1, a "triggering restored awareness" at time t_2, and a (tortuously) ensuing "terminal emergence" of repressed anxiety content at time t_3.

As Timpanaro (1976: 51) has noted, Freud did not hesitate to intervene occasionally in the flow of AJ's associations. Hence, Timpanaro has charged that Freud thereby subtly steered the associations in a manner akin to the Socratic method of eliciting answers to leading questions.

But let us grant here, at least for argument's sake, that there is some kind of *uncontaminated causal linkage* between the restored awareness of *aliquis* at time t_2, which triggers the labyrinthine sequence of associations, on the one hand, and the emerging anxiety thought with which this sequence terminated at time t_3, on the other. Yet we must now ask the following *first question*: on what grounds does Freud, or anyone else, take *this* assumed causal linkage to be *evidence* at all for the further claim that the repressed thought harbored by AJ before t_1 was the *cause* of his memory lapse at time t_1? More explicitly, why should the ultimately ensuing elicitation of AJ's previously repressed pregnancy fear, via circuitous intermediate associations starting from the restored *aliquis*, bespeak that this very fear—while as yet being repressed—had *caused* him to forget this word, as well as to invert *nostris ex*? Why indeed should the *repressed* fear be held to have caused the *forgetting* of *aliquis* at the outset just because meandering associations starting out from the restored memory of *aliquis* issued in the conscious emergence of the fear?

It would be untutored, besides being uncharitable, to suppose that Freud did not draw on some auxiliary hypotheses to fill the prima facie glaring inferential gap to which our questions have called attention. Indeed, he *extrapolated* from his repression etiology of neuroses, much as he had already done quite explicitly when claiming to explain manifest dream content (S.E. 1900, 4: 101 and 5: 528). Thus, he postulated that the compromise-formation model of neurotic symptoms—in which *repressed* contents are deemed *causally necessary* for symptom formation—may also be legitimately extrapolated to cover parapraxes. Once these bungled actions had thus been conceptualized as mini-neurotic symptoms, Freud felt entitled to make a further assumption: if a repression emerges into consciousness via free associations triggered by the subject's awareness of his parapraxis, then the prior presence of *that* repression was the cause of the parapraxis. *Mutatis mutandis*, he had already taken both of these hypotheses to apply to manifest dream contents, as we shall see in some detail later on.

Yet I maintain that the reasoning by which Freud thought he had supported these important postulates is grievously flawed. Note first that it was Freud's correct statement of the quotation from Virgil, but *not* the undoing of AJ's repression of his pregnancy fear, which served to *remove* the mnemonic lacuna of *aliquis* in the young man's awareness. Hence, it would plainly be altogether wrongheaded to credit the lifting of the repression of AJ's fear with filling the quite *different* memory gap constituting AJ's "slip." Indeed, let us suppose that Freud had *not* filled this gap for AJ by supplying the omitted *aliquis* to him. Assume further that AJ had taken *other* words in his defectively recalled Latin line as the point of departure for his associations. Then let us even postulate *without* evidence that the *latter* associations would have eventuated in AJ's recall of the forgotten word *aliquis* only *after* the conscious emergence of his repressed fear of the pregnancy. Even then, it would be quite unclear that the posited unaided filling of AJ's memory gap can be credited causally to the lifting of his repressed fear! In any case, Freud did not adduce any evidence that the permanent lifting of a repression to which he had attributed a parapraxis will be "therapeutic" in the sense of enabling the person himself to correct the parapraxis *and* to avoid its repetition or other parapraxes in the future. While the hypothesized repression "etiology" of parapraxes thus lacked "therapeutic" support, it was precisely such prima facie impressive support that Breuer and Freud had marshaled to show that the removal of neurotic symptoms is attributable to the lifting of repressions, so that repressions are presumably pathogens. In short, there is a striking disparity in regard to the adduced evidential support between the hypothesis that parapraxes are the result of repressions, on the one hand, and that repressions are the pathogens of neurotic symptoms, on the other.

Yet once Freud's postulational abandon was no longer daunted by Breuer's known theoretical restraint, Freud unabashedly enunciated his repression theory of parapraxes. He did so despite the lack of any counterpart to the evidential support from therapeutic outcome on which Breuer and he had emphatically grounded their repression etiology of neurotic afflictions. Instead of taking pause in this patent discrepancy, in 1900 and 1901 Freud assimilated manifest dream content, and then also parapraxes, to neurotic symptoms by construing them alike as compromise formations engendered by repressions (see S.E. 1900, 4: 144). Hence, I view his theory of parapraxes and of dreams as *misextrapolations* of the generic repression etiology of neurotic symptoms, which had at least had prima facie therapeutic support.

But, as I argued earlier, this very etiology, with its compromise model of symptoms, is itself devoid of adequate clinical credentials. We saw that, by the same token, Freud failed to sustain the investigative utility of lifting repressions (via "free" associations) in the conduct of etiologic inquiry. *A fortiori*, he has given us no *cogent* reason to infer that lifting repressions is a means of fathoming the causes of parapraxes and of dreaming, for the repression "etiology" of parapraxes just turned out to be a gratuitous extrapolation from the compromise-formation model of neurotic symptoms. Thus, even bona fide repressions uncovered by means of free associations can be presumed to be causally *irrelevant* to parapraxes and dreams, at least until and unless *additional* grounds for such relevance are shown to exist in particular cases.

This presumption of causal irrelevance has recently been further strengthened by the detailed and well-supported *alternative* causal explanations of parapraxes that have been put forward by Timpanaro (1976) in his important book *The Freudian Slip*. The highly instructive *non*-Freudian psychological hypotheses employed by him were evolved by philologists to carry out textual criticism. The various "etiologic" categories of errors he employs fully allow for causation by unconscious mechanisms. But instead of having the status of Freudian *repressions*, these hypothesized mental processes qualify technically as "preconscious" in the vocabulary of psychoanalysis. Timpanaro (1976: 95) expects a deepening of his non-Freudian psychological explanations of slips from the currently developing study of the physiological mechanisms underlying memory, forgetfulness, and concentration as well as of their liability to emotional influences. Let us give a digest of the rival explanations of parapraxes proposed by Timpanaro.

One task of textual critics is to investigate the conditions that contribute to the corruption of a text in the course of its successive written transcriptions or oral transmissions, including quotations learned by heart. Furthermore, philologists are concerned to delineate the linguistic patterns of the errors that result from these tendencies to make alterations. The various "etiologic" categories of such errors that they have evolved include the following:

1. "Banalization," which is the unconscious replacement of a word or group of words by an actual or supposed synonym whose usage is *more familiar* to the copyist in the context of his or her linguistic and cultural patrimony (Timpanaro 1976: 21). This kind of error takes various forms. One of these is just the sort of syntactic and stylistic alterations that AJ effected when quoting from Virgil (chap. 3), for the construction of the original line is highly anomalous in Latin, and virtually untranslatable into the native German spoken by AJ, who was hardly a professional Latinist. Again, AJ's inversion of *nostris ex* is a banalization both with respect to Latin usage and German word order, although this transposition may have been induced by his attempt to cope with his memory gap, as Freud himself points out. The tendency to banalize may well be a matter of mental economy (p. 97). Incidentally, the word *aliquis*, which AJ omitted, is relatively superfluous, since its omission does not destroy the polemical message that AJ wished to express by means of the line, whereas the deletion of *exoriare, nostris ossibus*, or *ultor* would have done so. The tendency to omit the superfluous may well be a matter of mental economy no less than banalization.

2. Errors inspired by influences from the *context* in which they occur: unlike banalizations, they are the result of assimilations to preceding or subsequent words belonging to the same phrase, rather than to the subject's linguistic patrimony (p. 97). Thus, a speaker or writer who is preoccupied with what he is *about* to say or write can readily distort a given word or phrase under the influence of his anticipation of a succeeding one. Furthermore, other preoccupations or loss of interest may tax our finite mnemonic capacity and issue in forgetting or omissions.

3. The common substitution of words of an equal number of syllables that also have a strong phonetic similarity, such as rhyming, and that refer to conceptually alike items (chap. 6). The case of Freud's trying to remember the name of the Renaissance painter Signorelli and thinking instead of Botticelli (S.E. 1901, 6: 2), who is another such painter, falls into this category. Freud had no sooner thought of Botticelli when he rejected it as incorrect and then thought of the name of the lesser painter Boltraffo, which he also knew at once to be wrong. As Timpanaro explains (pp. 70-71), in the catalog of errors familiar from textual criticism, the second error is no less recognized than the first. In the philological perspective, the second error—unlike the first—is *not* a memory slip. Instead, it is an unsuccessful attempt to correct the first error: having failed to pinpoint his initial substitution of "Bottic" for "Signor" in "Signorelli," Freud had mistakenly retained the syllable "Bo" from that initial substitution, but he then compounded or "disimproved" his error by dropping the authentic "elli," thereby coming up with nothing better than "Boltraffo." German textual critics call such disimprovements *Schlimmbesserung*, and French philologists refer to them as *fautes critiques*.

4. "Polar errors," consisting in the substitution of words having an opposite significance. Freud attributed such errors to the id's getting even with the mendacious ego (S.E. 1916, 15: lecture 3). But non-Freudians, such as the linguist Rudolf Meringer, whom Freud cites (e.g., S.E. 1901, 6: chap. 5), have held (Timpanaro 1976: 147-150, 151-153) that conceptual complementarity—such as between the words "omitted" and "inserted"—of itself can be the source of erroneous word substitutions.

5. Haplography and haplology: the coalescing of double letters or sounds in writing or speaking, respectively. Repeated instances of haplography in typesetting by the same printer may betoken a personal penchant to commit such errors (Timpanaro 1976: 136-137, 141).

6. Omissions effected when the glance of a copyist jumps from one group of letters, typically at the beginning or end of a word, to a similar group of letters in an adjacent or nearby word, as in mistranscribing the Italian word *teleologico* to become *teologico*. This sort of error is known as *saut du même au même* (p. 36).

7. Dipthography, the common, seemingly mechanical mistake of improperly *repeating* parts of words, whole words, or entire sequences of words (pp. 143-145). For example, a writer's thoughts and his putting them on paper do not always remain coordinated, so that he may mistakenly write down something that he has already written; copyists or printers may look back to a point in the text that is further back than the one at which they left off.

In largely much more sketchy form, "etiologic" categories of this sort were used by some psycholinguists and physiologists during Freud's time to give nonpsychoanalytic explanations of "slips." But, as Timpanaro stresses, textual critics are much more alert than these students of errors to the complex joint operation of a variety of such "etiologic" factors in the production of a particular slip. The "textual critic... demands an effort to understand how various general tendencies contribute on any given occasion to the production of a single and particular error" (p. 84). Yet Timpanaro (1976: 98-99) acknowledges that, at least in the current state of knowledge, such explanations are stochastic or, at any rate, yield only statistical predictions.

Thus, it is quite impossible to predict that, for example, a given text will be corrupted by a given error at a given point in a given copy. But the situation is very different at the statistical level. While I can in no way commit myself to the prediction that the word *cultuale* will be banalized to *culturale* by a particular typist or printer, I am able to predict that in all probability if the passage is given to a hundred typists or printers to reproduce, the majority of them will fall into the error. The same can be said of the banalization of *teleologico* ["*teleological*"] to *teologico* ["*theological*"]. Here the *saut de même au même* operates as an additional cause in conjunction with the tendency towards banalization, while the latter is further assisted by the fact that the two adjectives, though their meanings are significantly different, are often appropriate enough to the same context: belief in a finalism of nature is obviously related to a conception which can loosely be termed religious or "theological."

Additional non-Freudian psycholinguistic explanations for errors in linguistic performance are offered in Fromkin (1980).

Freud discusses some of the nonpsychoanalytic approaches to an understanding of slips made by his own contemporaries, but he belittles the causal factors singled out by them as merely generic and shallow (S.E. 1901, 6: 21-22, 80-81). Indeed, he indicts them for being satisfied with accepting factors that merely *favor* the commission of a parapraxis in lieu of causally necessary or sufficient conditions (S.E. 1916, 15: 45-46, 61). Scornful of the stochastic causation inherent in mere tendencies, he declares:

Such psycho-physiological factors as excitement, absentmindedness and disturbances of attention will clearly help us very little towards an explanation. They are only empty phrases, screens behind which we must not let ourselves be prevented from having a look. The question is rather what it is that has been brought about here by the excitement, the particular distracting of attention. And again, we must recognize the importance of the influence of sounds, the similarity of words and the familiar associations aroused by words. These facilitate slips of the tongue by pointing to the paths they can take. But if I have a path open to me, does that factor automatically decide that I shall take it? I need a motive in addition before I resolve in favour of it and furthermore a force to propel me along the path. So these relations of sounds and words are also, like the somatic dispositions, only things that *favour* slips of the tongue and cannot provide the true explanation of them. [S.E. 1916, 15: 46]

Prompted by this, I say: whatever the incompleteness or other defects of the more recent nonpsychoanalytic explanations of slips offered by Timpanaro or by psycholinguists, their deficits are not remedied at all by the psychoanalytic explanations. Thus, these deficits do not redound to the credibility of Freud's thesis, that all parapraxes are the result of repressions. For, to take Freud's earlier example, let it be granted that AJ's chain of associations from his corrected parapraxis issued causally in the disclosure of the repressed anxiety afflicting him, *and* that this unconscious fear of pregnancy had been clamoring for overt expression. How, then, does this assumed motive serve to explain even probabilistically why AJ committed any parapraxis at all, let alone why he forgot *aliquis*? *A fortiori*, how does Freud's claim that AJ's unconscious anxiety is the "*sense*" or *intention* behind his slip (S.E. 1916, 15: 40) even match, let alone excel, Timpanaro's explanation, which invoked the tendencies to effect mental economies by syntactic

and stylistic banalization coupled with the elimination of the superfluous? Yet Freud downgrades psycholinguistic explanations generically.
He remarks that, after such explanations were offered, "on the
whole... we were further than ever from understanding slips of the
tongue" (S.E. 1916, 15: 34), and he claims that the purported motives of
parapraxes are "more interesting than... the circumstances in which
they come about" (S.E. 1916, 15: 40). Furthermore, he maintains that,
unlike psychophysiological accounts, his motivational elucidations
address the question of "why it is that the slip occurred in this particular way and no other" (S.E. 1916, 15: 32; see also p. 36).

More fundamentally, suppose that Freud did use AJ's repressed
anxiety to give a hypothetico-deductive explanation of his slip. Then
the *causal nexus* between the repression and the slip asserted in its
explanans would have been *epistemically unacceptable*. For, as I have
argued above and also indicated elsewhere (Grünbaum 1980: 377-378),
Freud has offered nothing better than *post hoc ergo propter hoc* toward
the evidential support needed for *that* causal nexus, even if we grant
him that the sequence of AJ's associations was an uncontaminated
causal chain.

The *aliquis* example is representative of other cases in which Freud
fallaciously trades on the genuineness of a fear (or wish) with which
the subject is preoccupied, and on its elicitation by associations initiated by a given parapraxis, to gain plausibility for the causal attribution
of that parapraxis to the elicited fear (or wish). Even the unique
elicitation capacity presumed for these particular associations can be
spurious. As Timpanaro (1976: 143) has rightly stressed, genuine
preoccupations or obsessions tend to be evoked by a great *many*
stimuli, even or especially when they are devoid of any foundation.
Unmindful of these pitfalls, Freud compounds the logical defect of the
aliquis case by reporting Jung's brief analysis of a corpulent German
male who was not a student of German literature and omitted the
words *mit weisser Decke* ("with a white sheet") when reciting a well-
known poem by Heine. The man told Jung that the white sheet made
him think of a shroud, and thereby of an acquaintance who had
recently succumbed to a heart attack, which in turn evoked his fear that
he himself might meet the same fate. Here again, there is not the
slightest reason to attribute the parapraxis to the evoked fear (of
death), even if the anxiety was unconscious in Freud's dynamical
sense. In a similar vein, Timpanaro (1976: 90) has aptly remarked: "Nor
is it enough, in order to substantiate an avowed determinism, to assert
that every 'slip' has a cause and thereupon present extravagant causal
connexions as certain."

The psychoanalytic theory of slips, which offers explanations based on repressions unearthed via free associations, ought *not* to be allowed to benefit from such credibility as is possessed by other explanations having only a spurious similarity to them. One species of such different explanations features mental states of which the subject who committed the slip was clearly *conscious*. Another species features mental states that, though not at the *focus* of the subject's consciousness, were readily available to his conscious awareness. These states were "preconscious" in Freud's parlance, as opposed to being repressed (*dynamically* unconscious). Being the adroit pedagogue and even deft expository promoter that he was, Freud exemplifies both of these sorts of slips by way of *didactic prolegomena* (e.g., in S.E. 1916, 15: 64-65). But neither of these two species can be credited to psychoanalytic theory because, as Timpanaro (1976: 122) put it concisely:

The truly Freudian "slip" or instance of forgetting presupposes the existence of psychic material which my conscious ego has repressed because it proved *displeasing* — or, given it was desirable from a hedonistic point of view, because my moral inhibitions prevented my confession of it even to myself, let alone to others.

Thus, suppose that in the course of giving a lecture on human sexuality, a person misspeaks himself by saying "orgasm" instead of "organism." It is *not* a bona fide "Freudian" explanation to remark that conceptual preoccupation with the overall topic of the lecture combined with phonetic similarity to generate the slip. By the same token, Freudians should not trade on cases in which a slip may be plausibly held to bespeak the presence of a *conscious* thought that the subject wishes to conceal; nor on instances of slips in which there is little evidence for the prior repression of a thought that a speaker tried unsuccessfully to hide. An example of this, which I owe to Rosemarie Sand, would be the man who turns from the exciting view of a lady's exposed bosom muttering, "Excuse me, I have got to get a *breast* of *flesh* air!"

Since these embarrassing losses of control appear to have psychological causes, they do call for corresponding psychological explanations. Hence, they indeed militate *against* the view, which Freud decried as widely avowed, "that a mistake in speaking is a *lapsus linguae* and of no psychological significance" (S.E. 1901, 6: 94). To the contrary, these cases of misspeaking do qualify as "serious mental acts; they have a sense [motive]" (S.E. 1916, 15: 44). Furthermore, as Benjamin Rubinstein has pointed out illuminatingly, these sorts of "slips" — though *not* bespeaking repressions — share two significant features of the genuinely "Freudian" ones: (1) they exhibit intrusions upon the agent's control of his own behavior, and (2) the intruding element is a wish or an affect. But despite being psychologically revealing, such cases are not supportive of the psychoanalytic theory of parapraxes, in which repression is held to play the cardinal explanatory role. For, in the concluding chapter of his magnum opus on slips, one of the three necessary conditions layed down explicitly by Freud for inclusion of a given slip in the purview of his theory is as follows: "If we perceive the parapraxis at all, we must not be aware in ourselves of any motive for it. We must rather be tempted to explain it by 'inattentiveness,' or to put it down to 'chance'" (S.E. 1901, 6: 239). Indeed, the avowed contribution of Freud's theory to our understanding of various sorts of "slips" is to explain those species "in which the parapraxis produces nothing that has any sense of its own" for either the subject who commits the slip or for others (S.E. 1916, 15: 41). Thus, when Freud lists parapraxes *violating* his requirement that they be devoid of a sense of their own, these violations furnish mere didactic prolegomena: they serve the explicitly stated "limited aim of using the study of these phenomena as a help towards a preparation for psychoanalysis" (S.E. 1916, 15: 55).

Freud's illustrations of such propaedeutic cases include instances of nonsensical misspoken words such that the speaker who uttered them knows at once, when asked, "what he had really meant to say" (S.E. 1916, 15: 42; see also p. 47). In fact, "the disturbing purpose is known to the speaker and moreover had been noticed by him before he made the slip of the tongue" (S.E. 1916, 15: 64). More generally, as Freud explains, "we shall find whole categories of cases in which the intention, the sense, of the slip is plainly visible" (S.E. 1916, 15: 40). In such instances "the parapraxis itself brings its sense to light" so as to be perspicuous to the subject no less than to others (S.E. 1916, 15: 41; see also p. 47). Emphasizing the propaedeutic role of all such perspicuous cases, Freud declares: "My choice of these examples has not been unintentional, for their origin and solution [motivational explanation] come neither from me nor from any of my followers" (S.E. 1916, 15: 47).

One such example features a German-speaking anatomy professor who misspoke in a lecture as follows: "In the case of the female genitals, in spite of many *Versuchungen* ["temptations"] — I beg your pardon, *Versuche* ["experiments"]..." (S.E. 1901, 6: 78-79; 1916, 15: 33). When the anatomist himself thus corrected his slip, he patently required no lifting of a repression to disclose to him that *erotic interest* was a possible contributing motive for his use of a sex-oriented term instead of the phonetically similar neutral term he had expected to utter. Yet in an article entitled "On the Freudian Theory of Speech," the psycholinguist A. W. Ellis (1980: 124) overlooks the propaedeutic role of the anatomist's slip and of all the other motivationally perspicuous illustrations given by Freud. Drawing an exegetically incorrect conclusion from these transparent examples, Ellis asserts: "It is not necessary that the speaker should be unaware of the activity of the disturbing purpose [motive] within him before it reveals itself in the slip." But, qua characterization of the scope of the *psychoanalytic* theory of slips, this formulation contravenes Freud's aforecited restriction as to the purview of this theory, for he demanded that the speaker *not* be aware of any motive for his slip (S.E. 1901, 6: 239, condition C). Hence, the inferred perturbing intention had to be sequestered in the speaker's unconscious. Having overlooked Freud's restriction, Ellis violates it anew when he proceeds to give purported illustrations of "Freud's mode of explanation" (1980: 124). Thus, his *prime* example is the anatomist's perspicuous temptation slip rather than one "in which the parapraxis produces nothing that has any sense of its own" (S.E. 1916, 15: 41).

Yet Ellis does inquire as to whether "depth-analytic explanations are needed in addition to the mechanical-psycholinguistic explanations proposed more recently" (1980: 123). His domain of inquiry consists of fifty-one word-substitution slips, which he selected from Freud's 1901 index of speech lapses. The closest he comes to considering whether *repressed* ideation might generate slips is in his remarks on word-blend errors, which result from the blending of two words (1980: section 5). Ellis notes that the speaker can attest introspectively to the prearticulatory presence of thoughts that he wished to conceal, and Ellis allows that the word the speaker intended to utter blended with a lingering phonemic trace of the disturbing thoughts, thereby betraying their presence. But, as he hastens to point out, "those thoughts could not have been truly unconscious prior to manifesting themselves in the slip" (1980: 129). Indeed, since he took a word-blend example in which the subject's unaided introspection did disclose a prearticulatory disturbing motive, it was evident from the start that this motive did not qualify as repressed.

Unfortunately, Ellis does not reveal whether *any* of the fifty-one word-substitution slips examined by him were of the *opaque* sort required by Freud's restriction. But unless this requirement is demonstrably met, it is at best unclear whether Freud's repression theory of parapraxes is damaged by Ellis's findings. Yet Ellis claims such damage in virtue of the feasibility of giving psycholinguistic explanations of a *non*motivational kind for the fifty-one substitution slips he had selected. Thus, he notes that the erroneously substituted words are either phonetically similar to the target words, semantically closely related to them, or perseverations from prior utterances in the given lexical context.

Even psychoanalysts have rightly complained that the theoretically sympathetic experimental psychologist Saul Rosenzweig simply failed to test Freud's 1915 conception of repression when Rosenzweig claimed to have found experimental support for it in 1934 (see the first section of this article). Alas, the same type of complaint is appropriate to M. T. Motley's (1980) interpretation of his ingenious laboratory investigations. He did furnish telling experimental evidence for the *causal relevance* of cognitive-affective mental sets, and even of personality dispositions, to the production of verbal misreadings. These influences acted via prearticulatory semantic editing of the words to be read. Thus, semantic influences external to the speaker's intended utterance effected verbal slips that were "closer in meaning to those semantic influences than to the originally intended utterance" (Motley 1980: 145). The pertinent misreadings were phoneme-switching errors of the sort known as "spoonerisms" (Fromkin 1980: 11; Motley 1980: 134).

But, like Ellis, Motley misconstrues the probative relevance of his otherwise valuable findings to Freud's psychoanalytic theory of slips. In Motley's case, the crucial question is whether the cognitive-affective mental sets and/or personality dispositions he manipulated as the independent variable in his experiments qualify as *repressed*, rather than as focally conscious or preconscious. I shall argue that, in all three of his experiments, the answer is plainly negative. The semantic prearticulatory editing manifested in these experiments occurs at three corresponding levels as follows: consonance with the immediate verbal context in experiment 1, with the speaker's sociosituational context in experiment 2, and with one of the speaker's specified personality traits in experiment 3. Motley (1980: 136) views these three experiments sequentially as *ascendingly* qualified to serve as bona fide tests of Freud's own theory of parapraxes. By contrast, I claim that none of them reaches even the threshold of being a test of psychoanalytic theory, as distinct from a rival theory that *denies* the causal relevance of repressed ideation. For Motley's findings could *all* be explained by the sort of rival psychological theory that countenances *only conscious* motivational influences as generators of slips. To substantiate my claim that Motley's results are probatively irrelevant in the stated sense, let me comment briefly on the pertinent salient features of his three experiments in turn.

1. Motley himself describes experiment 1 as only a partial realization of Freud's initial conditions (1980: 138-139), but he nonetheless invokes it as generic support for psychoanalytic theory. And his grounds for this tribute are that, in Freud's account, the adduced motives operate in the production of slips via prearticulatory editing of a kind that is *generically* semantic rather than just phonological (p. 136). But note that the semantic interfering stimuli in this experiment are word pairs, each of which is presented tachistoscopically for one second. Such exposure is long enough for conscious, not to mention preconscious, cognitive registration. Furthermore, Motley gives no evidence at all for the prearticulatory *repression* of these interfering semantic stimuli.

True enough, his experiment 1 does attest that semantic influences from the immediate verbal context of a slip are causally relevant to the commission of the slip. But, as we just observed, in this experiment these influences are preconscious, if not outright focally conscious. Hence, I deem the causal relevance demonstrated in Motley's first experiment to be probatively unavailing as distinctive support for the psychoanalytic theory of slips, in the sense of being support for those of its consequences that are *not* likewise consequences of *any* rival theories eschewing repressed motives. For brevity, I shall speak of such distinctive support as support for psychoanalytic theory *"as such."*

2. Motley regards experiment 2 as "virtually a direct test of Freud's theory" (p. 139). Yet in this second experiment no less than in the first, the cognitive-affective situational sets Motley manipulated in the treatment groups can hardly be claimed to have been repressed by the subjects. In one group, the situational mental set was a conscious anticipation of experiencing an electric shock on the part of subjects who had been told explicitly to be prepared for it, and who were *ostensibly* connected to electrodes (p. 139). In another group, there was no electrical set, but the male subjects were pointedly stimulated sexually by "a female confederate experimenter who was by design attractive, personable, very provocatively attired, and seductive in behavior" (p. 140). The ensuing arousal was all too present in the subjects' conscious awareness. (There was a third "neutral set" control group.)

True enough, "Experiment 2 demonstrates that subjects' speech encoding systems were sensitive to semantic influence from their situational cognitive set [electric or sex stimulation]" (p. 141). And, as in Freud's theory, that influence originated *outside* the total semantic context of the intended utterance. All the same, since the influence was not repressed, the results of experiment 2, no less than those of experiment 1, are seen to be probatively unavailing as support for psychoanalysis as such. Hence, there is no foundation for Motley's conclusion that "Experiment 2 provides strong support for Freud's view of verbal slips" (p. 141).

3. Motley sees experiment 3 as the best of his three purported tests of Freudian theory. Male heterosexual anxiety was manipulated as the independent variable, and the experiment did succeed in exhibiting the influence of the subject's personality on his verbal slips. But, qua support for Freud, that demonstration is futile, unless the relevant personality disposition bespeaks the operation of repressed ideation. Motley gives us every reason to claim that it does not.

As Motley explains, the personality trait of sex anxiety "was operationalized as Mosher Sex-Guilt Inventory scores" (p. 142). Using these scores, Motley selected three treatment groups of high, medium, and low sex anxiety. But Mosher used a sentence-completion questionnaire filled out by the subjects *themselves* to develop scales for sex guilt, hostility guilt, and morality guilt. Thus, if the subjects who rate high, medium, and low on the sex-guilt scale are to furnish responses probatively relevant to the repression theory of parapraxes, these ratings would need somehow to betoken degrees of (sexual) repression, perhaps inversely or directly.

Yet I submit that the true-false and forced-choice answers given by the subjects on the questionnaire fail as a gauge of (sexual) repression. Plainly one reason for this failure is that a person with guilt feelings that qualify psychoanalytically as repressed will not consciously know of or admit the presence of such feelings when simply asked. Indeed, he or she will even deny such feelings in good faith, sometimes vehemently! Motley seems to have overlooked that insofar as the Mosher scores can be held to measure "psychodynamic conflict," what they measure is *conscious* conflict, *not* psychoanalytically pertinent conflict. It is as if one had devised a questionnaire to measure the *conscious* "income-tax conflict" experienced by a person torn between the conscious temptation to cheat on his tax return and the equally conscious fear of legal prosecution for having done so. By contrast, Freudian psychodynamic conflict is a clash between a repressed thought clamoring for conscious recognition, on the one hand, and the ego or superego, which denies that thought entry into awareness, on the other. When depicting Mosher sex-guilt scores as measures of "psychodynamic conflict," Motley (1980: 144) unfortunately pays no heed to the crucially pertinent difference between the conscious and the Freudian sorts of conflict: he gives no reason at all to suppose that the subjects who scored high, medium, and low on Mosher's sex-guilt

scale had repressed the sexual impulse aroused in them by the provoc-
ative, voluptuous female experimenter. Hence, by using the Mosher-
scale ratings as a gauge of personality disposition, Motley forfeited the
probative relevance of his otherwise valuable findings for the repression theory of slips.

Motley did find (1980: 142) that high Mosher-guilt subjects committed more sex-error spoonerisms than medium-guilt ones, whose
errors, in turn, exceeded those of the low-guilt subjects. And, as he
rightly maintains (p. 143), he has thereby shown that—within the
given situational cognitive set of sex arousal—personality disposition
can issue in verbal slips via semantic prearticulatory editing. Thus,
Motley's results emerge as quantitatively modulated instances of the
same motivational genre as the speech error of the consciously aroused
man who declared that he wanted "to get a *breast* of *flesh* air." By the
same token, Motley's findings are just as probatively unavailing for
buttressing the psychoanalytic theory of parapraxes as this "breast-
flesh" slip. Indeed, despite claiming support for Freudian theory from
the outcome of experiment 3, Motley issues the following concluding
disclaimer, among others: "Whereas Freud would claim that ALL
verbal slips are semantic manifestations of a speaker's private cognitive-affective state, the present study makes no such claim (and this
writer would expect such manifestations to be rare)" (p. 145). As I have
argued, the design of Motley's three experiments lends substance to
the complaint that experimental psychologists tend to overlook the
initial conditions required by a genuine test of Freud's theory. Yet, in
addition to yielding otherwise interesting results, these imaginative
designs seem to point the way to devising genuine tests.

The restricted purview that Freud enunciated for the *psychoanalytic*
contribution to the motivational elucidation of parapraxes has often
been overlooked, especially because Freud genuinely psychoanalyzes
only some parapraxes, as in the *aliquis* case, but essentially merely
reports others and largely lets them speak for themselves, as it were. In
this way, the reader is tempted to conclude incorrectly that if these
others are of the plausible sort that I have exemplified, then they
automatically bespeak support for Freud's theory. Thus, Freud (S.E.
1901, 6: 95) relates how a speaker in the German parliament asked for a
demonstration of "unreserved" (*rückhaltlos*) loyalty to the Kaiser, but
betrayed the hypocrisy of his subservience by saying "spineless"
(*rückgratlos*) instead. Another case of self-betrayal of a *conscious*
thought, which was reported to Freud by Theodor Reik, is that of a
young girl who did not intend to reveal to her parents her antipathy
toward the young man whom they wished her to marry. But when

asked by her mother how she felt about him, she described him by coining the neologism *sehr liebens*widrig ("very love-repelling"), though she had meant to be insincere and say *sehr liebens*würdig ("very worthy of love") (S.E. 1901, 6: 91). As Timpanaro (1976: 151-153, 144-145, 178-179) has shown illuminatingly, Freud describes other episodes in which a slip *might* be the result of the cunning of a repression but assumes *tout court* that it definitely *must* be, especially if the interpretation depicts individual motivations as misanthropic. Hence, Timpanaro (pp. 126-127) concludes that "all the really persuasive examples" in Freud's writings are what, *faute de mieux*, he calls "gaffes":

"Slips" of this kind certainly presuppose that something has been suppressed, but the speaker is fully conscious of, and currently preoccupied with, whatever it is that he wants to conceal from those to whom he is speaking. It is not something which has genuinely been "repressed" (forgotten) and re-emerges from the depths of his unconscious. [p. 127]

As Timpanaro remarks perceptively (p. 105), Freud's explanations increasingly forfeit cogency to the extent that the slips to which they pertain differ from the "gaffe" type, and are alleged to have a more recondite, unconscious genesis. Indeed, he points out (p. 104) that, as Freud fully appreciated, nonpsychoanalytic accounts of gaffes have long been clichés in the folklore of commonsense psychology. For instance, such expressions as "he gave himself away" betoken the recognition that, lacking complete control of what we do say, we sometimes fail to conceal from others what is not meant for them and we would even prefer not to know ourselves, although we *are* conscious of it. The vexation that often accompanies the slip may well be the result of the unexpected realization of just this incomplete control, rather than of the unconscious appreciation of the tainted origin of the slip, as claimed by Freud (Timpanaro 1976: 157n).

But the important conclusion is this: *if there are any slips that are actually caused by genuine repressions, Freud did not give us any good reason to think that his clinical methods can identify and certify their causes as such*, no matter how interesting the elicited "free" associations might otherwise be. As is apparent from my arguments, this adverse upshot seems indefeasible even if one were to grant that the analyst does not influence the subject's "free" associations. Besides, such an absence of influence would be utopian, as I shall argue shortly.

The psychoanalytic explanations of other species of parapraxes by means of repressed motivations are just as tenuously founded as in the cases we have discussed. For example, the same unfavorable verdict applies to Freud's account of *misreadings*. For, as he explains:

If we want to discover the disturbing purpose which produced the misreading, we must leave the text that has been misread entirely aside and we may begin the analytic investigation with the two questions: what is the first association to the product of the misreading? and in what situation did the misreading occur? [S.E. 1916, 15: 70]

And, as he explains further:

What we ought to read is something unwished-for, and analysis will convince us that an intense wish to reject what we have read must be held responsible for its alteration. [p. 71]

I do not deny that "an intense wish to reject what we have read" *may* be "responsible for its alteration"; but I do deny that Freud's reliance on the method of free association furnished a sound reason even for making this causal attribution, let alone for concluding—as he did— that the wish to reject "must" be held responsible. Hence, I claim that his method for identifying and certifying the purported motive ought *not* to "convince us," as he thinks. Yet I *allow*, of course, that genuinely probative methods of causal inquiry may turn out to vindicate, at least in some cases, Freud's imputations of unconscious motivations for the commission of parapraxes.

Can any of the above array of doubts as to the *repression* genesis of a slip be validly gainsaid by claiming, as Freud did, that the alleged cause of the slip is established to *be* its cause by the *introspective* confirmation of the subject who committed it? As he put it: "You shall grant me that there can no doubt of a parapraxis having sense if the subject himself admits it" (S.E. 1916, 15: 50). Thus, when an examinee attributed his own penchant to forget Gassendi's name to a guilty conscience, Freud took it for granted that this "very subtle motivation" had to be responsible, because it was one "which the subject of it has explained himself" (S.E. 1901, 6: 27). And he reports parapraxes by Storfer, himself, and Andréas Salomé, claiming that self-observation was able to certify the actual repressed cause of the bungled action in each case (S.E. 1901, 6: 118, 163, 168; cf. Timpanaro 1976: 146, for a rival account of Storfer's slip by reference to linguistic banalization, as well as phonic and conceptual similarity). But it is probatively unavailing that AJ can confirm having put his genuine anxiety about the Neapolitan woman's pregnancy out of his mind—if indeed he had—at least temporarily, when he discussed his resentment of religious discrimination with Freud just before quoting Virgil. It is similarly unhelpful that Jung's corpulent German interlocutor can attest to the authenticity of his cardiac fear, whether repressed earlier or not. For such confirmation is patently a far cry from certifying the alleged *causal nexus* between the given fear and the slip. Even if the person who "slipped" were not under the suggestive, intimidating influence of the analyst, how could the subject possibly know any better than any of the rest of us that the pertinent unconscious fear had actually caused his slip?

On the face of it, it would seem that the privileged epistemic access that introspection afforded these subjects to the existence of their anxieties hardly extends to the certification of the wholly unvalidated causal nexus. More significantly, this indictment of Freud's appeal to introspective confirmation is well supported, for substantial evidence recently marshaled by cognitive psychologists tells against a subject's privileged epistemic access to the identification of the causes of his own behavior (Grünbaum 1980: 354-367). I had prior occasion to adduce this evidence against Robert Waelder's accolade to introspection in psychoanalytic validation. True, near the very end of his career, Freud held that a subject's assent to a psychoanalytic interpretation does not guarantee its correctness. And, as will become clear in a later section, he thereby implied some weakening of his 1916 probative tribute to the subject's introspective confirmation of the alleged "sense" of a slip. But, in any case, there is every reason to conclude that this confirmation is spurious and hence cannot gainsay the array of objections that I have leveled against the psychoanalytic theory of slips.

So far, we have been granting, merely for the sake of argument, that the analyst does not significantly influence the patient's "free" associations. Furthermore, we took it for granted that the thought content in which the associative process issued was actually one that the subject had previously consciously entertained or registered but had subsequently repressed. But, as we saw, even if these associations actually were causally uncontaminated, it would still be unavailing to Freud. For even such undistorted associations *cannot* certify that the repressions brought to light by means of them qualify as any of the following: (1) the pathogens of the patient's neurosis, (2) the motive forces of his dream constructions, or (3) the causes of his slips.

But it now behooves us to address a *second* question: does the patient's adherence to the fundamental rule of free association indeed safeguard the *causally uncontaminated* emergence of actually existing repressed wishes, anger, guilt, fear, etc.? Or is the process of association contaminated by the analyst's injection of influence of one sort or another? Clearly, the answer will depend, at least partly, on just what the analyst does while the patient is busy fulfilling his share of the analytic compact. This answer is also likely to depend on the antecedent beliefs that patients going into analysis bring into the analytic situation, for many an intelligent analysand is consciously aware of the sort of material that his Freudian therapist does expect from his free associations. For example, male patients are expected to have repressed castration anxiety, and females are to have unconscious penis envy. While dealing with our question, we shall need to be mindful of another, since it likewise pertains to the epistemic effects of the analyst's *intervention*: if a plethora of unconscious thoughts surface, by what criteria does the analyst decide when to call a halt to the surfeit of associations, while investigating parapraxes and dreams? Hence, let us canvass in what respects overt and subtle interventions by the analyst affect the data yielded by the patient's associations.

The limitations of the analytic hour alone require that the patient's associations not be allowed to continue *indefinitely*. But suppose that one were to disregard the epistemically irrelevant expedient of this hour and allow the patient to continue unimpeded, even if he pauses off and on. If the intelligent and imaginative analysand is permitted to associate in this way long enough, his unfettered ruminations will, in due course, presumably yield almost any kind of thematic content of which he had at least recently not been conscious: thoughts about death, God, and indeed cabbages and kings. But, if so, how does the analyst avoid an antecedently question-begging *selection* bias in the face of this *thematic elasticity* of the associations, while unavoidably limiting their duration? Thus, if the associations do flow apace and the analyst somehow interrupts them at a certain point, he is interfering in their spontaneous causal dynamics. By what criterion does he do so? But in the case of, say, a parapraxis or a given element of manifest dream content, when the associations are faltering and the analyst demands their continuation, how does he manage *not* to load the dice by ever so subtly hinting to the patient what kind of material he expects to emerge? After all, his demand for continuation will convey his suspicion that it was censorial resistance to a related repressed content that brought the flow of associations to a halt *at that particular point*, and his attempt at overcoming that resistance may well convey his expectation.

Let me illustrate the problem of selection bias resulting from thematic elasticity. Suppose that Freud had allowed AJ to continue well past the disclosure of the pregnancy fear. Perhaps it would then have emerged that AJ's parents had taught him early that the Romans had crucified Jesus, but that Christians had then unfairly blamed the Jews for deicide. It might furthermore have emerged that AJ had repressed his ensuing hatred of the Romans when Virgil, Horace, and other Roman poets were shown great respect in his Austrian educational environment. Now let us recall Freud's criterion of "suitability as a determinant," which he invoked in the study of hysteria to give *etiologic* primacy to an earlier repression over a later one, even though the *memory* of the earlier one emerged later in the chain of the patient's associations (S.E. 1896, 3: 193-196) than the memory of the subsequent one. Would AJ's hypothesized repression of his hatred for the Romans not have had greater thematic "suitability as a determinant" of his *aliquis* slip than his anxiety about the pregnancy, even though the former assumedly emerged only later in his associative chain? After all, Virgil was a Roman, and AJ was citing the line from the *Aeneid* to express his conscious resentment of Christian anti-Semitism. What a golden opportunity to punish the unconsciously resented Romans simultaneously by spoiling Virgil's line! Although the repressed hatred for the Romans is, of course, purely hypothetical in the case of AJ, it does lend poignancy to the complaint of selection bias, which is given substance generally by the thematic elasticity of the associations I have emphasized.

Thus, as I indicated only briefly elsewhere à propos of parapraxes (Grünbaum 1980: 377-378), the clinical use of free association features epistemic biases of selection and manipulative contamination as follows: (1) the analyst *selects thematically* from the patient's productions by means of interrupting the associations — either explicitly or in a myriad more subtle ways — at points of his or her own theoretically inspired choosing; and (2) when the Freudian doctor harbors the suspicion that the associations are faltering because of evasive censorship, he uses verbal and also subtle nonverbal promptings to induce the continuation of the associations *until* they yield *theoretically* appropriate results; for surely not any and every previously repressed thought that emerges will be deemed a *relevant* repression for the purpose of etiologic inquiry, dream interpretation, or the analysis of a slip.

Experimental studies by L. Krasner, G. Mandler, W. K. Kaplan, and K. Salzinger, which are summarized by the analyst Marmor (1970), do bear out empirically the actual contamination of the products of free association by the analyst. As will be recalled, Freud had credited free association by saying: "it [free association] guarantees to a great extent that... nothing will be introduced into it by the expectations of the analyst" (S.E. 1925, 20: 41). Commenting on precisely this statement of Freud's, Marmor (1970: 161) writes: "Clinical experience has demonstrated that this simply is not so and that the 'free' associations of the patient are strongly influenced by the values and expectations of the therapist" (reprinted in Marmor 1974: 267). He then cites an earlier article of his (1962: 291-292), where he had written:

In face-to-face transactions the expression on the therapist's face, a questioning glance, a lift of the eyebrows, a barely perceptible shake of the head or shrug of the shoulder all act as significant cues to the patient. But even *behind* the couch, our "uh-huhs" as well as our silences, the interest or the disinterest reflected in our tone of voice or our shifting postures all act like subtle radio signals influencing the patients' responses, reinforcing some responses and discouraging others. That this influence actually occurs has been confirmed experimentally by numerous observers [reference omitted]. Krasner [reference omitted] has recently prepared a comprehensive and impressive review of the evidence in this area.

Indeed, recalling a finding from that earlier article, Marmor (1970: 161) concludes:

As a result, depending on the point of view of the psychoanalyst, patients of every psychoanalytic school tend, *under free association*, "to bring up precisely the kind of phenomenological data which confirm the theories and interpretations of their analysts! Thus each theory tends to be self-validating."

This report derives added poignancy from the studies marshaled by A. K. Shapiro and L. A. Morris (1978: 384) as support for claiming that therapists may subtly and unwittingly "communicate information to patients, such as hypotheses, expectations, attitudes, cultural values, and so on." They emphasize how this state of affairs issues in the *spurious* clinical confirmation of psychological hypotheses via the effects of suggestion: "The returned communication is then regarded as an independent confirmation of the therapist's theory [reference omitted]. This increases the credulity and suggestibility of both" (p. 384). This epistemological difficulty is, of course, compounded by the operation of those phenomena that Freud termed "countertransference" phenomena after shrewdly discerning them: the distorting effects of the therapist's feelings toward the patient on the accuracy of the former's perception of the latter's behavior (S.E. 1910, 11: 144–145).

It is evident from the current literature, as I shall illustrate presently, that even nowadays *some* analysts do intervene unabashedly in the associations of their patients. And, as my illustration will show, it is then pretended that the products of the ensuing associations are the subject's previously unconscious ideas, which have surfaced in unbiased fashion. Thus, it would be wrong to suppose that Freud's own "activist" handling of a patient's associations when giving interpretations is a thing of the past in psychoanalytic research and practice. The recognized analyst Benjamin Rubinstein, however, has pointed out to me that there surely are contemporary analysts who—mindful of the effects of overt, covert, and even *unconscious* suggestions on the patient—do indeed make a conscious effort to be far less "activist" than either Freud or the authors I am about to cite. But however sincere that effort in these quarters, it is at best unclear, I submit, to what extent this endeavor can be successful in coping with the serious data contaminant of patient compliance. How, for example, can the analyst guard against *unintended* yet potent suggestive influences? Thus, unless the mere effort to avoid them is *typically* successful when actually made, the epistemic sophistication that inspires it is surely not an adequate safeguard to assure noncontamination. In any case, there is telling evidence in the current literature that the effort is not even properly made among some influential practitioners.

Thus, a rather recent book by two respected teaching analysts (Blanck and Blanck 1974), recommending how analysis ought to be practiced, instructively reveals how at least some analytic patients are currently being coaxed, if not urged, to fulfill prior theoretical expectations. These authors present their recommendation by drawing on the case history of a patient who was unduly anxious about her general appearance, notably her skin, and who was being seen by a woman psychoanalyst. The excerpt from the paradigmatic case history provided by them is noteworthy, partly because they *interpret* their portrayal as showing that the therapist is testing her analytic interpretations quite *non*suggestively at every turn, while the patient gradually comes to discover penis envy in herself after two years of analysis. Yet precisely this methodologically favorable verdict is belied throughout by their own account.

To be specific, let us even disregard that today's typical female patient, if motivated to seek out a Freudian therapist and intelligent enough to be accepted for analysis, is likely to know a fair bit about the hypothesis of female penis envy even before going into treatment. Hence, even without the patent prompting shown in the following excerpt, such a patient may well realize that she is probably expected to give evidence of resenting her phallic deficit and of envying men their anatomical endowment. Thus, if she is minded to be a good patient, she will probably wish to accommodate her analyst by reporting such feelings of deficit. But, in any case, let us see how the Drs. Blanck relate the avowedly exemplary exchange between the analysand and her therapist.

The patient says: "Today I feel that I should see a dermatologist about my skin." The therapist responds: "You think constantly about your appearance because you are not sure that your body is always as it should be" (Blanck and Blanck 1974: 320). Note that the patient neither avowed nor implied any such motivation. This assertion is not based on data furnished by the patient but originates in the envy hypothesis.

The suggestion, "You are not sure that your body is as it should be" is subtly preparing the way for the penis envy notion. It is particularly insidious because many people do feel that they would like to be more attractive than they are. Hence, the patient may readily agree at this point that her body "is not as it should be." Yet her specific worries about her skin are not pursued in the analysis, which reportedly (p. 320) now proceeds like this *for two years*!

Thus, when the patient says, "Sometimes I think I look better than at other times," the therapist tells her, "You are not always certain that your body is the same." And when the patient complains, "I always feel there is something wrong," the therapist immediately concludes that "this is a classical phallic statement" (p. 321). Furthermore, when the patient dreams about one of these interpretations, the analyst considers the dream a confirmation of the interpretation (p. 321).

Finally, in response to a question from the analyst, the patient says, "Yes, men are always more admired" (p. 321). The analyst then comments beguilingly, "They have something more to be looked at," to which the patient then associates "freely": "Oh, you mean a penis." Flushed with this supposed further confirmation that women are not only anatomically envious *but also can be made ill by this unconscious feeling*, the Blancks promptly infer that their patient's two years of analysis were scientifically serendipitous. As they put it, "When the patient says, 'You mean' to her own association, it is a projection which represents the last defense against allowing the thought into consciousness" (p. 322). But once the analysand has thus been initiated into engaging in penis talk about herself, she is likely to believe in this alleged self-discovery afterward, thereby furnishing her analyst with ever more spurious confirmation.

This analytic disposition of the dermatologically discontented female patient is perhaps modeled after Freud's diagnosis of a male patient who was afflicted by a severe skin problem and had become withdrawn (schizophrenic): "Analysis shows that he is playing out his castration complex upon his skin" (S.E. 1915, 14: 199). Indeed, upon comparing the account given by the Blancks to how Freud handled the patients in many of his case histories, one can only conclude: *Plus ça change, plus c'est la même chose*. In the same vein, the present-day female analysts Bernstein and Warner (1981: 47) adduce their clinical experience and the study of the literature to conclude: "we are convinced that there is penis envy." No wonder that the renowned traditional analyst Kurt Eissler (1977) deplored the inhospitality of the current emancipatory, sexually egalitarian climate to the purported discovery of female penis envy.

MANIFEST DREAM CONTENTS AS MINI-NEUROTIC SYMPTOMS

So far, the criticism I have offered of Freud's theory of dreams has been largely just a corollary, generated *mutatis mutandis* from the failure of free associations to validate the psychoanalytic theory of parapraxes. But the psychoanalytic interpretation of dreams calls for some further scrutiny in its own right, if only because Freud regarded it as "*the royal road to a knowledge of the unconscious activities of the mind* [emphasis in original]" (S.E. 1900, 5: 608).

As Freud tells us, "the idea that *some* dreams are to be regarded as wish-fulfillments" had been commonplace in *pre*psychoanalytic psychology (S.E. 1900: 4: 134). Hence, Freud propounded a distinctive and exciting thesis about dreaming only when he *universalized* this commonsensical idea: "the meaning [motive force for the formation] of *every* dream is the fulfillment of a wish." And, as he is the first to recognize, prima facie this completely general thesis is impugned by sundry wish *contravening* and distressing manifest dream contents (e.g., anxiety dreams). Besides nightmares and examination dreams, for instance, "nonsensical" dreams also challenge Freud's account.

Even in the prepsychoanalytic dream theories mentioned by Freud, the claim that a *particular* dream is "wish fulfilling" goes beyond maintaining that the specifics of the dream's content *depict* the realization of some antecedent hope or desire. For, in the case of such a dream, these preanalytic psychological theories maintain furthermore that once the pertinent desires are not satisfied in waking life, they *cause* the formation of a dream content in which they achieve vicarious consummation. Perhaps the commonsense credibility of this preanalytic causal attribution of *some* dreams to wishes derives from those familiar *waking fantasies* in which unrequited love and other desires find vicarious consummation. In any event, Freud relies on this commonsense credibility of the motivational role of wishes in the formation of some dreams. Thus, in the case of one of his specimen dreams—the Irma dream—he plainly trades on the conviction carried by just this credibility when attempting to authenticate the trustworthiness of his method of free association as a means of identifying the motivational causes of *any and all* dreams. His reason for endeavoring to establish this trustworthiness was that free association seemed to him to yield repressed wishes as the motives of even those dreams whose manifest contents are anything but wish fulfilling. In this way, he thought he had legitimated his universalization of wish fulfillment as being the formative cause of any and all manifest dream contents.

True, in 1933, he acknowledged the existence of some exceptions to this universal claim (S.E. 1933, 22: 28-30), and he thus modified his wish fulfillment hypothesis. While retaining wish fulfillment as the function of dreaming, he acknowledged that it does miscarry with fair frequency. Hence, he then concluded that "the dream may aptly be characterized as an *attempt* at the fulfillment of a wish" (S.E. 1925, 20: 46n; this footnote was added in 1935). In short, the motive for dreaming is still held to be a wish, but the dream that actually ensues is no longer claimed to qualify universally as its fulfillment. But let us defer comment on this rather minor modification and deal with Freud's earlier unqualified generalization first.

Freud relies on two avenues to ascertain the purported motivational cause (or "meaning") of a dream: (1) the free associations of the individual dreamer, which originate at the separate elements of the manifest content (usually visual images), and (2) dream symbolism, whose unconscious motivational significance is claimed to be independent of individual and even cultural differences. Freud does explain that when gleaning the "sense" of a dream, the translation of interpersonal dream symbolism complements the method of free association (S.E. 1900, 5: 341-342, 359; 1916, 15: 150). But he emphasizes that the interpersonally significant symbols play only an auxiliary, subordinate role in dream interpretation vis-à-vis the "decisive significance" of the dreamer's free associations (S.E. 1900, 5: 360; 1916, 15: 151).

Indeed, in the magisterial digest of the dream theory he gave in his "Autobiographical Study," which he revised in 1935, he even seems to deny the probative value of dream symbolism by implication. True, he there makes passing mention of the role of symbolism in the dream work (S.E. 1925, 20: 45). But he does so after having told us that the "manifest content was simply a make-believe, a façade, which could serve as a starting point for the associations but not for the interpretation" (S.E. 1925, 20: 44). Thus, when interpersonal dream symbolism is present in the manifest content, its interpretative translation can yield only *bits* for the interpretation. Hence, for the purpose of examining the credentials of his interpretation of dreams, it will suffice to confine our comments to his reliance on the method of free association as an epistemic avenue to the purported motivational cause of dreaming.

As he claims, free associations setting out from the manifest content of any dream *always* yield a repressed wish and other assorted repressed content, commingled with miscellaneous thoughts that qualify as "preconscious" in his familiar technical sense (S.E. 1900, 5: 552-553; 1916; 15: 224-226; 1923, 19: 114; 1925, 20: 44, 46). Being the presumed residues of the dreamer's waking life before the dream, the emerging preconscious thoughts may well *happen* to include a *non*repressed wish. He then identifies the repressed wish, which is purportedly universally yielded by the associations, as the agency to which the dream owes its initial formation: "This impulse is the actual constructor [cause] of the dream: it provides the energy for its production and makes use of the day's residues as material" (S.E. 1925, 20: 44). Yet it is "often of a very repellent kind, which is foreign to the waking life of the dreamer and is consequently disavowed by him with surprise or indignation."

I shall now examine Freud's interpretation of his Irma dream. This scrutiny will hardly vindicate his claim that this specimen dream authenticates free association as a reliable means of fathoming the formative causes of *all* dreams (S.E. 1900, 4: chap. II) Far from supplying such vindication, I shall maintain that even when commonsense psychology regards a given dream as patently wish fulfilling, psychoanalytically conducted free association does not have the probative resources to *underwrite* this verdict!

In a preamble to his own dream about his patient Irma, Freud details the events of the previous day that avowedly provided its point of departure (S.E. 1900, 4: 106). It is clear from this account that these events left him with *conscious* feelings of frustration and aggressive desires, which clamored for expression: annoyance with Irma because she had rejected Freud's conjecture as to the unconscious cause of her hysterical symptoms; frustration because, as the presumed consequence of her rejection of his "solution," her somatic symptoms had persisted; irritation by his junior colleague Otto, who had implied censure of his handling of Irma's therapeutic expectations; and the desire "to justify" his treatment of Irma for the benefit of his respected senior colleague Dr. M, who has since been revealed to be his mentor Breuer (Grinstein 1980, chap. 1).

The aggressive wishes that had remained unfulfilled by the end of the day in question are then patently acted out or realized in the manifest dream content that Freud goes on to report (p. 107); for early within the dream, Freud avowedly rebukes Irma for her resistance to his "solution," and he explicitly blames *her* for the persistence of her pains. Then, at the end of the dream, Dr. M. and he condemn Otto for negligently causing Irma to become infected by his use of a dirty syringe. Thus, after recapitulating the conscious motives specified in the preamble, and the manifest content, Freud tells us convincingly that the following motivational interpretation "leapt to the eyes" from these data: the dream "*content was the fulfillment of a wish and its motive was a wish* [emphasis in original]" (S.E. 1900, 4: 119).

Now, if a dreamer remembers on the day after a dream what *conscious* thoughts he had on the day before his dream, it is true enough that this recollection *may* occur *in the wake* of thinking of the dream, thereby qualifying as a kind of association with the dream. Yet this sort of association clearly differs from the recovery of a *repressed* thought, first achieved if the dreamer takes elements of the manifest content as points of departure *and* is careful to heed the demanding injunctions of Freud's "fundamental rule" of "free association" (S.E. 1923, 18: 238). This distinction does indeed matter in the context of Freud's attempted use of the Irma dream to authenticate free association as a trustworthy avenue for identifying repressed wishes as the formative causes of manifest dream contents; for he traded on the label "association" to insinuate the falsehood that the plainly *conscious* aggressive wishes of the prior day, which he specifies in his preamble, were first excavated associatively in the manner of a repressed thought. That this suggested conclusion is mere pretense is evident from his own report. For when speaking of the events on the day and evening *before* the dream, he says: "The same evening I wrote out Irma's case history, with the idea of giving it to Dr. M. (a common friend [of Otto's and Freud's] who was at that time the leading figure in our circle) in order to justify myself" [in the face of Otto's implied reproof] (S.E. 1900, 4: 106).

In sum, though the aggressive conscious wishes that Freud had on the day before his Irma dream were then patently fulfilled in its manifest content, free association played *no excavating role* in his recall of these wishes after the dream, for he had been avowedly conscious of them the evening before. Hence, for this reason alone, the purportedly paradigmatic Irma dream cannot serve to authenticate free association as a trustworthy avenue for certifying that *repressed infantile* wishes are the formative *causes* of manifest dream content, as claimed by Freud's theory. Yet he relies on free association to make just this claim (S.E. 1900, 5: 546, 548-549, 552-554, 567-568, 583-584). For example, he does so to make the following assertions: "*a conscious wish can only become a dream-instigator if it succeeds in awakening an unconscious wish with the same tenor and in obtaining reinforcement from it.* . . . *A wish which is represented in a dream must be an infantile one* [emphasis in original]" (S.E. 1900, 5: 553). Fully *thirty years* after he had had a childhood dream at about age seven whose dominant theme was anxiety, he was satisfied that his analysis of this dream warranted the following conclusion: "The anxiety can be traced back, when repression is taken into account, to an obscure and evidently sexual craving that had found appropriate expression in the visual content of the dream" (S.E. 1900, 5: 584). Since he invoked free association crucially to draw these causal inferences, I maintain that *Freud had indeed failed to sustain the major thesis of his dream theory*, a theory in which he took special pride. Yet even in a quite recent article, the analysts Frank and Trunnell (1978) describe a training procedure based on the assumption that an archaic wish is the universal motive force of dreaming.

Thus, to this day, Freudians claim that repressed *infantile* wishes are the primogenitors of *all* dreams. Yet, judging by Freud's own report on his celebrated Irma dream, there is no evidence at all that he ever carried his analysis of the dream far enough to extend to his childhood wishes (S.E. 1900, 4: 120-121). Hence, if one of his infantile wishes was to have been the instigator of the Irma dream, Freud's own published analysis of this dream cannot possibly underwrite the principal substantive tenet of his dream theory. How, then, can his disciples justify hailing it as *the* dream specimen of psychoanalysis, instead of demoting it to a mere popularized example? Over fifty years after the publication of *The Interpretation of Dreams* in 1900, Erik Erikson made a strenuous effort to rise to this challenge in an article entitled "The Dream Specimen of Psychoanalysis" (1954). In this way, *Irma* was supposed to retain pride of place as the prototype dream of psychoanalysis.

But if it was thus not until fifteen years after Freud's death that an orthodox interpretation of the Irma dream was even proposed, how did Freud himself justify using this particular dream "specimen" to *introduce* his analysis of dreams? The answer is encapsulated in the word *method* found within the title of the pertinent chapter 2 of his magnum opus on the subject: "The Method of Interpreting Dreams: An Analysis of a Specimen Dream" (S.E. 1900, 4: 96). Early in this chapter (pp. 100-102), he states clearly in what manner his "knowledge of that procedure [method of dream interpretation] was reached" (p. 100). As he explains there, it was a matter of *simply enlarging* the epistemic role of *free association* from being only a method of *etiologic* inquiry aimed at therapy to serving likewise as an avenue for interpreting dreams:

> My patients were pledged to communicate to me every idea or thought that occurred to them in connection with some particular subject; amongst other things they told me their dreams and so taught me that a dream can be inserted into the psychical chain that has to be traced backwards in the memory from a pathological idea. It was then only a short step to treating the dream itself as a symptom and to applying to dreams the method of interpretation that had been worked out for symptoms. [S.E. 1900, 4: 100-101]

Note here how Freud makes light of the epistemically dubious nature of this momentous extension by vastly understating its gaping pitfalls as "only a short step." Yet he apparently wanted this step to carry conviction for his readers as well.

Thus, his initial accent in the opening presentation of his dream theory was on authenticating the *method* of interpreting dreams; for even if one grants that the method of free association ("fundamental rule of psychoanalysis") can fathom and certify the pathogens of neuroses as such, it is anything but obvious that this method can reliably perform the same epistemic service in identifying the causes (motives) of our dreams. And it would beg the question to *assume outright* that any dream can be regarded as a kind of neurotic symptom. Hence, Freud's strategy was to argue first that, in the case of the Irma dream, the use of free association does yield motives independently countenanced by commonsense psychology as having patently engendered *this* dream. Thereafter, he is prepared to rest his *substantive* theory of dreams as *universally* wish fulfilling on the deliverances of the method purportedly authenticated by the analysis of his Irma dream. This order of argument is recapitulated in the very last sentences of the pertinent chapter, which read:

For the moment I am satisfied with the achievement of this one piece of fresh knowledge. If we adopt the method of interpreting dreams which I have indicated here, we shall find that dreams really have a meaning and are far from being the expression of a fragmentary activity of the brain, as the authorities have claimed. *When the work of interpretation has been completed, we perceive that a dream is the fulfillment of a wish* [italics in original]. [S.E. 1900, 4: 121]

Accordingly, as I already indicated, this dream earned its laurels as "*the* dream specimen of psychoanalysis" on methodological rather than substantive grounds. The more so since the wishes that had been *shown* to be fulfilled by it were hardly repressed infantile ones but *only* adult conscious desires!

As for the substantive conclusions derived from the published analysis of this paradigmatic dream, Freud issues a disclaimer in regard to the completeness of his account of it:

I will not pretend that I have completely uncovered the meaning of this dream or that its interpretation is without a gap. I could spend much more time over it, derive further information from it and discuss fresh problems raised by it. I myself know the points from which further trains of thought could be followed. [S.E. 1900 4: 120-121]

Given the principally methodological basis of the exemplar status accorded to the Irma dream, it is very disappointing that psychoanalysts have not *scrutinized* its purported authentication of free association as the method of dream analysis. One's disappointment is the greater because, of all of Freud's own dreams, the Irma dream has spawned the largest literature (see Grinstein 1980: 22, for some citations). Though the aforementioned paper by Erikson (1954) is just as insouciant epistemologically as the rest of this literature, it warrants comment, for its avowed burden is to give the Irma dream the *infantile* motivational underpinning required by orthodox doctrine. Thus, Erikson sees himself as having made good on his conclusion that "the latent infantile wish that provides the energy... for the dream is embedded in a manifest dream structure which on every level reflects significant trends of the dreamer's total situation" (1954: 55). Let us examine his reasoning.

After quoting from Freud's own lengthy summary of the Irma dream, Erikson (p. 15) points out that it does not contain any *repressed* motive: "We note that the wish demonstrated here is not more than preconscious." Furthermore, the conscious wishes detailed by Freud are all adult rather than infantile ones. Indeed, nowhere in his magnum opus on dream interpretation does Freud explicitly offer a repressed wish for *this* dream, let alone an infantile one. Hence, Erikson (pp. 15-16) proposes to supply a missing latent dream motive satisfying both of these theoretical desiderata and featuring sexual themata.

Erikson develops the hypothesized sexual origin by pointing to colloquial, sexually allusive overtones ("double meanings") of several German words in Freud's original. In the 1938 English translation cited by Erikson, the rendition of these German words was "so literal that an important double meaning gets lost" (1954: 24). The original German words, he tells us, "allude to sexual meanings, as if the Irma Dream permitted a complete sexual interpretation alongside the professional one—an inescapable expectation in any case" (p. 26).

Our focus is on Erikson's quest for the purported "infantile meaning of the Irma Dream" (p. 27), *not* on the *pansexual* significance that he claimed for it as well. Hence, I shall forgo making a methodological complaint against the alleged inescapability of the expectation that "a complete sexual interpretation" of the dream is feasible. What does matter is that *only* the sexual allusion of the German word *Spritze* figures in Erikson's account as a clue to the conjectured infantile meaning of the Irma dream. Stressing the unique allusive role of this one word in Freud's original, Erikson explains: "The recognition of this double meaning is absolutely necessary for a pursuit of the infantile meaning of the Irma Dream" (p. 27).

What, then, is the presumed sexual significance of *Spritze* on which Erikson rests his entire case for an infantile interpretation? He articulates the sexual and infantile overtones of *Spritze*, in turn, before they can be seen to merge.

First he explains the phallic-urinary tinge of the word's colloquial allusion:

The German word..."*Spritze*"...is, indeed, used for syringes, but has also the colloquial meaning of "squirter"...Squirter is an instrument of many connotations; of these, the phallic-urinary one is most relevant, for the use of a dirty syringe makes Otto a "dirty squirter," or "a little squirt," not just a careless physician.

It is undeniable that this sexual overtone is one of Erikson's *own* associations to the word *Spritze*. But, according to the psychoanalytic methodology of dream interpretation, the interpretively relevant associations are those of the dreamer *himself*; for if a repressed infantile wish is to emerge as the motive for a given dream, it can be *certified* as its primogenitor only by probing the dreamer's *own* associations to elements of the manifest content. And it was Freud, not Erikson, who had the Irma dream. Hence, even according to the inferential standards countenanced by psychoanalytic theory, the sexual allusion of *Spritze* has probative merit only if it was one of Freud's *own* associations. But that is still not enough. If a thought revealed by an association is to be adduced as a motive for the Irma dream, it must be shown to be one of Freud's associations to *this* particular dream. Therefore, those of Freud's associations that he himself linked to elements of *other* dreams, as far as we know, cannot be adduced as motives for *this* dream.

Yet Erikson's phallic-urethral association to *Spritze* is conspicuously absent from Freud's own account of the associations evoked in *him* by Otto's syringe as part of the manifest content of the Irma dream. As Freud himself explains:

And probably the syringe had not been clean. This was yet another accusation against Otto, but derived from a different source. I had happened the day before to meet the son of an old lady of eighty-two, to whom I had to give an injection of morphia twice a day [footnote omitted]. At the moment she was in the country and he told me that she was suffering from phlebitis. I had at once thought it must be an infiltration caused by a dirty syringe. I was proud of the fact that in two years I had not caused a single infiltration; I took constant pains to be sure that the syringe was clean. In short, I was conscientious [emphasis in original]. [S.E. 1900, 4: 118]

So far, at any rate, Erikson has come up empty-handed. But the success of his endeavor to legitimate the Irma dream as a doctrinal centerpiece does not turn on finding a sexual overtone for the dream motive. Mindful of the theory's call for a repressed infantile theme, Erikson offers "the dream's [sexual] allusion to a childhood problem"

(p. 27) as his clincher. But unfortunately, he relies on speculation instead of clear evidence that Freud himself ever linked Dr. Otto's *Spritze* associatively to the memory of the childhood episode in question.

In the section entitled "Infantile Material as a Source of Dreams" (S.E. 1900, 189-219), Freud does indeed relate the episode adduced by Erikson to a dream. But one looks in vain for a reference to the Irma dream in the whole series of dreams he interprets there. Nor is there even any passing mention of Irma, let alone of Dr. Otto's *Spritze*. When the childhood episode invoked by Erikson is discussed near the end of the section (p. 216), its explicit associative context (pp. 215-216), is a dream relating to the revolution of 1848 (pp. 209-211) in central Europe.

At best, Freud's own report of the associative linkages of the given episode to dreams allows Erikson to *speculate* as follows: Freud *may* perhaps *also* have associated that childhood scene with repaying Otto in kind by having him malpractice with a dirty syringe. Notice Freud's own wording:

When I was seven or eight years old there was another domestic scene, which I can remember very clearly. One evening before going to sleep I disregarded the rules which modesty lays down and obeyed the calls of nature [in a chamber pot] in my parents' bedroom while they were present. In the course of his reprimand, my father let fall the words: 'The boy will come to nothing.' This must have been a frightful blow to my ambition, for references to this scene are still constantly recurring in my dreams and are always linked with an enumeration of my achievements and successes, as though I wanted to say: 'You see, I *have* come to something.' [S.E. 1900, 4: 216]

It is, of course, quite true that there is a great deal of *thematic* affinity between this humiliating paternal rebuke for immodest urination and the Otto syringe motif in the Irma dream. But surely this thematic affinity alone is not evidence that the memory of the childhood scene was the motivational primogenitor of having dreamt the Irma injection dream in particular. Thematic affinity alone fails to bespeak such primogenesis, if only because it is not a reason for giving *psychodynamic priority* to the childhood memory over the actual *adult* thought of a syringe, which Freud himself gave as the explanation for the dream syringe! Flawed though it is as a method of *certifying causes*, free association does not even give epistemic sanction to Erikson's psychodynamic attribution on the flimsy basis he uses. For even if one deems the method of free association competent to identify the agencies of dream formation for any given dream, Erikson's use of Freud's reported associations is too speculative to sustain the hypothesized motivational origin of the Irma dream.

As if to acknowledge the tenuous character of his documentation, Erikson proceeds gingerly when he conjectures what infantile experience engendered the Otto syringe motif:

If his father told little Freud under the embarrassing circumstance of the mother's presence in the parental bedroom, that he would never amount to anything, i.e., that the intelligent boy did not hold what he promised — is it not suggestive to assume that the tired doctor [Sigmund Freud] of the night before the dream had gone to bed with a bitter joke in his preconscious mind: yes, maybe I did promise too much when I said I could cure hysteria; maybe my father was right after all, I do not hold what I promised. [p. 42]

Here the interrogative phrase "is it not suggestive to assume" has a commendably tentative tenor. But ironically, Erikson himself undermines the probative value of the childhood memory, even if its genetic relevance is granted, as he explicitly places it in the dreamer's "preconscious mind" on the eve of the dream. Though Freud's wish to prove his father wrong meets the requirement of being a childhood vestige, it does not lend support to the *psychoanalytic* dream theory, unless it was also *repressed* when Freud was on the verge of having the Irma dream.

Yet despite having declared Freud's childhood memory to have been preconscious on the eve of the dream (p. 42), Erikson does not hesitate to transform it into a *latent* infantile wish in the concluding paragraph of his essay (p. 55). And unmindful of his initial caution in proposing *infantile* primogenesis, he goes on to affirm it categorically in the metapsychological idiom of "energy" (p. 55): "The Irma Dream," he maintains, "illustrates how the latent infantile wish that provides the energy for . . . the dream, is imbedded in a manifest dream structure." But for all of Erikson's impressive sensitivity to associative nuances, he offers nothing to justify thus giving *psychodynamic priority* to the infantile urination experience over the waking adult thought of a *dirty syringe*, which Freud reported from the day before the dream. Indeed, even as regards mere thematic affinity to the Otto syringe motif, the thoughts Freud reported having on the day before the dream seem closer than the childhood memory adduced by Erikson.

Moreover, the temporal priority of the infantile wish over the adult one hardly vouches for a corresponding *psychodynamic* primacy. Why, then, does Erikson, no less than other Freudians, insist (p. 34) that dreams owe their very occurrence dynamically to "an id wish and all of its infantile energy"? Let me suggest that this strained insistence on infantile causes becomes more intelligible — albeit *not* cogent — if one bears in mind that Freud explicitly modeled his interpretation of dreams on his repression etiology of neuroses (S.E. 1900, 4: 100-101; 5:

528). As I recounted earlier, when Breuer postulated the *adult* occasioning traumata to be the primogenetic pathogens of hysteria, this etiologic version was discredited by therapeutic failures. Yet Freud was determined to retain a repression etiology in some form. Hence, he was driven to demote the *adult* occasioning traumata etiologically to mere *precipitators* of neurosis, and to claim that childhood repressions were the *essential* pathogens. But, as he explained (S.E. 1900, 4: 100-101), he developed his theory of dreams by assimilating manifest dream content to neurotic symptoms at the outset. And having downgraded adult occasioning traumata etiologically in favor of childhood pathogens, he presumably felt entitled, by analogy, to give repressed *infantile* wishes psychodynamic primacy over adult ones.

Perhaps we should assume that the conclusion of this rationale was a tacit premise of Erikson's account, for in the absence of such an assumption, Erikson's entire case for attributing the occurrence of the Irma dream to the "energy" from a childhood motive dangles ever so precariously from the thin thread of the colloquial *Spritze* allusion. Indeed, it appears as a product of scraping the bottom of the epistemic barrel, unless infantile motives *generically* have psychodynamic primacy over adult ones. But, as I have argued, Freud's analogical rationale is not viable. Hence, it cannot serve to underwrite the psychodynamic primacy of infantile wishes. So much, then, for Erikson's imaginative but abortive attempt to provide a doctrinally orthodox infantile underpinning for Freud's own interpretation of the Irma dream.

It so happens that in the case of the Irma dream, there are actually grounds from commonsense psychology for regarding the aggressive motives reported in Freud's preamble as having engendered the manifest dream content. But free association did not first uncover these motives. Hence, their commonsense causal credentials cannot serve at all as evidence that, for any and all dreams, if certain repressed wishes reentered consciousness via a tortuous causal chain of free associations initiated by the manifest content, then *the latter emergence* would *itself* reliably identify these wishes as the initial motivational causes of the dream. Yet it is presumably just this probative reliance on free association that Erikson extolls, in the context of interpreting the Irma dream, by speaking breezily of "the necessity to abandon well-established methods of sober investigation (invented to find out a few things exactly and safely to overlook the rest) for a method of self-revelation apt to open the floodgates of the unconscious" (1954: 54).

Nor did Freud offer a *cogent* reason, in the case of dreams, for resting the *interpretive* use of free association on an extrapolation from the repression etiology of neuroses. The reasoning he does offer begs the question as follows: "We might also point out in our defense that our procedure in interpreting dreams [by means of free association] is identical with the procedure by which we resolve hysterical symptoms; and there the correctness of our method is warranted by the coincident emergence and disappearance of the symptoms" (S.E. 1900, 5: 528). More specifically, as we saw in detail in an earlier section, Freud had *hypothesized* from the *therapeutic* results of the cathartic method that affect-laden, conflict-ridden *repressed* thoughts are the pathogens of the neurotic disorders. Hence, he saw the excavation of the pertinent repressed ideation as the *sine qua non* of discovering the specific etiologies of the neuroses, and besides as indispensable to their therapeutic conquest. But once he became convinced that repression is the hallmark of pathogenesis, he was willing to postulate further that even the parapraxes and dreams of "normal" people are the telltale outcroppings of particular repressions. In brief, he viewed even such episodic events in the lives of healthy persons as the symptoms of (temporary) *mini*-neuroses, initiated and sustained by a repression. Thus, in his compromise model of manifest dream content, that content is seen as a compromise between the repressed (forbidden) wish and the mind's censorship, which distorts its expression in the dream (S.E. 1900, 4: 144).

But this assimilation of manifest dream content and parapraxes to the status of "compromise formations" had an important corollary: their adequate *causal explanation*, no less than that of full-fledged neurotic symptoms, could be furnished only by ferreting out the repressions that had purportedly engendered them. And, as Freud had argued, the method of free association is unmatched in achieving just such fathoming. Hence, it was the protean causal role he had bestowed on repression—generating "slips," actuating dream construction, and being generically pathogenic—that secured pride of place epistemically for free association in his theory.

But, as I have already explained in conjunction with my criticism of Freud's repression theory of parapraxes, his compromise model of manifest dream content rests on a *misextrapolation*; for he does not even try to adduce any counterpart to the *therapeutic* support that Breuer and he had claimed to have for the repression etiology of hysteria and for the *investigative* utility of lifting repressions via free associations to fathom the pathogens. Therefore, I conclude that *Freud's reliance on free association as a means of fathoming the causes of dreams is just as grievously flawed epistemically as his use of free association to identify the causes of parapraxes.*

One must deplore some of the transparent inconsistency demonstrated by Freud in offering the Irma dream to underwrite his epistemic trust in free association as a *causally* probative tool of inquiry. Thus, first he tells us (S.E. 1900, 4: 107) that the Irma dream is *unusual* in the sense that "it was immediately clear [from his preamble] what events of the previous day provided its starting point." And three chapters later, he acknowledges: "the connection with the previous day is so obvious as to require no further comment" (p. 165). Having himself pointed out this transparency, he declares all the same: "Nevertheless no one who had only read the preamble and the [manifest] content of the dream could have the slightest notion of what the dream meant" (p. 108). One is immediately taken aback by this puzzling declaration of obscurity precisely because, as we saw, the preamble clearly reveals that the events of the preceding day had left Freud with *conscious* aggressive desires (wishes), which are then patently fulfilled in the manifest dream content reported by him. Even on the heels of claiming that without free association, the dream's wish motives would be utterly obscure, he belies this claim as follows: "the words which I spoke to Irma in the dream showed that I was specially anxious not to be responsible for the pains which she still had" (p. 108). But worse, he waits until after he detailed his associations to *contradict* flatly his declaration of *initial* obscurity as to the dream's motive. For he then tells us convincingly that the wish character of that motive had "leapt to the eyes" (p. 119) from the conscious motives specified in the preamble and the description of the manifest content.

How, I must ask, by the way, can the critique I gave of Freud's dream theory possibly be seen as an *illicit* extrapolation of standards of appraisal appropriate *only* to the *physical* sciences? I am prompted to ask this rhetorical question, because the inveterate complaint of just such methodological transgression has again been leveled in a recent article by Jane Flax (1981: 564), which is directed against my views on psychoanalysis.

A second specimen dream discussed by Freud is one whose manifest content clearly depicts the *thwarting* of the very wish consciously felt by the dreamer in the dream itself (S.E. 1900, 4: 146-149). Freud presents the analysis of this dream to illustrate his contention that the manifest content of the dream is wish fulfilling despite its distressing content.

The dreamer, "a clever woman patient," challenged Freud to show how his wish-fulfillment theory can accommodate the thwarting of just the desire she felt within the dream itself. She dreamt that on a Sunday afternoon, she found herself wishing to give a dinner party.

Having nothing but a little smoked salmon in the house, she had to buy some food. Yet, since it was Sunday, the stores were closed. The attempt to enlist the service of some caterers failed, since the telephone was out of order, thus aborting the plan to give the dinner party.

The frustrated hostess reported to Freud that in her waking life, she had had a long-standing craving to "have a caviare sandwich every morning but had grudged the expense" (p. 147). On the day before the dream, she had asked her husband *not* to indulge this desire of hers, although he would readily have done so. Allegedly, she had made this request "so that she could go on teasing him about it," as she was wont to do generally. Furthermore, as Freud relates:

The day before she had visited a woman friend of whom she confessed she felt jealous because her (my patient's) husband was constantly singing her praises. Fortunately this friend of hers is very skinny and thin and her husband admires a plumper figure. I asked her what she had talked about to her thin friend. Naturally, she replied, of that lady's wish to grow a littler stouter. Her friend had enquired, too: "When are you going to ask us to another meal? You always feed one so well." [p. 148]

When Freud asked her how she would account for the presence of the smoked salmon in the manifest dream content, she replied that this delicacy is her female friend's favorite dish.

Initially, Freud identified the dream motive as the wish to lessen the rival's chances of becoming plumper, since that would have made her still more attractive to the dreamer's husband. Thus, the inability to give a dinner party is conducive to the fulfillment of the patient's aim. But Freud appreciates that this account has not dealt with an uncomfortable detail: since the rival had expressed the wish to gain weight,

it would not have been surprising if my patient had dreamt that her friend's wish was unfulfilled; for my patient's own wish was that her friend's wish (to put on weight) should not be fulfilled. But instead of this she dreamt that one of her *own* wishes was not fulfilled. [p. 149]

How, then, does he propose to deal with this recalcitrant datum?

An auxiliary hypothesis is brought to the rescue. Freud postulates that instead of being the patient herself, the person who figures in the dream is actually her rival, with whom she had "identified" herself to the extent of putting herself into the rival's place. He seems to be well aware that a rescuing auxiliary can be indicted as *ad hoc*, unless it is buttressed by *independent* evidential support. Thus, he goes on to claim at once (p. 149) that just such support is supplied by the patient's request to her husband in waking life *not* to cater to her craving for caviar. For, under the collateral hypothesis that the patient can assume her rival's identity even in waking life, her avowed conscious desire to deprive the rival of food would make sense of her renunciatory request to her husband.

In this way, Freud believed he had shown that even a dream depicting the *thwarting* of a wish felt in the dream does qualify, after all, as the fulfillment of another wish, which is only latent, being a residue from the day before. As he sees it, his auxiliary hypothesis of interpersonal identification contributed to an understanding of a datum from the patient's behavior in waking life, besides enabling his major postulate of wish fulfillment to explain the initially refractory feature of the manifest dream content.

Glymour (unpublished) has discussed the aborted dinner party dream as an illustration of Freud's device "to confirm an interpretation by finding two or more elements of the dream which are independently associated with a key figure in the interpretation of the dream." This dream illustrates such a device, because after Freud had inferred the aim to thwart the dreamer's rival as the dream motive, he said: "All that was now lacking was some coincidence to confirm the solution" (S.E. 1900, 4: 148). When his patient reported her rival's fondness for smoked salmon, he had seized on the role of this delicacy in the manifest dream content as the confirming coincidence.

Glymour challenges this claim of confirmation as spurious. As he points out, Freud's conclusion as to the motivational cause had asserted an order of cause and effect that is the *reverse* of the causal order exhibited by the free associations, for associations generated by two manifest dream elements (the dinner party and the salmon) had *each* prompted his patient to think of her rival. But Freud took this to be evidence that the affect bound to that rival was the motivational cause for the thematic occurrence of both a dinner party and salmon in the manifest dream content. Glymour objects that "evidence for the first causal model is not necessarily evidence for the second," a causal reversal he indicts as "one of Freud's favorite fallacies." Hence, Glymour (unpublished) rejects Freud's invocation of the "coincidence" that both a dinner party and salmon figured in the manifest dream content: "the coincidence is manufactured: one associates, at Freud's direction, until one thinks of something which has connections with several elements in one's dream; the several elements cause the common thought, not vice-versa, and the coincidence requires no further explanation. The method of manufacture is all the explanation required." Indeed, Freud thus argues fallaciously from the confluence of associations to a causal reversal in *explicitly generalized* form (S.E. 1900, 5: 528).

As the reader will recall from my earlier discussion, it was in the context of my critique of Freud's theory of parapraxes that I argued for the rejection of his inference of causal reversal, *and emphasized its fallacious origination in his repression etiology of the psychoneuroses*. As a corollary to my historico-logical discreditation of his causal inference, I objected to his commission of the same fallacy in his theory of dreams. Glymour independently uncovered the fallacy in the context of Freud's dream theory by pointing out illuminatingly that it lurked behind Freud's reliance on a coincidence in the manifest dream content to *confirm* his analysis of the dream. But, as I showed earlier, Freud's fallacious causal inference is not quite the glaringly crude blunder that it appears to be. This flagrant appearance results from seeing that inference in the context of the dream theory alone, as Glymour did.

Such an *isolated* appraisal neglects that Freud speaks of dreams as being "like all other psychopathological structures" (S.E. 1900, 4: 149). Twenty-five years later, he stressed this assimilation of manifest dream content to his compromise model of neurotic symptoms: "dreams are constructed like a neurotic symptom: they are compromises between the demands of a repressed impulse and the resistance of a censoring force in the ego" (S.E. 1925, 20: 45). Thus, as I explained earlier, Freud did believe that the legacy of Breuer's method vouches for free association as an avenue to the identification of repressed dream motives. And, as I showed furthermore, Freud was led to this conclusion by misextrapolation from a flawed repression etiology of the neuroses. All the same, it emerges that Freud's causal reversal inference in his dream theory is not quite as devoid of a plausible rational motivation as Glymour makes it appear to be.

The objections I have raised so far against Freud's dream theory would hold, even if the method of free association were not flawed epistemically by the analyst's overt and covert interventions. But this method is considerably impaired by the defects I have charged against it: manipulative adulteration as well as selection bias. In fact, these liabilities vitiate it, regardless of whether the repressions it yields are deemed the pathogens of neurotic symptoms, the causes of slips, or the motives for dream constructions. Indeed, as we shall see later, this conclusion bespeaks the spuriousness of the consilience of clinical inductions that Freud adduced late in life (S.E. 1937, 23: 257-269) to validate analytic interpretations.

Clark Glymour (unpublished) has rightly complained that the contrived manner of selecting from the products of free association has enabled Freud's method to function *ad hoc* when generating the elements belonging to the purported *latent* dream content. For, as Glymour argues cogently, Freud so selected the latent content as to preserve his wish-fulfillment hypothesis from refutation by such prima facie counterexamples as nightmares and diffuse anxiety dreams. Freud gave no justificatory criteria in advance for weaving *particular* associations together to make *one* sort of story. Instead, he begged the question by tailoring his selections from the patient's associative output *ad hoc* to the preservation of his wish-fulfillment hypothesis, whenever the manifest dream content was anything but wish fulfilling. A suitably different set of selections from the associations could have been made to yield other motives, such as fear or disgust. Thus, Freud failed to sustain his account of the latent content by *warrantedly* selected evidence. But since this account was *essential* to evading refutation by anxiety dreams, Glymour concludes reasonably enough that the universal wish-fulfillment hypothesis of psychoanalytic dream theory ought to be presumed false rather than unfalsifiable.

Even more censoriously, Timpanaro (1976: 115) points especially to Freud's lecture "The Dream Work" (S.E. 1916, 15: 179-183) as evidence for the following indictment: "Perhaps most capricious and scientifically dishonest of all is Freud's 'proof' that all dreams, even anxiety dreams, are the expressions of a repressed wish." Timpanaro (1976) illustrates his accusation:

Does someone have an anxiety dream about the death of a beloved person? Have no fear; this too is a wish-fulfillment, for it represents a resurgence of archaic psychic material which reveals that at some point in the infantile life of the dreamer the death of that person was indeed desired. The anxiety dream is concerned with the dreamer's *own* death? Another case of a wish — this time for self-punishment because of a guilt complex. [p. 218]

Freud did not come to grips with any of the array of objections to his dream theory that we have put forward so far. These were of three sorts: (1) his infantile wish genesis of all dreams is causally unfounded; (2) equally unfounded is his claim that the motivational cause of dream construction, if unconscious, must be present among the free associations triggered by the manifest content; and (3) the method of free association yields probatively defective data. But, to his credit, Freud did address another epistemic challenge to his dream theory.

The latter misgiving leaves aside the methodological pitfalls of free association. Instead, it arises from the presumed likelihood that patients compliantly produce corroborative dreams under the analyst's suggestive influence (S.E. 1911, 12: 96; 1923, 19: 115). In essence, Freud is being called upon to rule out that the patient obligingly generates repressed wishful impulses, because he is aware, at least unconsciously, of the analyst's belief in their presence. Freud optimistically denied just such adulteration in 1923 (S.E. 1923, 19: 114-115).

He first points out that since the *manifest* contents of dreams are indeed susceptible to the influence of waking life, it is small wonder that those powerful impressions of waking life that the patient obtains from his analyst likewise affect what will be the foci of his manifest dream content (p. 114). Also, as he tells us, even thoughts that *happen* to be unconscious at a given time but that might readily become conscious—i.e., "preconscious" thoughts as *contrasted* with *repressed* wishes—may ingress into the latent dream content in response to the analyst's suggestive influence (p. 114). But Freud then emphasizes that the dream also "contains indications of the repressed wishful impulses to which it owes the possibility of its formation" (p. 114). Having said this, he is adamant that these wishful impulses are immune to the analyst's expectations. Freud rebuffs the skeptic: "The doubter will reply that they appear in the dream because the dreamer knows that he ought to produce them—that they are expected by the analyst. The analyst himself will rightly think otherwise" (pp. 114-115).

But why is the analyst right in thinking otherwise? Freud gives a mere analogy in which the interpretative task in psychoanalysis is likened to solving a jigsaw puzzle that has a *unique* solution (p. 116). Yet astonishingly, he concedes on the very next page that "most of the dreams that can be made use of in analysis are obliging dreams and owe their origin to suggestion." For there, he explains first that one of the patient's unconscious motives is "compliance towards the analyst which is derived from his parental complex—in other words, the positive portion of what we call the transference" (p. 117). Then he goes on at once to say quite serenely:

In fact, in many dreams which recall what has been forgotten and repressed, it is impossible to discover any other unconscious wish [than obliging the analyst] to which the motive force for the formation of the dream can be attributed. So that if anyone wishes to maintain that most of the dreams that can be made use of in analysis are obliging dreams and owe their origin to suggestion, nothing can be said against that opinion from the point of view of analytic theory. [p. 117]

Thus, here Freud concedes that the repressed wishes to which the patient's dreams purportedly owe their formation are indeed often induced by "compliance toward the analyst." But he does not let on that only a couple of pages earlier he had denied that the analyst wields just such suggestive influence. He sidetracks this unacknowledged inconsistency at once by moving on to invoke the defunct Tally Argument in support of the following claim: the patient's unconscious wish to oblige the analyst by dreaming only mobilizes the uncontaminated disclosure, via the emerging *latent* dream content, of "what has been forgotten and repressed," largely from the patient's preanalytic life.

Freud also maintained repeatedly that the "dream *work*" is impervious to any kind of outside influence, be it from the analyst or any other quarter (S.E. 1916, 15: 238; 1923, 19: 114). Jones (1955: 221) relates Freud's reactions to a telling criticism of this thesis:

> He discussed the objection raised that the dreams of a patient often depended on which analyst he attended, that there was a similarity in the dreams of a given analyst's patients. This also may happen, but the inference sometimes drawn from it was again due to the same confusion between manifest and latent content. Remarks made by an analyst could often be the stimulus to a dream, just as those made by anyone else or, for that matter, any bodily stimulus. But how the patient's dream-making activity worked up such stimuli was a purely internal matter that was not susceptible to any outside influence.

But, as Rosemarie Sand has remarked, the immunity of the dream work to outside influence claimed by Freud and Jones is incompatible with the avowed malleability of the *manifest* dream content by external influences; for the dream work is the machinery that produces the manifest dream from the latent content, and any outside influence on the manifest content must clearly be effected by means of the dream work. Thus, even if the latent content were entirely endogenous, this would not assure that its transformation into the manifest content is similarly endogenous.

We can now conclude our appraisal of the clinical credentials of the dream theory by making a deferred comment on the qualification to which Freud was driven in his "Revision of the Theory of Dreams" (S.E. 1933, 22: 28-30). As he sees it there, he had "completely disposed of" the ever-recurring "lay" objection that anxiety dreams refute his wish-fulfillment hypothesis. He adds that "punishment-dreams, too, are fulfillments of wishes, though not of wishes of the instinctual impulses but of those of the critical, censoring and punishing agency in the mind [the superego]" (p. 27). But then he notes that two, and "only two," serious difficulties have arisen for the wish-fulfillment theory. Of these, only one seems insurmountable to him, and it is posed by the dreams of the victims of traumatic hysteria.

Those afflicted by this neurosis—for example, soldiers who endured a severe psychical trauma in combat— *regularly* relive their traumatic experiences in their dreams. "What wishful impulse," Freud asks, "could be satisfied by harking back in this [recurrent] way to this exceedingly distressing traumatic experience?" Hence, he acknowledges: "According to our hypotheses about the function of dreams this should not occur" (p. 28). Furthermore:

We should not, I think, be afraid to admit that here the function of the dream has failed. . . . But no doubt the exception does not overturn the rule. You can say nevertheless that a dream is an *attempt* at the fulfillment of a wish. In certain circumstances a dream is only able to put its intention into effect very incompletely, or must abandon it entirely. Unconscious fixation to a trauma seems to be foremost among these obstacles to the function of dreaming. [p. 29].

From the standpoint of our earlier strictures on the wish-fulfillment hypothesis, this important, if limited, modification is only to be welcomed, for the dreams of the war neurotics are chronic and intense anxiety dreams. And, for the reasons I have stated, I claim that Freud never succeeded in rebutting the "lay" objection to his handling of ordinary, nonchronic anxiety dreams. One is all the more disappointed by Ernest Jones's (1957: 269) lame attempt to show that even the dreams of the war neurotics may well not require Freud's qualification after all:

It may be pointed out, however, that none of these dreams were quite confined to an accurate presentation of the traumatic experience. One always found in them some other irrelevant feature which called for analysis, and which may well have signified a tendency to manipulate the traumatic memory in the direction of a wish-fulfillment, even if the patient waked in terror before this could be accomplished. Indeed it would seem possible to bring all the examples mentioned above under the broad tendency of abreaction.

So much for the clinical credentials of the dream theory, which was predicated epistemically on the purported imperviousness of the products of free association to the analyst's suggestive influence.

Besides attributing such freedom from adulteration to the analysand's associative output, Freud maintained that there is even some safeguard against the patient's compliant assent to the analyst's interpretations: "in general the arousing of resistances is a guarantee against the misleading effects of suggestive influence" (S.E. 1923, 18: 251). But what is Freud's evidence that the patient's resistance in actually a guarantee against the regimentation of the analysand's responses by suggestion from his doctor? It can readily be granted that the patient's resistance prevents his uncritical, *automatic* acceptance of *all* of the analyst's interpretations. But, as Freud himself conceded some years later (S.E. 1937, 23: 257-265), this fact can hardly assure that when there is such acceptance after the resistance has been *overcome*, the given interpretation may be presumed correct and hence uncontaminated; for after resisting initially, the patient may acquiesce in a false interpretation after all. Besides, the docility of patients *even under free association*, which the analyst Marmor (1970: 161) adduced to argue for the *self-fulfilling* function of clinical hypotheses, likewise impugns Freud's reliance on patient resistance as a safeguard against spurious validation.

That the patient's acceptance can hardly vouch for lack of distortion by the analyst is attested by the following summary:

Research evidence has consistently indicated that a patient's belief in interpretations and his consequent anxiety reduction do *not* depend on the accuracy of the interpretations. Investigators have found that individuals will enthusiastically accept bogus interpretations as accurate descriptions of their own personalities. [Fisher and Greenberg 1977: 364]

For example, aggressive people accept descriptions of themselves as being shy. As these authors note further:

In fact, Heller [reference omitted] points out that therapy systems emphasizing ambiguity and limited therapist responsiveness (such as analysis) create situations that are the most susceptible to the subtle interpersonal influence described in the studies of verbal conditioning. [pp. 363-364]

This seems to me to belie what I call "the myth of catalyticity" espoused by those analysts who conceptualize themselves as quite *non*directively interpretative: they see themselves as mere catalysts, expeditors of the unadulterated emergence of repressions previously bottled up by the walls of censorship.

The spuriousness of clinical confirmation in psychoanalysis is *not* lessened by the now well-recognized fact that epistemological distortions are definitely *not* confined to the responses of patients undergoing psychotherapy. Expectations entertained by *experimental* psychologists can strongly color their purported observational findings even in tests of the learning skills of laboratory rats (Shapiro and Morris 1978: 382-383). Yet psychologist Robert Rosenthal (1976: part 2, sec. 19-24) and others have provided careful accounts of how to *control* for experimenter expectancy effects. Nonetheless, the need for vigilance in regard to expectancy effects has been heeded less often than one would like. Thus, as Merrilee Salmon has pointed out to me, Bertrand Russell (1960: 32-33) declared himself discouraged because studies of animal learning have yielded the following results:

All the animals that have been carefully observed have behaved so as to confirm the philosophy in which the observer believes before his observations began. Nay, more, they have all displayed the national characteristics of the observer. Animals studied by Americans rush about frantically, with an incredible display of hustle and pep, and at last achieve the desired result by chance.

Animals observed by Germans sit still and think, and at last evolve the solution out of their inner consciousness.

In any case, one wonders how Freud could have persuaded himself to put much stock in patient resistance as insurance against adulteration by suggested compliance. For he himself maintained that when the patient's transference toward the analyst is positive, "it clothes the doctor with authority and is transformed into belief in his communications and explanations" (S.E. 1917, 16: 445). Interestingly, Freud's aforecited reliance on patient resistance is introduced by the following tribute to the analyst's purported ability to winnow the bona fide memories from the fancied ones: "Any danger of falsifying the products of the patient's memory by suggestion can be avoided by prudent handling of the technique" (S.E. 1923, 18: 251). But this particular assurance is especially unconvincing. Clearly the clinical authentication of the etiologically relevant early history in the lives of psychoneurotics must largely rely on the adult patient's memories of *infantile* and *childhood* experiences, and such early memories are surely more fragile epistemically than ordinary recollections from adult life! This is so especially since the analyst is doing exactly what a cross-examining attorney is forbidden to do in the courtroom: leading the witness. Freud makes no bones about this particular feature of analysis:

The treatment is made up of two parts — what the physician infers and tells the patient, and the patient's working-over of what he has heard. The mechanism of our assistance is easy to understand: we give the patient the conscious anticipatory idea [the idea of what he may expect to find] and he then finds the repressed unconscious idea in himself on the basis of its similarity to the anticipatory one. This is the intellectual help which makes it easier for him to overcome the resistances between conscious and unconscious [S.E. 1910, 11: 141-142; see also 1910, 11: 225-226, for further details]

Freud does not specify just how the "prudent handling of the technique," which he claims to have exercised in the psychoanalytic quest for the recovery of repressed memories (S.E. 1923, 18: 251), actually provided a safeguard against the suggestive elicitation of pseudo-memories ("paramnesias").

It can be granted, of course, that requirements of consistency or at least overall coherence do afford the analyst *some* check on what the patient alleges to be bona fide memories. But Freud's own writings attest to the untrustworthiness of purported adult memories of early childhood episodes that had presumably been repressed in the interim and then retrieved by analysis (see the documentation in Grünbaum

1980: 353). And as we had prior occasion to note, he conceded that even reliance on the slender reed of the patient's recall is sometimes disappointingly unavailable: "The patient cannot remember the whole of what is repressed in him, and what he cannot remember may be precisely the essential part of it" (S.E. 1920, 18: 18; see also 1937, 23: 265-266). To fill just this lacuna, the patient simply has to take the analyst's word for the soundness of the reconstruction of his past. Indeed, the malleability of adult memories from childhood is epitomized by a report from Jean Piaget (Loftus 1980: 119-121), who thought he vividly remembered an attempt to kidnap him from his baby carriage along the Champs Elysées. He recalled the gathered crowd, the scratches on the face of the heroic nurse who saved him, the policeman's white baton, the assailant running away. However vivid, Piaget's recollections were false. Years later the nurse confessed that she had made up the entire story, which he then internalized as a presumed experience under the influence of an authority figure. Yet, writing about Leonardo da Vinci's memories from childhood, Freud declared:

What someone thinks he remembers from his childhood is not a matter of indifference; as a rule the residual memories — which he himself does not understand — cloak priceless pieces of evidence about the most important features in his mental development. [S.E. 1910, 11: 84]

The early Freud had even been sanguine enough to declare that if he ever were to alter or falsify the reproduction of memories, or the connection of events, "it would inevitably have been betrayed in the end by some contradiction in the material" (S.E. 1895, 2: 295). Hence, he concluded insouciantly: "We need not be afraid, therefore, of telling the patient what we think his next connection of thought is going to be. It will do no harm"!

Apparently the analyst cannot justly claim to be a mere neutral expeditor or catalyst for the recovery of memories that can be *intra*clinically certified as authentic by virtue of his "prudent handling of the technique." Indeed, the help-seeking patient may well sense that the analyst expects confirmation of a conjecture by a memory, and the knowledge, authority, and help-giving potential he attributes to the analyst may well serve to make him compliant, no less than his desire to gain the analyst's approval qua parental surrogate. Such approval or disapproval manifests itself through the myriads of subtle nonverbal cues present in human communication.

That psychoanalytic treatment ought not to be regarded as a bona fide *memory-jogging* device emerges more generally as a corollary of at least three sets of recent research findings elaborated by Loftus (1980):

(1) the remarkable extent to which human memory is malleable, (2) the interpolative reconstruction and bending of memories by theoretical beliefs or expectations, and (3) the penchant, under the influence of leading questions, to fill amnesiac gaps by confabulated material. As for the first point, people have pseudomemories for events that never occurred (Loftus 1980: chap. 3). For example, under the influence of racial stereotypes, some experimental subjects who were shown a picture of several people on a subway car—including a black man with a hat and a white man with a razor in his hand—claimed to remember seeing the razor in the hands of the black man (Loftus 1980: 39).

The tendency characterized under the second point arises from taking various fragments of experiences and filling in details under the guidance of all sorts of suppositions, so as to create a new distorted or even fictitious "memory" (pp. 40, 76). As Loftus summarizes the evidence:

Human remembering does not work like a videotape recorder or a movie camera. When a person wants to remember something he or she does not simply pluck a whole memory intact out of a "memory store." The memory is constructed from stored and available bits of information; any gaps in the information are filled in unconsciously by inferences. When these fragments are integrated and make sense, they form what we call a memory. [p. 163]

Finally, Loftus's discussion (chap. 8) of confabulation in response to leading questions is likewise germane. For example, when people are asked to point out a previously seen culprit in a police lineup, worthless identifications can result in this *recognition test* unless care is taken *not* to steer them suggestively to a particular individual in the lineup. I claim that such pitfalls of memory-based recognition tests lurk even more when an analytic patient is asked to draw on his memory to *test* an interpretation offered him by his analyst. Such a memory test normally does *not* match the features of a *well*-designed police lineup recognition test, for the therapist tends to favor his own interpretations of the analysand's past, and this attitude will typically not be lost on the patient.

In this part of my essay, I have addressed the following key question: "Are clinical data probatively cogent even if uncontaminated?" Let us pause to recapitulate the results obtained so far from our endeavor to deal with that issue. In the first place, I argued that even if "free" association were actually free, the clinical responses yielded by it could validate neither the repression etiology of the psychoneuroses, nor the psychoanalytic theory of dreams, nor even Freud's theory of parapraxes. Yet Freud claimed just such clinical validation for these core hypotheses of his entire psychoanalytic enterprise, each of which is founded on the notion of compromise formations engendered by repressions. But in the second place, I canvassed solid evidence for the considerable epistemic contamination of three major kinds of clinical findings that Freud deemed either initially exempt from such adultera-tion or certifiably unmarred by it because of due precautions: the products of "free" association, the patient's assent to analytic interpre-tations that he or she had initially resisted, and memories recovered from early life.

Indeed, the epistemic adulteration I have documented seems to be *ineradicable* in just those patient responses that are supposed to lay bare repressions and disguised defenses after resistances have been over-come. Yet Freud attributed pride of place to these very data in the validation of his theory of repression, a doctrine that is avowedly "the cornerstone on which the whole structure of psychoanalysis rests, . . . the most essential part of it" (S.E. 1914, 14: 16). Thus, generally speaking, clinical findings—in and of themselves—forfeit the proba-tive value that Freud had claimed for them, although their potential heuristic merits may be quite substantial. To assert that the contamina-tion of intraclinical data is *ineradicable* without extensive and essential recourse to *extra*clinical findings is *not*, of course, to declare the auto-matic falsity of any and every analytic interpretation that gained the patient's assent by means of prodding from the analyst. But it *is* to maintain—to the great detriment of intraclinical testability!—that, in general, the epistemic devices confined to the analytic setting cannot reliably *sift* or decontaminate the clinical data so as to *identify* those that qualify as probative.

Though I have given an epistemic critique of the basic pillars of psychoanalysis, one might ask: why does my critique anachronistically focus on Freud's reasoning to the exclusion of the modifications and elaborations by those post-Freudians whose doctrines are recognizably psychoanalytic in content rather than only in name? Latter-day psy-choanalytic theoreticians that come to mind are the very influential Heinz Kohut, who pioneered the so-called "self-psychology," and the so-called "object-relations" theorists, who include not only the leading Otto Kernberg but also Harry Guntrip, W.R.D. Fairbairn, Donald Winnicott, and others. Thus, Heinz Kohut's "self-psychology," for example, downgrades Freud's Oedipal, *instinctual* factors in favor of even earlier, *environmental* ones as the sources of the purported *uncon-scious* determinants of personality structure (see Ornstein 1978; Meyers 1981: Basch 1980: chap. 11). More generally, insofar as these post-Freudian neo-revisionist theories are indeed recognizably psychoanalytic, they do of course embrace some version of the repression etiology. Furthermore, they rely epistemically on free association in the clinical investigation of purported pathogens and other unconscious determinants of behavior, and lift repressions to effect therapy.

But, I submit, precisely to the extent that these outgrowths of Freud's ideas are thus recognizably psychoanalytic in content as well as in method of inquiry and therapy, my epistemic critique of Freud's original hypotheses applies with equal force to the etiologic, developmental, and therapeutic tenets of these successors. How, I ask, for example, can Kohut possibly claim better validation for his species of unconscious determinants than Freud can for the sexual ones? Moreover, it is just ludicrous to pretend with Flax (1981: 564) that my focus on Freud in appraising psychoanalytic theory epistemically is akin to the anachronistic procedure of "throwing out physics because there are unresolved problems in Newton's theory," for this purported analogy suggests misleadingly that the epistemic difficulties that beset Freud's original formulations have been overcome by the much-vaunted post-Freudian formulations of neo-revisionist theory. It overlooks, as well, the logical incompatibility of the most influential of these versions: as Robbins (1980: 477) points out, Kohut's and Kernberg's views are "fundamentally antagonistic" to one another, being rooted in a schism between Melanie Klein and W.R.D. Fairbairn.

Indeed, there is not even agreement among the post-Freudians in regard to the probative value that may be assigned to *the same case-study material*: while Kohut claimed clinical support for his theory from his reanalysis of Mr. Z.—a patient whose prior analysis had been traditional—the contemporary Chicago analyst Gedo (1980: 382) harshly discounts the scientific quality of Kohut's case-study material, and he concludes that the "theoretical inferences" drawn by Kohut from his clinical observations "fail to carry scientific conviction." A similarly negative assessment is reached by the psychoanalytic psychologist F. J. Levine (1979), an ardent exponent of psychoanalytic methods of investigation and therapy. Ferguson (1981: 135-136), however, believes that Kohut's case history of Mr. Z. is "a crystalline example of the *fact* that a progressive theory change [in L. Laudan's sense] has taken place in psychoanalysis." But Ferguson then seems to damn it with faint praise, saying "the case of Mr. Z. provides something of a 'confirming instance' of the new theory." For all of the fundamental defects of Freud's clinical arguments, their caliber and amenability to scrutiny is mind-boggling as compared to the reasoning of these neo-revisionist epigoni, let alone of their apologists (Eagle, in press).

No wonder that the psychodynamically oriented psychologists

Fisher and Greenberg (1977: ix) reached the following verdict: "The diversity of the secondary elaborations of Freud's ideas is so Babel-like as to defy the derivation of sensible deductions that can be put to empirical test." For this reason alone, it will be most useful to focus the remainder of this essay on Freud's own formulations.

One must admire the strenuous and ingenious efforts made by Freud to legitimate his psychoanalytic method by arguing that it could *sift* clinical data so as to identify reliably those that are authentically probative. As we saw, these efforts included the attempt to vouchsafe the probity of free associations by secluding their *contents* in the bastion of *internal* causal relatedness, and his dialectical exertions culminated in the generic underwriting of clinical investigations by the Tally Argument. The NCT premise of this argument, we recall, was also to furnish the basis for a fundamental differentiation in regard to the *dynamics* of therapy between psychoanalysis, on the one hand, and *all* purely suggestive therapies, on the other. Hence, I submit that Freud's explicit avowal of this premise in his famous 1909 case of phobic Little Hans provides a *coherent rationale* for disregarding his seemingly equivocal, question-begging, and evasive handling of the suggestibility problem in that very case history (S.E. 1909, 10: 104-106, 120-121). There he *seems* to vacillate by adopting alternative postures as follows: (1) disclaiming the scientific reliability of patient assent and being content to secure practical therapeutic benefit, on the one hand (p. 104), and fairly soon thereafter, (2) excusing therapeutic failure by appeal to scientific gain, on the other (pp. 120-121).

If Freud's NCT were true, so that only veridical insight would have been dependably psychotherapeutic, that state of affairs would have been a tribute to the efficacy of human rationality fully on a par with the fact that "knowledge is power." And it would have supplied a rationale for the fact, reported by one of the pioneers of behavior therapy (Wolpe 1981), that analytic treatment still continues to dominate the clinical field in the United States, and that the teaching of psychotherapy is largely under the control of psychodynamically oriented clinicians. But the empirical untenability of the cardinal premise of the Tally Argument has issued in the latter's collapse, leaving intraclinical validation defenseless against all of the skeptical inroads from the massive evidence for the distortion and tailoring of its data by the mechanisms we have depicted.

Oblivious to the import of the whole array of doubts I have marshaled against Freud's NCT, Flax (1981: 566) sees herself entitled to reiterate NCT blithely as follows:

The only way to undo distorted relations with others is to reexperience them in a context in which the consequences of these relations are acted out [in the transference], can be interpreted [psychoanalytically!] and worked through [in the transference]. . . . But transference love and rational insight [as predicated on psychoanalytic etiology] are necessary for the patient's emancipation.

Indeed, despite my documentation of Freud's own keen appreciation of the *epistemic* challenge from suggestibility, his lifelong concern with this reproach was totally lost on Flax, who writes:

All the phenomena that Grünbaum counts as the clinical liabilities of psychoanalysis on empiricist grounds — epistemic contamination (i.e. [*sic*] intersubjectivity), suggestion, the placebo effect, etc. — are essential parts of the analytic process. Far from being liabilities, they are evidence that object-relations theory is correct. [pp. 566-567]

Here she completely fails to comprehend that precisely by being a *therapeutic* asset, the patient's transference attachment to the analyst may well be an *epistemic* liability for the purported clinical validation of the analytic theory of personality (S.E. 1917, 16: 446-447)! As Freud himself put this ominous challenge:

There is a risk that the influencing of our patient may make the objective certainty of our findings doubtful. What is advantageous to our therapy is damaging to our researches [i.e., damaging to the clinical validation of the general psychoanalytic theory of personality]. [S.E. 1917, 16: 452]

Believing he had met just this challenge by means of his NCT, Freud thought that he was warranted in confining the therapeutic role of suggestion in psychoanalytic treatment to that of a mere *catalyst* ("vehicle"). Hence, he declared: "It is perfectly true that psychoanalysis, like other psychotherapeutic methods, employs the instrument of suggestion (or transference). But the difference is this: that in analysis it is not allowed to play the decisive part in determining the therapeutic results" (S.E. 1925, 20: 43). Yet, as I was at great pains to explain in an earlier article (Grünbaum 1980: section 2), just this reply of Freud's to the charge of placebogenesis was gravely undermined by the demise of his NCT. Astonishingly enough, Flax simply ignores this damaging fact.

To boot, Flax (1981: 563) makes light of epistemic contamination by claiming that, in *every* field of inquiry, "All data are epistemically contaminated." But this reliance on a *tu quoque* argument is specious: while all data are indeed more or less theory-laden, their mere theory-ladenness hardly assures their *spurious confirmation* of the pertinent theory in the manner of a self-fulfilling prediction. Thus, Flax simply equivocates on the term "epistemic contamination," for she pretends that the mere theory-ladenness of a perceptual datum in any of the sciences is on a par with the spurious kind of confirmation by sugges- tion employed for psychoanalytic hypotheses, which even the analyst Marmor (1962: 289) decried as "self-validating." As will be recalled, Marmor did so by pointing to the striking effects of the analyst's communicated expectations on the character of the patient's clinical responses. Von Eckardt (1981: 572) has offered further telling objections to Flax's shoddy arguments.

In any case, since no viable substitute for the Tally Argument appears to be in sight, it is *unavailing* to take contaminated findings from the psychoanalytic interview more or less at face value, and then to try to employ them probatively in some testing strategy whose *formal* struc- ture is rational enough as such. Indeed, the seeming ineradicability of epistemic contamination in the clinical data adduced as support for the cornerstones of the psychoanalytic edifice may reasonably be presumed to doom any prospects for the cogent intraclinical testing of the major tenets espoused by Freud. Moreover, the clinical testing of *etiologic* hypotheses has *further* difficulties of its own.

These considerations can now be brought to bear in scrutiny of Glymour's defense of clinical testability, which was outlined in the first section of this essay.

CAN THE REPRESSION – ETIOLOGY OF PSYCHONEUROSIS BE TESTED RETROSPECTIVELY?

Glymour gives an illuminating reconstruction of Freud's account of the Rat Man case by means of the logical pincer-and-bootstrap strategy, which Glymour had teased out of that account. I have no reason to gainsay this strategy in general as far as it goes. But I shall now argue that, with or without it, strong reasons militate against the intraclinical testability of the specific etiologic hypothesis at issue in the case of the Rat Man, Paul Lorenz, who suffered from an obsessional fear of rats.

At the time of the Rat Man case, Freud had postulated that prema- ture sexual activity, such as excessive masturbation, subjected to severe repression is the specific cause of obsessional neurosis. As will be recalled from an earlier section, in his carefully defined usage of "specific cause," the claim that X is the specific cause of Y entails unilaterally that X is causally *necessary* for Y. The latter, in turn, unilaterally entails that all cases of Y were Xs. Thus, if *this particular consequence* of the conjectured sexual etiology is to get confirmation from Lorenz's psychoanalysis, the intraclinical data yielded by it need to be able to certify the following: Lorenz, who was an adult victim of obsessional neurosis, engaged in precocious sexual activity that was then repressed. Hence, let us inquire, first, whether intraclinical data produced by the adult patient can *reliably* attest the actual occurrence of a childhood event of the stated sort. But, as I shall argue, even if the answer to this question were positive, this much would be quite insufficient to support Freud's etiologic hypothesis that repressed precocious sexual activity is *causally relevant* to adult obsessional neurosis.

As Glymour (1980: 272) notes, "Freud had . . . arrived at a retrodicted state of affairs, namely, the patient's having been punished by his father for masturbation." Indeed, "the crucial question is whether or not Lorenz was in fact punished by his father for masturbation" (p. 273). But Freud's specific etiology of adult obsessional neurosis as such calls only for an early childhood event in which precocious sexual activity was repressed. Why, then, should it be probatively "crucial" whether it was the patient's *father* who was involved in the sexual event required by the hypothesized etiology?

As is clear from Freud's account, the elder Lorenz's involvement became probatively weighty, because of the unconscious significance that psychoanalytic theory assigns to the patient's recollection of recurring fears of his father's death, at least after the age of six. While having these fears, the child Paul bore his father deep conscious affection. Freud derived the presumed unconscious origin of the fears from a theoretical postulate of so-called precise contrariety, which he took pains to communicate to the patient, who then became "much agitated at this and very incredulous" (S.E. 1909, 10: 180). Freud both explains his reasoning and revealingly relates his indoctrination of the patient:

He was quite certain that his father's death could never have been an object of his desire but only of his fear. — After his forcible enunciation of these words I thought it advisable to bring a fresh piece of theory to his notice. According to psycho-analytic theory, I told him, every fear corresponded to a former wish which was now repressed; we were therefore obliged to believe the exact contrary of what he had asserted. This would also fit in with another theoretical requirement, namely, that the unconscious must be the precise contrary of the conscious. — He was much agitated at this and very incredulous. He wondered how he could possibly have had such a wish, considering that he loved his father more than any one else in the world. . . . I answered that it was precisely such intense love as his that was the necessary precondition of the repressed hatred. (S.E. 1909, 10: 179-180)

Having thus theoretically inferred the patient's deep childhood grudge against his father from the recurring fears of losing the father, Freud also conjectured that the grudge remained so durably unconscious only because it was a response to the father's interference with the patient's sensual gratification.

This conclusion was, then, serendipitous by suggesting that there had been an early event satisfying the specific etiology that Freud had hypothesized for Lorenz's obsessional neurosis. Since this etiology required precocious masturbation events, Freud retrodicted that the patient had been punished by his father for masturbation "in his very early childhood... before he had reached the age of six" (S.E. 1909, 10: 183). Clearly, the actual occurrence of an event having these attributes would *simultaneously* satisfy the initial condition of the postulated etiology and explain Lorenz's early dread of his father's death via Freud's principle of precise contrariety.

Let us now suppose, just for argument's sake, that Freud's avowedly well-coached adult patient had actually reported having a memory of the very early childhood event that Freud had retrodicted. Then I ask: could such a clinical event have reliably attested the actual occurrence of the distant event? I have framed this question hypothetically, because it so happened that Lorenz actually had no *direct* memory of any physical punishment by his father, let alone of a punishment for a *sexual* offense. He did remember having been *told* repeatedly by his *mother* that there had been *one* incident of angry conflict with his father at age three or four, when he was beaten by him. When the mother was consulted about whether this beating had been provoked by a misdeed of a sexual nature, her answer was negative. Furthermore, this was apparently the *only* beating the child had ever received from the father.

But for the purpose of our inquiry, we are positing that, at some point in his analysis, the patient had claimed to remember just the kind of early childhood event that Freud had retrodicted via his specific etiology of obsessional neurosis. Then I am concerned to show that, taken by itself, such a finding would be quite insufficient to lend any significant support to the hypothesized etiology of obsessional neurosis. My reasons for this claim will then enable me to argue quite generally for the following conclusion: given the demise of the Tally Argument, the intraclinical testing of the causal assertions made by Freud's specific etiologies of the psychoneuroses, and by his ontogenetic developmental hypotheses, is *epistemically quite hopeless*!

Let "N" (neurosis) denote a psychoneurosis such as the syndrome of obsessional neurosis, and let "P" (pathogen) denote the kind of sex-related antecedent event that Freud postulated to be the specific cause of N. Thus, I shall say that a person who had a sexual experience of the sort P "is a P," and if that person was then afflicted by N, I shall say that he was both a P and an N, or just a PN. It is taken for granted, of course, that *there are* both Ns and non-Ns, as well as Ps and non-Ps. To support Freud's etiologic hypothesis that P is causally necessary for N, evidence must be produced to show that being a P *makes a difference* to being an N. But such causal relevance is *not* attested by *mere* instances of Ns that were Ps, i.e., by patients who are both Ps and Ns. For even a large number of such cases does not preclude that just as many *non-Ps* would also become Ns, if followed in a horizontal study from childhood onward! Thus, instances of Ns that were Ps may just *happen* to have been Ps. Then being a P has no etiologic role at all in becoming an N. A telling, sobering illustration of this moral is given by the following conclusion from a review of forty years of research (Frank 1965: 191):

No factors were found in the parent-child interaction of schizophrenics, neurotics, or those with behavior disorders which could be identified as unique to them or which could distinguish one group from the other, or any of the groups from the families of the [normal] controls.

Hence, it is insufficient evidence for causal relevance that any N who turns out to have been a P does instantiate the retrodiction "All Ns were Ps," which is entailed by Freud's specific etiology. Thus, to provide evidence for the causal relevance claimed by Freud, we need to *combine* instances of Ns that were Ps with instances of non-Ps who are *non-Ns*. Indeed, since he deemed P to be causally necessary for N — rather than just causally relevant — his etiology requires that the class of non-Ps should not contain *any* Ns whatever, and the class of Ps is to have a positive (though numerically unspecified) incidence of Ns.

One can grant that since "All Ns are/were Ps" is logically equivalent to "All non-Ps are/will be non Ns," any case of an N who was a P will support the latter to whatever extent it supports the former. But this fact is unavailing to the support of Freud's etiology, for the issue is *not* merely to provide evidential support for "All non-Ps are/will be non-Ns," or for its logical equivalent, by some instance or other. Instead, the issue is to furnish evidential support for the (strong kind of) *causal relevance* claimed by Freud. But, for the reasons I have given, the fulfillment of that requirement demands that there be cases of non-Ps that are non-Ns, no less than instances of Ns that were Ps. Yet *at best*, the Rat Man could furnish only the *latter* kind of instance. In other words, if we are to avoid committing the fallacy of *post hoc ergo propter hoc*, we cannot be content with instances of Ns that were Ps, no matter how numerous. Analogously, suppose it were hypothesized that drinking coffee is causally relevant to overcoming the common cold. Consider, too, the case of a recovered cold sufferer who turns out to have been drinking coffee while still afflicted by the cold. Then such an instance, taken by itself, would hardly qualify as *supportive* of the hypothesized causal relevance.

Psychoanalytic theory and therapy have encouraged the disregard and even flouting of the elementary safeguards against the pitfalls of causal inference familiar since the days of Francis Bacon, not to speak of J. S. Mill. Yet even informed laymen in our culture are aware that such safeguards are indeed heeded *in medicine* before there is public assent to the validity of such etiologic claims as "heavy tobacco smoking causes cardiovascular disease." This double standard of evidential rigor in the validation of etiologic hypotheses even makes itself felt in current criminal law. Thus legal prohibitions—and so-called expert psychiatric testimony in courts of law—are sometimes predicated on such hypotheses even when they are no better than articles of faith given credence through blithe repetition. The recently publicized reiteration of the purported pathogenicity of child molestation in opposition to its decriminalization is a case in point. (A wealth of *other* documentation on the *unwarranted legal use* of purported psychiatric expertise predicated on theories of unconscious motivations is given by S. J. Morse [in press; 1982].)

In our society, the sexual molestation of children is often alleged to be pathogenic, even when it is affectionate and tender rather than violent. This allegation has been invoked to justify making such behavior illegal and fraught with substantial penalties. Yet recently, a number of sexologists have maintained that very young children should be allowed, and perhaps even encouraged, to have sex with adults, unencumbered by interference from the law. In their view, such activity itself is harmless to the child and becomes harmful only when parents raise a fuss about it. Indeed, *some* of these advocates have made the daring and quite unfashionable etiologic claim that unless children do have early sex, their psychological development will go awry. Even the less daring champions of harmlessness are opposed to jailing affectionate pedophiles.

Reasons of elementary prudence and also of humaneness make it a good policy, in my view, to put the burden of proof on those who maintain that affectionate and tender child molestation is *not* distressing to the child, let alone pathogenic. But a cautionary basis for a legal prohibition is a far cry from the confident assertion of demonstrated pathogenicity, and the difference between mere caution and authenticated causation of neurosis may, of course, be relevant to the severity of the punishment appropriate for violations of the interdiction.

In a recent issue of *Time* magazine, John Leo (1981: 69) inveighs etiologically *against* the demand to legalize tender pedophilia, which he sees as a thinly disguised manifesto for child-molesters' liberation. The justification offered by him for his indictment is as follows:

Unfortunately, few responsible child experts have reacted...so far to the radical writing on child sex. One who has is Child Psychiatrist Leon Eisenberg of Children's Hospital Medical Center, Boston: "Premature sexual behavior among children in this society almost always leads to psychological difficulties because you have a child acting out behavior for which he is not cognitively or emotionally ready."

Psychotherapist Sam Janus, author of a new book, *The Death of Innocence*, says that people who were seduced early in life "go through the motions of living and may seem all right, but they are damaged. I see these people year after year in therapy." U.C.L.A. Psychiatrist Edward Ritvo also says that much of his work is with children who have been involved in catastrophic sexual situations. His conclusion: "Childhood sexuality is like playing with a loaded gun."

But the etiologic reasoning of those whom Leo cites to document the pernicious effects of child molestation is just as shoddy as the causal inferences of those advocates of pedophilia who claim dire psychological consequences from the *failure* of infant boys to act on their erections, and of infant girls to utilize their vaginal lubrications. For the findings adduced by Leo do not answer either of the following two questions:

1. Is the occurrence of childhood seduction not equally frequent among those who are well enough never to see a psychotherapist? In the parlance of John Stuart Mill, this question calls for the use of the *joint* method of agreement and difference, rather than just the heuristic method of agreement.

2. Would a representative sample of those who were *not* seduced in childhood have a significantly *lower* incidence of adult neurosis than those who *were* seduced? By the same token, we must ask those who claim seduction to be *beneficial* psychologically to show that those who were indeed seduced *fared better* psychologically than those who were not sexually active in this way. Without the appropriate answers to these questions, the respective assertions of causal relevance remain gratuitous.

Thus, we must ask those who *condemn* childhood seduction the foregoing questions, because it may be that childhood seduction just *happens* to be quite common among neurotics, even though it has no etiologic role in the production of neurosis. In that case, the same people would have become neurotics anyway, without early seduction. Without answers to these questions, the evidence given by those whom Leo invokes as authorities merely suggests the bare *possibility* that childhood seduction is pathogenic. By the same token, psychoanalysts have overlooked that repressed homosexual feelings cannot be shown to be the pathogen of adult paranoia by merely pointing to the frequency of homosexually tinged themes in the associative output of paranoiacs during analysis. This finding does not tell us whether homosexual themes would not likewise turn up to the same extent in the so-called free associations of nonparanoiacs who lead well-adjusted lives and who never see a therapist. Here, no less than in the case of the Rat Man, the invocation of J. S. Mill's heuristic method of agreement is not enough to lend support to the hypothesis of etiologic relevance.

Hence, even if the Rat Man did in fact have the sexually repressive experience *P* retrodicted via Freud's etiology of obsessional neurosis, this alone would hardly qualify as evidential support for that etiology. And there is a further reason for concluding that even if the child Paul Lorenz had actually been punished by his father for masturbating, as retrodicted via Freud's etiology, this putative occurrence would confer little, if any, support on this etiology. For, as Ronald Giere has remarked (private communication), the occurrence of this sort of event is to be routinely expected in the Victorian child-rearing culture of the time on grounds *other than* psychoanalytic theory.

Moreover, Freud had made the adult Rat Man patient well aware, as we saw, of the inferences that Freud had drawn about his childhood via psychoanalytic theory. Given the massive evidence I adduced earlier for the notorious docility of patients in analysis, I submit that one ought to discount Lorenz's *putative* early childhood memory as too contaminated to attest reliably to the actual occurrence of the retrodicted early event. Such discounting is hardly a general derogation of the reliability of adult memories in ordinary life, but in the clinical context, the *posited* memory is simply not sufficiently dependable to qualify as evidence for the retrodicted event. Thus, the retrospective intraclinical ascertainment of the actual occurrence of the retrodicted distant event is just too unreliable. Furthermore, in general, the patient's memory may simply fail to recall whether the pertinent event did occur, as Freud himself stressed (S.E. 1920, 18: 18; 1937, 23: 265-66). Indeed, even in survey studies of lung cancer patients who are asked about their prior smoking habits, and of heroin addicts who are questioned about previous use of marijuana, the retrospective ascertainment of the actual occurrence of the suspected causal condition is epistemically flawed (Giere 1979: 216, 265).

Have I provided adequate grounds for maintaining that long-term *prospective* studies, which employ control groups and spring the clinical confines of the usual psychoanalytic setting, must supplant the *retrospective* clinical testing of etiology defended by Glymour? Not just yet. For suppose that analysts could secure reasonable numbers of patients who, though presumed to need analysis for some affliction or other, are certifiably free of the *particular* neurosis N (say, obsessional neurosis) whose etiology is currently at issue. Since neuroses usually occur in mixed rather than pure form, this is a generous assumption. All the same, let us operate with it. Then if we are given such patients who, though neurotic, are non-N, Freud's pertinent specific etiology does *not* retrodict whether patients of *this* sort were Ps or non-Ps. For his hypothesized pathogenesis allows given non-Ns to have been Ps no less than to have been non-Ps, although it does require any non-P to become a non-N. Now postulate, for argument's sake that, though retrospective, psychoanalytic inquiry *were* typically able to ascertain *reliably* whether a given case of non-N was indeed a non-P or a P. If so, then non-Ns who putatively turn out to have been Ps would merely be compatible with Freud's etiologic hypothesis instead of supporting it, since this hypothesis allows these instances without requiring them.

But what of patients who are *neither* Ns nor Ps? Would such people, together with other persons who are both Ns and Ps, jointly bespeak that P is pathogenic for N (*obsessional* neurosis) within the class of all persons?

Note that the clinical testing design I have envisaged for scrutiny is *confined* to the class of neurotics. For even the non-Ns of this design are presumed to be afflicted by some neurosis other than N. The reason is that persons who have practically no neuroses of any sort are hardly available to analysts in sufficient numbers to carry out the putative retrospective determination of whether they were non-Ps or Ps. But, as Mr. Blake Barley has noticed, the confinement of this retrospective clinical determination to the class of neurotics has the following consequence: Even if every observed non-N (non-obsessive neurotic) is a non-P while every observed N is a P, these combined instances lend credence only to the hypothesis that, *within* the class of neurotics, P is etiologically relevant to N. But these putative combined instances do not support the Freudian claim of such etiological relevance within the wide class of persons.

In short, the Freudian clinical setting does *not* have the epistemic resources to warrant that P is *neurotogenic*! And this unfavorable conclusion emerges even though it was granted, for argument's sake, that the retrospective methods of psychoanalytic inquiry can determine *reliably* whether adult neurotics who are non-obsessives were non-Ps in early life. But is it reasonable to posit such reliability? It would seem not.

For clearly, even if the patient believes he has the required memories, the retrospective clinical ascertainability of whether a given non-N was actually a non-P is epistemically on a par with the psychoanalytic determination of whether a given N was a P. And, as we saw, the latter is unreliable. Moreover, as Freud himself acknowledged: "The patient cannot remember the whole of what is repressed in him, and what he cannot remember may be precisely the essential part of it" (S.E. 1920, 18: 18).

Now contrast the stated epistemic liabilities of the retrospective psychoanalytic inference that a given adult patient was or was not a P during his early childhood with the assets of *prospective* controlled inquiry: a *present* determination would be made, under suitably supervised conditions, whether children in the experimental and control groups are Ps and non-Ps, respectively; again, during long-term follow-ups, later findings as to N or non-N would be gathered and would pertain to the then state.

Recently, experimental validations of therapeutic efficacy have been carried out by using the response history of single individuals *without* control groups drawn from other individuals (Hersen and Barlow 1976; Kazdin 1981; Kazdin forthcoming). Thus, in these validations, the *causal* claims inherent in the pertinent assertions of therapeutic efficacy have been validated by single-case experimental designs. Hence, it behooves us to ask whether these "*intra*subject" validations could become prototypic for using a given analysand to test *intra*clinically the causal assertions made by the long-term etiologic hypotheses of psychoanalytic theory and by such claims of efficacy as are made for its avowedly slow therapy. To answer this question, let us first look at situations in physics in which the *probative equivalent* of controlled experiments is furnished by other means.

When a billiard ball initially at rest on a billiard table suddenly acquires momentum upon being hit by another billiard ball, we are confident that the acceleration of the first ball results from the impact of the second. Even more strikingly, astronomers made sound causal claims about the motions of planets, binary stars, etc., before they were able to manipulate artificial earth satellites, moon probes, or interplanetary rockets. What took the probative place of control groups in these cases? In the case of the billiard ball, Newton's otherwise well-supported first law of motion gives us background knowledge as to the "natural history" of an object initially at rest that is not exposed to external forces: such an object will remain at rest. This information, or the law of conservation of linear momentum, enable us to point the finger at the moving second billiard ball to furnish the cause of the change in the momentum of the first. A similar reliance on otherwise attested background knowledge supplies the probative equivalent of experimental controls in the astronomical cases.

Turning to the *single*-case validations of therapeutic efficacy, they pertain to the following sort of instance:

A seven-year-old boy would beat his head when not restrained. His head was covered with scar tissue and his ears were swollen and bleeding. An extinction procedure was tried: the boy was allowed to sit in bed with no restraints and with no attention given to his self-destructive behavior. After seven days, the rate of injurious behavior decreased markedly, but in the interim the boy had engaged in over ten thousand such acts, thus making the therapists fearful for his safety. A punishment procedure was subsequently introduced in the form of one-second electric shocks. In a brief time, the shock treatment dramatically decreased the unwanted behavior. [Erwin 1978: 11-12]

Here the dismal prospects of an untreated autistic child are presumably known from the natural history of other such children. In the light of this presumed background knowledge, the dramatic and substantial behavior change ensuing shortly after electric shock, allowed the attribution of the change to the shock without control groups, for, under the circumstances, the operation of *other* causal agencies seems very unlikely. More generally, the *paradigmatic* example of an *intra*subject clinical validation of the causal efficacy of a given intervention is furnished by the following *variant* of using the single patient as his own "historical" control: (1) the natural history of the disorder is presumably otherwise known, *or* (2) the therapist intervenes only in on-off fashion, and this intermittent intervention is found to yield alternating remissions and relapses with dramatic rapidity.

Can the causal validation designs employed in these intrasubject clinical tests of therapeutic efficacy become prototypic for using an individual analysand to validate Freud's *long*-term etiologic hypotheses, or to furnish evidence that an analysis whose typical duration extends over several years deserves credit for any therapeutic gain registered by the patient after, say, four years? To ask the question is to answer it negatively. The natural history of a person *not* subjected to the experiences deemed pathogenic by Freudian theory is *notoriously* unknown! As for crediting therapeutic gain to analytic intervention on the basis of an intrasubject case history, how could such an attribution possibly be made in the face of Freud's own aforecited acknowledg-ment of the occurrence of *spontaneous* remissions? At best, Freudians can hope to show that the incidence of therapeutic gain in groups of patients who undergo analysis exceeds the spontaneous remission rate in untreated control groups belonging to the same nosologic category (Rachman and Wilson 1980). In short, the stated intrasubject validation by means of dramatic therapeutic gains can hardly be extrapolated to underwrite the prospective single-case evaluation of slow analytic therapy, let alone to vindicate the *retrospective* testing of a Freudian etiology in the course of an individual analysis.

Though Freud's specific etiologies did not specify numerically the percentage of Ps who become Ns, it is noteworthy that only prospec-tive investigation can yield the information needed for such a statistical refinement. For let us suppose that retrospective data confirm the retrodiction of Freud's specific etiology that the incidence of Ps within the sample group of Ns is 100 percent; then this incidence clearly does not permit an inference as to the percentage incidence of Ns within the class of Ps. Yet such information is clearly desirable, if only in order to estimate the probability that a child who was subjected to P will become an N. More generally, when P is not deemed causally neces-sary for N but merely causally relevant, retrospective data simply do not yield any estimates of P's degree of causal effectiveness (Giere 1979: 274, 277).

Our inquiry into the Rat Man case so far has operated with a *counterfactual* posit in order to discuss the reliability of clinical data in the context of this case. The *hypothetical* clinical datum we used was that the patient *had* reported having a memory of the early childhood event retrodicted by Freud. As against Glymour's generic thesis that the specific psychoanalytic etiologies can be cogently tested "on the couch," I have argued that, at least typically, such testing is epistemi-cally quite hopeless. Hence, it would seem that Paul Lorenz's psycho-analysis would have completely failed to furnish evidential support for the *etiologic relevance* of childhood sexual repression to obsessional neurosis, even if Paul's father had reliably reported having repeatedly punished his young son for masturbation. Incidentally, when Waelder (1962: 625-626) defended the clinical confirmation of the psychoana-lytic etiologies, he overlooked precisely that their substantiation requires evidential support for the *causal relevance* of the purportedly pathogenic experience, and not merely the historical authentication of the bare occurrence of that experience.

Let us return to Glymour's account of the testing strategy in Paul Lorenz's analysis, which was predicated on Lorenz's failure, in fact, to have any *direct* recall of receiving a punishment from his father, let alone a castigation for a sexual offense. Therefore, let us now see how Glymour evaluated the probative significance of this finding. I shall be concerned to stress the scope that Glymour does give to *essential* reliance on *extra*clinical data for probative purposes. Indeed, it will turn out that the entire testing procedure in the Rat Man case comes out to be probatively *parasitic* on an extraclinical finding. Hence, I wonder how Glymour imagines that he has rebutted Eysenck's denial of intraclinical testability, although he does succeed in impugning the demand that all extraclinical disconfirmation be *experimental*.

By Glymour's own account of the Rat Man case, the probatively "crucial" data came from the *extra*clinical testimony of the patient's mother. On Glymour's reading of Freud, at the time of Lorenz's analysis, Freud still postulated *actual* rather than fancied early sexual experiences to be the pathogens of obsessional neurosis (Glymour 1980: 274-275). As Glymour explains lucidly, what made Lorenz's case a *counterexample* to this etiology was *not* the mere failure of the patient to recall the event retrodicted by Freud. Instead, it was the *extra*clinical testimony from the *mother* that had this negative probative import (p. 273). For it was her testimony that supplied the probatively crucial datum by contravening Freud's retrodiction when she answered the question that Glymour characterized as "the crucial question." He himself characterizes "the memory of an adult observer" — in this case that of the mother — as "the most reliable available means" for answering this decisive question as to the character of the offense for which the child Paul had been punished (p. 273). How, then, in the face of the *extra*clinical status of the *decisive* datum, can Glymour justify his description of the testing rationale used in the Rat Man case as "a strategy that relies almost exclusively on clinical evidence" (Glymour 1974: 287)?

It is true enough that, as we know from the case history of the Wolf Man, Freud regarded stories told by older members of the family to the patient about the patient's childhood to be generally "absolutely authentic" and hence, admissible as data (S.E. 1918, 17: 14, n. 2). But Freud completes this assertion by cautioning that responses by relatives to pointed inquiries from the analyst — or from the patient while in analysis — may well be quite contaminated by misgivings on their part:

So it may seem tempting to take the easy course of filling up the gaps in a patient's memory by making enquiries from the older members of his family; but I cannot advise too strongly against such a technique. Any stories that may be told by relatives in reply to enquiries and requests are at the mercy of every critical misgiving that can come into play. One invariably regrets having made oneself dependent upon such information; at the same time confidence in the analysis is shaken and a court of appeal is set up over it. Whatever can be remembered at all will anyhow come to light in the further course of analysis. [S.E. 1918, 17: 14, n. 2]

In the same vein, the present-day analyst W. W. Meissner (1978: 155) writes: "Parental recollections are noteworthy for their propensity to distortion."

Even if one were to discount Freud's and Meissner's caveat, several facts remain: (1) It is misleading to claim intraclinical testability if, as in the Rat Man case, the avowedly crucial datum does *not* come from "the couch." (2) What makes the reliance on extraclinical devices important is that, far from being marginal epistemically, its imperativeness derives from the typically present probative defects of the analytic setting, defects that are quite insufficiently acknowledged by Glymour. And, in my view, it does not lessen the liabilities of intraclinical testing that the compensations for its deficits from *outside* the clinical setting *may occasionally* be available *in situ* (e.g., from family records) and thus do not necessarily have to require the experimental laboratory. For even when supplemented by such nonexperimental extraclinical devices, the thus enlarged "clinical" testing procedure is not adequate or epistemically autonomous. For example, when it becomes necessary to resort to extraclinical information for the sort of reason that was operative in the Rat Man case, it will be a matter of mere happenstance whether suitable relatives are even available, let alone whether they can *reliably* supply the missing essential information. Why, then, dignify as a "clinical testing strategy" a procedure of inquiry that depends on such contingent good fortunes and hence, when luck runs out, cannot dispense with experimental information? (3) The real issue is whether the clinical setting *typically* — rather than under contingently favorable circumstances — does have the epistemic resources for the cogent validation of the etiology at issue in the Rat Man case, and of other analytic etiologies. In dealing with that issue, Glymour's otherwise illuminating account has not demonstrated the existence of a cogent intraclinical testing strategy, even if he succeeded in showing that extraclinical compensations for its lacunae need not be wholly experimental.

Indeed, the extent of his essential epistemic reliance on extraclinical findings can now be gauged from his view of the effect that Freud's modifications of the specific sexual etiology of obsessional neurosis (and of other neuroses) had on the *testability* of these evolving etiologic hypotheses. Glymour (1980: 276-277) recounts this evolution:

After the turn of the century and before 1909, . . . there is no statement of the view that sexual phantasies formed in childhood or subsequently, having no real basis in fact, may themselves serve *in place of* sexual experiences as etiological factors. . . . Yet after the Rat Man case the view that either infantile sexual experiences *or* phantasies of them may equally serve as etiological factors became a standard part of Freud's theory. In *Totem and Taboo*, four years after the Rat Man case appeared, Freud emphasized that the guilt that obsessional neurotics feel is guilt over a happening that is physically real but need not actually have occurred [footnote omitted]. By 1917 Freud not only listed phantasies themselves as etiological factors alternative to real childhood sexual experiences, but omitted even the claim that the former are usually or probably based on the latter [footnote omitted]. The effect of these changes is to remove counterexamples like that posed by the Rat Man case, but at the cost of making the theory less easily testable. For whereas Freud's theories, until about 1909, required quite definite events to take place in the childhood of a neurotic, events that could be witnessed and later recounted by adults, Freud's later theory required no more than psychological events in childhood, events that might well remain utterly private.

Thus, Glymour attributes the diminishing testability of Freud's modified etiologies quite rightly to the lessening *extra*clinical ascertainability of the sorts of events that Freud successively postulated as etiologic. But if the testability of the psychoanalytic etiologies is in fact "almost exclusively" intraclinical, as Glymour told us, why should it be *vital* for their testability that the etiologic events required by Freud's later theory are just mental states of the patient to which only the patient himself and his analyst become privy?

Incidentally, the problem of testing Freud's sexual etiology of the neuroses—either clinically or extraclinically—became less well defined after he gave up the quest for qualitatively *specific* pathogens of nosologically distinct psychoneuroses in favor of a generic Oedipal etiology for all of them. In fact, he used the analogy of explaining the great qualitative differences among the chemical substances by means of quantitative variations in the proportions in which the same elements were combined. But having thus dissolved his prior long-standing concern with the problem of "the choice of neurosis," he was content to leave it at vague metapsychological remarks about the constant intertransformation of "narcissistic libido" and "object libido" (S.E. 1925, 20: 55-56).

What of Glymour's reliance on *intra*clinical data? In that context, he seems to have taken much too little cognizance of even the evidence furnished by analysts that intraclinically the suggestibility problem is radically unsolved, if not altogether insoluble, because there is no viable substitute for the defunct Tally Argument. Can we place any stock in Glymour's aforecited aspiration that "clinicians can hopefully be trained so as not to elicit by suggestion the expected responses from their patients"? In view of the evidence for the *ineradicability* of suggestive contamination, it would now seem that this hope is sanguine to the point of being quite utopian. In an afterword to his 1974 article published in a second edition of the Wollheim volume in which it first appeared, Glymour has reacted to some of these particular doubts as follows:

I do not see . . . that the experimental knowledge we now have about suggestibility requires us to renounce clinical evidence altogether. Indeed, I can imagine circumstances in which clinical evidence might have considerable force: when, for example, the clinical proceedings show no evident sign of indoctrination, leading the patient, and the like; when the results obtained fall into a regular and apparently law-like pattern obtained independently by many clinicians; and when those results are contrary to the expectation and belief of the clinician. I do not intend these as *criteria* for using clinical evidence, but only as indications of features which, in combination, give weight to such evidence.

To this I say the following:

1. I do *not* maintain that any and all clinical data are altogether irrelevant probatively. Instead, I hold that such findings cannot possibly bear the probative burden placed upon them by those who claim, as Glymour did, that psychoanalysis can *typically* be validated or invalidated "on the couch," using a clinical testing strategy that is mainly confined to the analytic setting.

2. The existence of *some* circumstances under which we would be warranted in not renouncing clinical evidence "altogether" is surely not enough to sustain clinical testing as a largely cogent and essentially autonomous scientific enterprise. As for Glymour's illustrations of such circumstances, I cannot see that absence of evident indoctrination, or regular concordance among the results obtained independently by many clinicians, exemplifies circumstances under which "clinical evidence might have considerable force." For—apart from the arguments I gave against these illustrations, if only à propos of "free" association—it seems to me that their utopian character as a step toward solving the compliance problem is epitomized by the following sobering results, which are reported by the analyst Marmor (1962: 289):

Depending upon the point of view of the analyst, the patients of each [rival psychoanalytic] school seem to bring up precisely the kind of phenomenological data which confirm the theories and interpretations of their analysts! Thus each theory tends to be self-validating. Freudians elicit material about the Oedipus Complex and castration anxiety, Jungians about archetypes, Rankians about separation anxiety, Adlerians about masculine strivings and feelings of inferiority, Horneyites about idealized images, Sullivanians about disturbed interpersonal relationships, etc.

3. I do not deny at all that *now and then* clinical results "are contrary to the expectations and belief of the clinician." But as a step toward vindicating clinical inquiry qua epistemically autonomous testing strategy, I can only say, "One swallow does not a summer make."

What seems to me to emerge from Glymour's interesting reconstruction is that, on the whole, data from the couch *acquire* probative significance when they are independently corroborated by extraclinical findings, or when they are inductively consilient with such findings in Whewell's sense of joint accreditation. Thus, I do not maintain that any and all clinical data are altogether irrelevant probatively. But this much only conditionally confers *potential* relevance on intraclinical results beyond their heuristic value, and surely this is not enough to vindicate testability on the couch in the sense claimed by its Freudian exponents, and countenanced by Glymour heretofore.

CLINICAL CREDENTIALS AND THE FUTURE APPRAISAL OF PSYCHOANALYTIC THEORY

Even some recognized analysts have largely conceded that the clinical method of investigation cannot be credited with normally yielding the kinds of veridical insights that analysts have traditionally been wont to claim for it in concert with Freud. Thus, in an avowedly "irreverent" article about the future of analysis, both as a theory and qua therapy, Kurt Eissler (1969: 462) writes:

As the model of what analysis of a neurosis should be, *qua* analysis of the infantile neurosis — the dissolution of which remains the ultimate goal of classical analysis — Freud's record of the Wolf Man's analysis has always impressed me as paradigmatic. The crux of that analysis was the reconstruction of the chief events and processes taking place during the infantile period. It is not a question here of speculating as to whether Freud was right or wrong in his reconstruction in that particular instance (he himself was ready to withdraw one part of it), but rather of the requirements that an analyst would have to fulfill if he were to attempt to live up to what Freud there outlined as a goal.

I am certain that a significantly high percentage of the interpretations offered today to patients in all parts of the world have to do with the infantile period. But I doubt that they are true reconstructions, in the sense in which Freud meant that activity. . . . When they have to do with a later stage of the infantile period, they are, I fear, in most instances either intellectualizations on the part of both the analyst as well as the patient, or else generalizations obtained by way of screen memories. It is not difficult, of course, to demonstrate to a patient that he once harboured aggressive feelings against a beloved father; but a true reconstruction goes beyond the mere unearthing of a hidden impulse and includes those specific details of time, place, environment and inner processes that conjoined to produce a trauma. Yet to take hold of these is a formidable task.

As Eissler emphasizes, this epistemic task is nearly Sisyphean, even if one abjures the usual ambitious therapeutic objectives, i.e., "even if the task of psychoanalysis is not considered—as the tendency is at present—extensive enough to include the restructuring of the personality, but is instead limited to the uprooting of the neurosis, with its deepgoing ramifications" (p. 462).

Speaking of the dream *laboratory*, Eissler points out that it is one of the *extra*clinical sources that has yielded "data that do not fit psychoanalytic theory in its present form" (p. 467). Then he gives another example bearing on the poverty of clinical data as *dis*confirmations:

Masters & Johnson [reference omitted] have proven that, during clitoridean orgasm, vaginal spasms occur that are identical with those that occur during vaginal orgasm. For obvious reasons, the psychoanalytic theory has been that absence of vaginal orgasm is caused by lack of vaginal responsiveness. In view of the new data, however, one has to say that such a lack is not due to any defect in physiological functioning but rather to a suppression of sensations that the organ itself is quite ready to provide. . . . Once again we encounter the situation we encountered in relation to the new data about the dream. The error in the previous theory was by no means caused by erroneous observation, for the relevant data could never have been derived from the psychoanalytic situation. [p. 468]

The moral he draws from these cases of extraclinical disconfirmation goes well beyond the particular analytic hypotheses to which they pertain: "The fact that observations that cannot be expected to be made in the psychoanalytic situation and are gained outside the psychoanalytic situation lead to data that require new psychoanalytic paradigms is of the greatest historical importance" (p. 467). Prognostically, Eissler sees this historical importance as follows: "The fact that the dream laboratory has introduced a paradox makes me more certain that the next phase of progress in psychoanalysis will come about through the supply of data obtained from outside the psychoanalytic situation proper" (p. 470). In short, the limitations of clinical *dis*confirmations are portentous and are even more significant than the liabilities of clinical confirmations.

Despite these exhortations to expand the investigative horizons of

Freud's theory well beyond the clinical setting, the lesson that Eissler derives from the limitations of clinical findings acknowledged by him does not go nearly far enough. Thus, he hails the epistemic yield from the use of Freud's method of free association in wanton terms:

I shall be discussing the methodology of psychoanalysis only in terms of the method of free association. This method is one of those glorious inventions that can hold its own with Galileo's telescope... [p. 461]. It is breathtaking to review what Freud extracted, during the course of four decades, from the free associations of eight subjects who each lay on a couch for 50 minutes per day. [p. 465]

Here Eissler depicts the yield of Freud's eight case histories as results that Freud "extracted...from the free associations" of these eight patients. In this depiction, Eissler is undaunted even by Wilhelm Fliess's 1901 challenge that Freud had no safeguard against reading his own thoughts into those distilled from his patients' "free" associations (Freud 1954, letter #145: 334; letter #146: 337).

Similarly, Eissler no less than our present-day psychohistorians is unchastened by the need to provide adequate evidential validation of psychoanalytic principles before their *application* to other fields can be creditable. Unencumbered by such hesitations, Eissler (1969: 461) claims that

if society, science and research were organized in accordance with the principle of maximal investment returns, then an Academy of Man would long since have been founded along the lines indirectly suggested by Freud. It is apparent that all the various branches of the humanities have to be rewritten in accordance with the new knowledge that psychoanalysis has brought to light about man's psychic existence.

In a similarly exuberant vein, Eissler disregards his initial misgiving that "there are many reasons" for concluding that "psychoanalysis as a therapy... does not have a bright future" (p. 462). For nonetheless, he states, "I believe the psychoanalyst of the future may have to devote a large portion of his practice to the repair of the damage that is done in psychotherapy and drug treatment" (p. 463, n. 3). But Eissler gives no hint of how he knows that analysis is generally far less psychonoxious than rival interventions.

In sum, one can only welcome Eissler's refreshing anticipation that the future validation and/or disconfirmation of Freudian theory will come very largely from extraclinical findings. But one may not gloss over the serious epistemological liabilities of intraclinical testing that were set forth in the preceding section. The import of these fundamental drawbacks for the current credibility of psychoanalysis is dismal, for its credentials are avowedly almost entirely *intra*clinical, and hence quite weak. Yet, as we pointed out early in this essay, Freud, Ernest Jones, and a host of other orthodox spokesmen claimed their theory to be well supported precisely on the strength of data from the psychoanalytic interview. So much so that Freud claimed "certainty" for the *clinically* inferred etiology of a patient's affliction, and then relied on that very etiology to: (1) *explain* therapeutic failure (S.E. 1920, 18: 147, 152, 156-157, 164, 168), and (2) justify dismissing the patient's dissent from an etiologic interpretation as unquestionably the result of neurotic resistance, which will be conquered, he says, "by emphasizing the unshakable nature of our convictions" (S.E. 1898, 3: 269).

CAN THE CONSILIENCE OF CLINICAL INDUCTIONS SERVE AS A CHECK ON THE PROBATIVE VALUE OF PATIENT ACCEPTANCE OR REJECTION OF THE ANALYST'S INTERPRETATIONS?

As we saw earlier, Freud explicitly assured the potential falsifiability of his etiology of anxiety neurosis in his 1895 reply to Löwenfeld. To the further detriment of Popper's mythological exegesis, Freud was no less alert to the need for safeguarding the falsifiability of the analyst's interpretations and/or reconstructions of the patient's past. Indeed, this methodological exigency and its implementation is the theme of his very late paper "Constructions in Analysis" (S.E. 1937, 23: 257-269), because it might seem that patient *dissent* from an interpretation could always be *discounted* as inspired by neurotic resistance. Hence, it is Freud's aim to show just how the analyst deals with patient assent and dissent such that "there is no justification for accusing us of invariably twisting his remarks into a confirmation" (S.E. 1937, 23: 262). He had already adumbrated this problem by reference to the etiology of paranoia (S.E. 1915, 14: 265-266).

Freud begins his paper by reporting that "a certain well-known man of science," who treated psychoanalysis fairly at a time when most of the people felt themselves under no such obligation," had nonetheless been "at once derogatory and unjust" on one occasion as follows:

He said that in giving interpretations to a patient we treat him upon the famous principle of "Heads I win, tails you lose" [footnote omitted]. That is to say, if the patient agrees with us, then the interpretation is right, but if he contradicts us, that is only a sign of his resistance, which again shows that we are right. In this way we are always in the right against the poor helpless wretch whom we are analysing, no matter how he may respond to what we put forward. [S.E. 1937, 23: 257]

Yet Freud grants that this charge of nonfalsifiability of analytic interpretations by dissent from the patient needs to be addressed, because "it is in fact true that a 'No' from one of our patients is not as a rule enough to make us abandon an interpretation as incorrect." He therefore proceeds "to give a detailed account of how we are accustomed to arrive at an assessment of the 'Yes' or 'No' of our patients during analytic treatment—of their expression of agreement or of denial" (p. 257). This evaluation is to be carried out as an essential step in the quest for "a picture of the patient's forgotten years that shall be alike trustworthy and in all essential respects complete" (p. 258).

Since the analysand "has to be induced to remember something that has been experienced by him and repressed," the analyst's task of *reconstruction*

resembles to a great extent an archaeologist's excavation of some dwelling-place that has been destroyed and buried or of some ancient edifice. The two processes are in fact identical, except that the analyst works under better conditions and has more material at his command to assist him, since what he is dealing with is not something destroyed but something that is still alive— and perhaps for another reason as well. [p. 259]

In Freud's view, the material at the analyst's disposal that "can have no counterpart in excavations" includes "the repetitions of reactions dating from infancy and all that is indicated by the transference in connection with these repetitions" (p. 259). But this does not exhaust the decided epistemic advantages that the psychic researcher enjoys over the archaeologist:

it must be borne in mind that the excavator is dealing with destroyed objects of which large and important portions have quite certainly been lost. . . . No amount of effort can result in their discovery and lead to their being united with the surviving remains. The one and only course open is that of reconstruction, which for this reason can often reach only a certain degree of probability. But it is different with the psychical object whose early history the analyst is seeking to recover. . . . All of the essentials are preserved; even things that seem completely forgotten are present somehow and somewhere, and have merely been buried and made inaccessible to the subject. Indeed, it may, as we know, be doubted whether any psychical structure can really be the victim of total destruction. It depends only upon analytic technique whether we shall succeed in bringing what is concealed completely to light. [pp. 259-260]

Freud tempers this paean to retrodictability in psychoanalysis only to the following extent:

There are only two other facts that weigh against the extraordinary advantage which is thus enjoyed by the work of analysis: namely, that psychical objects are incomparably more complicated than the excavator's material ones and that we have insufficient knowledge of what we may expect to find, since their finer structure contains so much that is still mysterious. [p. 260]

But this qualification, though sobering, does not go nearly far enough for at least two reasons: (1) on the whole, the physical regularities on which the archaeologist relies to make his retrodictions are incomparably better tested and supported than the etiologies and other hypotheses invoked by the analyst retrodictively to vouchsafe his reconstructions, and (2) the archaeological data secured from the excavated relics are uncontaminated by any epistemic counterpart to suggestion in analysis. Freud's comparison of psychoanalytic and archaeological reconstruction is disappointingly silent in regard to these two major drawbacks to his theory. But in the next section of his paper, just before turning to the central issue of how false constructions allegedly "drop out" in the course of the analysis, he plays down the problem of suggestibility by appealing to the analyst's good character:

The danger of our leading a patient astray by suggestion, by persuading him to accept things which we ourselves believe but which he ought not to, has certainly been enormously exaggerated. An analyst would have had to behave very incorrectly before such a misfortune could overtake him; above all, he would have to blame himself with not allowing his patients to have their say. I can assert without boasting that such an abuse of "suggestion" has never occurred in my practice. [p. 262]

Freud now proceeds to explain (pp. 262-265) that the analyst no more takes a patient's assent to a construction at face value than he accepts without question a dissent from it. He does so in the course of giving two main reasons for contending that "there is no justification for accusing us of invariably twisting his [i.e., the patient's] remarks into a confirmation" (p. 262):

1. Though a patient's verbal assent may indeed result from genuine recognition that the analyst's construction is true, it may alternatively be spurious by springing from neurotic resistance as readily as his dissent. Assent is thus "hypocritical" when it serves "to prolong the concealment of a truth that has not been discovered." The criterion of whether assent is genuine or hypocritical is that there be *inductive consilience* of the patient's verbal assent with new memories as follows: "The 'Yes' has no value unless it is followed by indirect confirmations, unless the patient, immediately after his 'Yes,' produces new memories which complete and extend the construction" (p. 262).

2. Just as assent may be *either* genuine or a mere cover for resistance, so also dissent. Though the analysand's dissent thus "is quite as ambiguous as a 'Yes' " (p. 262), his "No" is of even less face value; for a "No" response may betoken the *incompleteness* of a construction rather than that the patient is actually disputing it. In fact, incompleteness may prompt apparent dissent just as frequently as neurotic resistance does. Therefore, "the only safe interpretation of his 'No' is that it points to incompleteness" (p. 263). It is only "in some rare cases" that avowed dissent "turns out to be the expression of legitimate dissent." Hence, "a patient's 'No' is no evidence of the correctness of a construction, though it is perfectly compatible with it" (p. 263). The criterion of genuineness or legitimacy for dissent, no less than for assent, is that there be *inductive consilience* with other pieces of evidence.

Indeed, as Freud explained, he placed very much greater epistemic reliance on patient responses *other than* verbal assent or dissent as "indirect confirmations" or disconfirmations of analytic constructions. For after concluding that "the direct utterances of the patient after he has been offered a construction afford very little evidence upon the question whether we have been right or wrong," Freud declares that "it is of all the greater interest that there are indirect forms of confirmation which are in every respect trustworthy" (p. 263). As one illustration of these allegedly dependable clinical data, he mentions the patient's having a mental association whose content is similar to that of the construction. Moreover, he claims that such *content*-related associations are good predictors of "whether the construction is likely to be [further] confirmed in the course of the analysis" (p. 264). As a particularly striking example of a further clinical datum that is thus inductively consilient, he recalls a case in which the patient committed a parapraxis as part of a direct denial. Indeed, when a masochistic patient is averse to the analyst's therapeutic efforts, an incorrect construction will not affect his symptoms, but a correct one will produce "an unmistakable aggravation of his symptoms" (p. 265).

Freud sums up by denying any pretense that "an individual construction is anything more than a conjecture which awaits examination, confirmation or rejection," and insisting that the subsequent course of the analysis has epistemic prospects that are decidedly upbeat (p. 265).

It is patent that Freud appealed to a Whewellian consilience of clinical inductions to assess the probative value of the patient's acceptance or rejection of his analyst's interpretations. In particular, he invoked the patient's neurotic resistance to discount the latter's dissent *only* when the analyst had what he took to be consilient support that the interpretation was nonetheless true. Hence, the epistemic conduct of an analyst who follows this recipe for testing his constructions intraclinically can certainly not be accused of simply having immunized them against falsification by the facile device of pleading that the patient is being neurotically resistant.

Nonetheless, I submit that in view of the demise of the Tally Argument, the purported consilience of clinical inductions has the presumption of being *spurious,* and this strong presumption derives from the fact that the *independence* of the inferentially concurring pieces of evidence is grievously jeopardized by a *shared* contaminant: the analyst's influence. For *each* of the *seemingly* independent clinical data may well be more or less alike confounded by the analyst's suggestion so as to conform to his construction, at the cost of their epistemic reliability or probative value. For example, a "confirming" early memory may be compliantly produced by the patient on the heels of giving docile assent to an interpretation. But, more fundamentally, it is precisely in the context of the claimed consilience that the epistemic defects of free association that I have discussed come home to roost; for these liabilities *ingress alike* into *each* of the three major areas of clinical inquiry in which *free association serves to uncover purported repressions*: etiologic clinical investigation of the pathogens of the patient's neurotic symptoms, and the interpretation of his dreams as well as of his parapraxes. By depending alike on free association, the clinical data from these three areas forfeit the independence they require, if their prima facie consilience is to be probatively cogent. Thus, the consilience among the seemingly distinct sets of data is likely to be spurious, or at least cannot justly be claimed genuine. But even if the emergence of repressions were genuinely consilient, it would *not* show that such repressions are pathogenic or are the primogenitors of dreams and slips. This probative failure was one moral of my scrutiny above.

In a very recent article on reconstructions in analysis, the analyst Greenacre (1981) recapitulates Freud's 1937 paper and emphasizes the fundamental epistemic role of free association in effecting psychoanalytic reconstructions. Avowedly, Greenacre wrote her article to help young analysts understand the task of retrieving the patient's past, but she gives no hint of awareness that the problem to which Freud addressed his 1937 paper remains unsolved, if only because of the liabilities of free association. Nor is there any appreciation of the epistemic failings of that paper in Walter Kaufmann's journalistic treatment of Freud's ideas (Kaufmann 1980: 87-88, passim).

According to the so-called "*hermeneutic*" construal of psychoanalysis, a "*scientistic misunderstanding*" vitiated Freud's life-long aspiration that his theory be accorded natural science status (Habermas, 1971: ch. 11; Ricoeur, 1981: ch. 10). Thus, as the hermeneuticians would have it, I have been applying inappropriate standards to the assessment of the credentials of Freud's theory of personality and therapy. In a lengthy introductory chaper of a forthcoming work of mine (1983), I have examined their theses in detail, with the following upshot: All of the pertinent misunderstandings were committed not by Freud, but by the hermeneuticians themselves, who have parlayed their egregiously untutored, primitive notion of the physical sciences into pseudo-constrasts between psychoanalytic explanations and the causal explanations given in the sophisticated natural sciences.

THE ROLE OF CLINICAL "CONFIRMATIONS" IN POPPER'S INDICTMENT OF INDUCTIVISM

Popper ignores that the inductivist legacy of Bacon and Mill gives no methodological sanction to the ubiquitous "confirmations" claimed by some of those Freudians and Adlerians whom he had encountered by 1919 (Grünbaum 1977: sec. 2; 1979a: 134). As he describes these partisans, they "saw confirming instances everywhere: the world was full of *verifications* of the theory. Whatever happened always confirmed it" (Popper 1962: 35). Indeed, Popper claims that, by *inductive* standards, both Freud's and Adler's psychology "were always confirmed" (p. 35). He then adduces this alleged universal confirmation of these theories, *come what may*, to indict both them and the inductivist methodology that purportedly countenances their credibility; for he characterizes them as follows: "It was precisely this fact—that they always fitted, that they were always confirmed—which in the eyes of their admirers constituted the strongest argument in favour of these theories. It began to dawn on me that this apparent strength was in fact their weakness" (p. 35). Having deemed it to be a "fact—that they always fitted, that they were always confirmed," he feels entitled to chide inductivism for probative laxity qua method of scientific theory validation, and to advocate its abandonment as a criterion of demarcation.

That Popper did regard inductivism as probatively promiscuous because he believed the ubiquitous confirmations claimed for psychoanalysis to be sanctioned by it is clear from his account of how he was led to enunciate his new criterion of demarcation in 1919-1920 (p. 36). In that account, he formulates the differences that he sees between his falsifiability criterion and its inductivist predecessor in a manifesto of seven theses, after explaining what considerations led him to them. The first of these theses was: "It is easy to obtain confirmations, or verifications, for nearly every theory—if we look for confirmations"

(p. 36). But the most emphatic of the considerations that avowedly led him to the tenets espoused in his manifesto was the following: whereas Einstein's gravitational theory is falsifiable, Freudian and Adlerian theory are not, *because* "it was practically impossible to describe any human behavior that might not be claimed to be a verification of these theories" (p. 36).

It is ironic that Popper should have pointed to psychoanalytic theory as a prime illustration of his thesis that inductively countenanced confirmations can easily be found for nearly every theory, if we look for them. Being replete with a host of etiological and other causal hypotheses, Freud's theory is challenged by neo-Baconian inductivism to furnish a collation of positive instances from *both* experimental and control groups, if there are to be inductively *supportive* instances. But, as we recall from our earlier discussion of the Rat Man case, if such instances do exist, the retrospective psychoanalytic method would find it extraordinarily difficult, if not impossible, to furnish them. Moreover, to this day, analysts have not furnished the kinds of instances from controlled inquiries that are *inductively required* to lend genuine support to Freud's specific etiologies of the neuroses. Hence, it is precisely Freud's theory that furnishes poignant evidence that Popper has caricatured the inductivist tradition by his thesis of easy inductive confirmability of nearly every theory!

Yet Popper concluded that *because* they are always confirmed, come what may, the two psychological theories "were simply non-testable, irrefutable" (p. 37). Then he hastens to add: "This does not mean that Freud and Adler were not seeing things correctly. . . . But it does mean that those 'clinical observations' which analysts naively believe confirm their theory cannot do this any more than the daily confirmations which astrologers find in their practice" (pp. 37-38). To this last sentence, Popper appends a very important footnote in which he gives his appraisal of the *clinical* confirmations claimed by analysts. Since I now need to scrutinize this appraisal thoroughly, let me cite it *in toto*:

"Clinical observations," like all other observations, are *interpretations in the light of theories* [reference omitted]; and for this reason alone they are apt to seem to support those theories in the light of which they are interpreted. But real support can be obtained only from observations undertaken as tests (by "attempted refutations"); and for this purpose *criteria of refutation* have to be laid down beforehand: it must be agreed which observable situations, if actually observed, mean that the theory is refuted. But what kind of clinical responses would refute to the satisfaction of the analyst not merely a particular analytic diagnosis but psycho-analysis itself? And have such criteria ever been discussed or agreed upon by analysts? Is there not, on the contrary, a whole family of analytic concepts, such as "ambivalence" (I do not suggest that there is no such thing as ambivalence), which would make it difficult, if not impossible, to agree upon such criteria? Moreover, how much headway has been made in investigating the question of the extent to which the (conscious or unconscious) expectations and theories held by the analyst influence the "clinical responses" of the patient? (To say nothing about the conscious attempts to influence the patient by proposing interpretations to him, etc.) Years ago I introduced the term "*Oedipus effect*" to describe the influence of a theory or expectation or prediction *upon the event which it predicts* or describes: it will be remembered that the causal chain leading to Oedipus' parricide was started by the oracle's prediction of this event. This is a characteristic and recurrent theme of such myths, but one which seems to have failed to attract the interest of the analysts, perhaps not accidentally. (The problem of confirmatory dreams suggested by the analyst is discussed by Freud, for example in *Gesammelte Schriften*, III, 1925, where he says on p. 314: "If anybody asserts that most of the dreams which can be utilized in an analysis . . . owe their origin to [the analyst's] suggestion, then no objection can be made from the point of view of analytic theory. Yet there is nothing in this fact," he surprisingly adds, "which would detract from the reliability of our results.") [p. 38, n. 3]

This series of charges prompts me to offer several corresponding comments:

1. Popper asks what sorts of clinical responses would count for Freud as adverse to his general theory. Early in this paper, I itemized a number of episodes of significant theory modification that eloquently attest to Freud's responsiveness to *adverse* clinical and even extraclinical findings. I can now add the lesson that Freud learned from the failure of his Rat Man case to bear out his etiological retrodiction. Furthermore, we need only recall the very theme of Freud's 1937 paper "Constructions in Analysis," namely, just how he assures the intraclinical falsifiability of those clinical reconstructions that are avowedly the epistemic lifeblood of his whole theory! When Popper asks, "what kind of clinical responses would refute to the satisfaction of the analyst . . . psychoanalysis itself?" I ask in return: what is "psychoanalysis itself"? Is it the theory of unconscious motivations, or the psychoanalytic method of investigation? As to the former, Freud stressed its conjectural nature by espousing Poincaré's view that the postulates of the theory are evidentially undetermined free creations of the human mind (S.E. 1914, 14: 77, 117). As to the latter, he stated explicitly that when his seduction etiology of hysteria collapsed, he considered giving up the psychoanalytic method of investigation itself as unreliable (S.E. 1914, 14: 17; 1925, 20: 34).

The bulk of the pertinent textual evidence was available to Popper in the German edition of Freud's collected writings from which he cited in the passage above. Popper's deplorable neglect of this telling evidence has issued in exegetical mythmaking. Indeed, the myth has crept even into elementary textbooks, where it is untutoredly repeated as if it were a matter of well-documented exegesis (Abel 1976: 162). Though its burial is long overdue, I fear that it has become so widespread that its ravages may well continue.

2. Does the psychoanalytic employment of Eugen Bleuler's concept of ambivalence epitomize a family of theoretical notions that make for nonfalsifiability? Here, too, I can refer to an earlier part of this essay where I have argued that this complaint of Popper's boomerangs.

3. Popper characterizes the analyst's suggestive effect on the patient's clinical responses as being a matter of "the influence of a theory or expectation or prediction *upon the event which it predicts* or describes." Then Popper makes the incredibly uninformed and grossly unfair claim that such self-fulfillment of predictions via mechanisms akin to suggestion "seems to have failed to attract the interest of the analysts, perhaps not accidentally." He reports, to boot, that it was he who, years earlier, had recognized the epistemic danger of specious validation by spurious data when he coined the generic term "Oedipus effect." Thus, he chides the Freudians for not having been aware, as he was, of the relevant moral of the Oedipus legend.

As against this, I must point out to begin with that as early as 1888— fourteen years before Popper was even born—Freud gave a sophisticated, incisive account of several kinds of suggestion and of their effects (S.E. 1888, 1: 75-85). In that year, he published a long preface to his German translation of H. Bernheim's book on the therapeutic use of suggestion. There Freud called attention to the *epistemic havoc* that may be wrought in psychiatry by the doctor's suggestive intervention, if one fails to allow for the potential suggestive production of *spurious* symptoms that are *not* characteristic of the syndrome under investigation. Bernheim charged precisely such a failure against J.-M. Charcot's report of a symptom complex called "major hypnotism." Charcot contended that unlike normal hypnotized subjects, *hysterical* patients exhibit *three* stages of hypnosis, each of which is distinguished by highly remarkable characteristic *physical* symptoms. But, as Freud explains, if the symptomatology of hysteria under hypnosis were first *generated* by mere suggestion as charged, then those students of hysteria who thought they were investigating an objective syndrome would have been duped as follows:

All the observations made at the Salpêtrière are worthless; indeed, they become errors in observation. The hypnosis of hysterical patients would have no characteristics of its own. . . . We should not learn from the study of major hypnotism what alterations in excitability succeed one another in the nervous system of hysterical patients in response to certain kinds of intervention; we should merely learn what intentions Charcot suggested (in a manner of which he himself was unconscious) to the subjects of his experiments—a thing entirely irrelevant to our understanding alike of hypnosis and of hysteria.

It is easy to see the further implications of this view and what a convenient explanation it can promise of the symptomatology of hysteria in general. If suggestion by the physician has falsified the phenomena of hysterical hypnosis, it is quite possible that it may also have interfered with the observation of the rest of hysterical symptomatology: it may have laid down laws governing hysterical attacks, paralyses, contractures, etc., which are only connected with the neurosis through suggestion and which consequently lose their validity as soon as another physician in another place makes an examination of hysterical patients.

Here we should have a splendid example of how neglect of the psychical factor of suggestion has misled a great observer into the artificial and false creation of a clinical type as a result of the capriciousness and easy malleability of a neurosis. [S.E. 1888, 1: 77-78]

As Freud notes, Bernheim's stricture of spuriousness against Charcot's major hypnotism will have the salutary effect that "in every future investigation of hysteria and hypnotism the need for excluding the element of suggestion will be more consciously kept in view" (p. 78). But Freud relates that, in this case, the bogus character of the symptomatology had been ruled out by telling evidence that Charcot had gathered; for this evidence shows that "the principal points of the symptomatology of hysteria are safe from the suspicion of having originated from suggestion by a physician" (p. 79).

Thus, even as early as 1888, Freud patently had a sophisticated grasp of the *epistemic* problem of spurious data as posed by the patient's susceptibility to the doctor's influence. Thereafter, in 1901, Freud broke with his longtime close friend Wilhelm Fliess when the latter objected that the psychoanalytic technique of free association was vitiated by its inability to prevent the production of specious findings. And, as we saw, Freud's 1917 Tally Argument was a brilliant effort to come to grips with the full dimensions of the challenge of epistemic contamination by adulterated clinical responses. Freud had remained alert to this challenge in the interim by addressing it in his 1909 case history of Little Hans. Thus, by the time Popper came on the philosophic scene in 1919, Freud's writings had long since resoundingly undercut Popper's accusation that analysts are oblivious to the contamination problem. Thereafter, the writings of such other distinguished analysts as Glover (1931) have continued to undermine it.

Popper compounds his exegetical legerdemain by the slur that the purported obliviousness of the Freudians occurred "perhaps not accidentally," thereby intimating that they are being intellectually evasive if not emotionally unable to face the challenge.

To *justify* a disparaging verdict on Freud's handling of the suggest-ibility problem, Popper ought to have impugned the *empirical* creden-tials of the NCT premise in the Tally Argument, as I have done here. What *is* fair to say, I claim, is the following: Freud unswervingly, brilliantly, but *unsuccessfully tackled* the contamination issue in his "Analytic Therapy" paper, though he failed pathetically for *empirical* reasons rather than for want of methodological sophistication.

4. Popper comments on Freud's explanation of why suggestively induced dream content does not spuriously confirm analytic interpre-tations. Very unfortunately, Popper's citation from Freud borders on a sheer travesty. Popper cites only an excerpt from the pertinent Freud-ian passage in his own translation from the German text in Freud's *Gesammelte Schriften* (1925, vol. 3: 134). The full passage is given in S.E. 1923, 19: 117.

Upon comparing Popper's excerpt to this original German wording, it becomes evident that Popper simply truncated Freud's crucial sen-tence in a highly misleading way *without* any indication of this omis-sion. Freud was responding to the criticism implied by the claim that most of the dreams that are interpreted in the course of an analysis are compliant dreams whose occurrence was induced by the analyst's expectation, and his response was as follows: "Then I only need to refer to the discussion in my 'Introductory Lectures [#28],' where the rela-tion between transference and suggestion is dealt with, and it is shown how little the recognition of the effect of suggestion in our sense detracts from the reliability of our results." Amid expressing surprise, Popper purports to be rendering this sentence in the following words: "Yet there is nothing in this fact [of compliant dreams] which would detract from the reliability of our results."

Thus, in just the initial portion of the sentence, which Popper mysteriously omits, Freud refers to his Tally Argument to contend that the role of suggestion in compliant dreams and analysis generally is *not* epistemically confounding after all. Having given no hint that Freud had *argued* for this conclusion, albeit unsuccessfully, Popper misrepresents him as having offered a mere *ipse dixit*. Thereupon, Popper declares himself puzzled by Freud's allegedly unreasoned assertion. Yet it would strain charity to attribute this weighty omission to the constraints imposed on Popper by writing within the confines of a footnote.

Since Freud's Tally Argument failed and no substitute for it is in sight, Popper is quite right that contamination by suggestion does undermine the probative value of clinical data. But I have argued that insofar as his case against the clinical confirmability of psychoanalysis *is* sound, it does *not* redound to the discredit of inductivism qua method of scientific theory validation. And I have documented that Freud had carefully addressed—albeit unsuccessfully—all of Popper's arguments against clinical validation well before Popper appeared on the philosophic scene.

NOTES

1. Sigmund Freud, "Notes upon a Case of Obsessional Neurosis," in *Standard Edition of the Complete Psychological Works of Sigmund Freud*, trans. J. Strachey et al. (London: Hogarth Press, 1955), vol. 10, pp. 155-318. This paper first appeared in 1909. Hereafter, any references to Freud's writings in English will be to this *Standard Edition* under the initials "S.E.," followed by the year of first appearance, the volume number, and the page(s), unless otherwise specified. Thus, the 1909 paper just cited in full would be cited within the text in abbreviated fashion as follows: S.E. 1909, 10: 155-318.

2. The English translation of the pertinent passage is unfortunately misleading. It renders Freud's German word *Vorkommen*—which means "incidence"—as "onset." The word *onset* is likely to mislead the reader into *misidentifying* a state that is likely to *contain* the underlying *specific* etiologic factor (e.g., coitus interruptus) with a mere "precipitating or releasing cause," which Freud was at pains to distinguish from the "specific cause" (S.E. 1895, 3: 135-136).

BIBLIOGRAPHY

Abel, R. *Man Is the Measure.* New York: Free Press, 1976.

Basch, M. *Doing Psychotherapy.* New York: Basic Books, 1980.

Bernstein, A. E., and Warner, G. M. *An Introduction to Contemporary Psychoanalysis.* New York: Jason Aronson, 1981.

Bird, B. "Notes on Transference: Universal Phenomenon and Hardest Part of Analysis." *Journal of the American Psychoanalytic Association* 20 (1972):267-301.

Blanck, G., and Blanck, R. *Ego Psychology: Theory and Practice.* New York: Columbia University Press, 1974.

Campbell, L. A. "The Role of Suggestion in the Psychoanalytic Therapies." *International Journal of Psychoanalytic Psychotherapy* 7 (1978):1-22.

Clark, R. *Freud: The Man and the Cause.* New York: Random House, 1980.

Colby, K. M. "On the Disagreement Between Freud and Adler." *American Imago* 8 (1951):229-238.

Cooper, A. M., and Michels, R. "An Era of Growth." In *Controversy in Psychiatry,* edited by J. P. Brady and H.K.H. Brodie. Philadelphia: W. B. Saunders, 1978.

Eagle, M. "Psychoanalysis and Modern Psychodynamic Theories." In *Personality and the Behavior Disorders*. Rev. ed., edited by N. S. Endler and J. McV. Hunt. New York: Wiley, forthcoming.

Eissler, K. R. "Irreverent Remarks about the Present and the Future of Psychoanalysis." *International Journal of Psycho-Analysis* 50 (1969):461-471.

——— . "Comments on Penis Envy and Orgasm in Women." *Psychoanalytic Study of the Child* 32 (1977):29-83.

Ellis, A. W. "On the Freudian Theory of Speech Errors." In *Errors in Linguistic Performance: Slips of the Tongue, Ear, Pen, and Hand,* edited by V. A. Fromkin, pp. 123-131. New York: Academic Press, 1980.

Erikson, E. H. "The Dream Specimen of Psychoanalysis." *Journal of the American Psychoanalytic Association* 2 (1954):5-56.

Erwin, E. *Behavior Therapy*. New York: Cambridge University Press, 1978.

Eysenck, H. *Uses and Abuses of Psychology*. Baltimore: Penguin, 1963.

Fancher, R. E. *Psychoanalytic Psychology*. New York: Norton, 1973.

Ferguson, M. "Progress and Theory Change: The Two Analyses of Mr. Z." *Annual of Psychoanalysis* 9 (1981):133-160.

Fisher, S., and Greenberg, R. P. *The Scientific Credibility of Freud's Theory and Therapy*. New York: Basic Books, 1977.

Flax, J. "Psychoanalysis and the Philosophy of Science: Critique or Resistance?" *Journal of Philosophy* 78 (1981):561-569.

Frank, A., and Trunnell, E. E. "Conscious Dream Synthesis as a Method of Learning about Dreaming: A Pedagogic Experiment." *Psychoanalytic Quarterly* 47 (1978):103-112.

Frank, G. H. "The Role of the Family in the Development of Psychopathology." *Psychological Bulletin* 64 (1965):191-205.

Freud, S. *Gesammelte Schriften.* Leipzig: Internationaler Psychoanalytischer Verlag, 1925.

———. *The Origins of Psychoanalysis.* New York: Basic Books, 1954.

Fromkin, V. A., ed. *Errors in Linguistic Performance: Slips of the Tongue, Ear, Pen, and Hand.* New York: Academic Press, 1980.

Fromm, E. *The Crisis of Psychoanalysis.* Greenwich, Conn.: Fawcett Publications, 1970.

Gedo, J. E. "Reflections on Some Current Controversies in Psychoanalysis." *Journal of the American Psychoanalytic Association* 28 (1980):363-383.

Giere, R. N. *Understanding Scientific Reasoning.* New York: Holt, Reinhart & Winston, 1979.

Gill, M. "The Analysis of the Transference: Discourse on the Theory of Therapy." In *Psychoanalytic Explorations of Technique,* edited by H. P. Blum, pp. 263-288. New York: International Universities Press, 1980.

Glover, E. "The Therapeutic Effect of Inexact Interpretation." *International Journal of Psychoanalysis* 12 (1931):397-411.

Glymour, C. "Freud, Kepler and the Clinical Evidence." In *Freud,* edited by R. Wollheim. New York: Anchor Books, 1974. An afterword appeared in the second edition. New York: Cambridge University Press, 1982.

———. *Theory and Evidence.* Princeton, N.J.: Princeton University Press, 1980.

———. "Lectures on Freud." Mimeographed, University of Pittsburgh, n.d.

Goldberg, A., ed. *The Psychology of the Self: A Casebook.* New York: International Universities Press, 1978.

Greenacre, P. "Reconstruction: Its Nature and Therapeutic Value." *Journal of the American Psychoanalytic Association* 29 (1981):27-46.

Grinstein, A. *Sigmund Freud's Dreams.* 2d ed. New York: International Universities Press, 1980.

Grünbaum, A. "Is Falsifiability the Touchstone of Scientific Rationality? Karl Popper Versus Inductivism." In *Essays in Memory of Imre Lakatos.* Boston Studies in the Philosophy of Science, vol. 38, edited by R. S. Cohen, P. K. Feyerabend, and M. W. Wartofsky, pp. 215-229. Dordrecht: D. Reidel, 1976.

――― . "How Scientific is Psychoanalysis?" In *Science and Psychotherapy*, edited by R. Stern, L. Horowitz, and J. Lynes, pp. 219-254. New York: Haven Press, 1977.

――― . "Is Freudian Psychoanalytic Theory Pseudo-Scientific by Karl Popper's Criterion of Demarcation?" *American Philosophical Quarterly* 16 (1979*a*): 131-141.

――― . "Epistemological Liabilities of the Clinical Appraisal of Psychoanalytic Theory." *Psychoanalysis and Contemporary Thought* 2 (1979*b*):451-526.

――― . "Epistemological Liabilities of the Clinical Appraisal of Psychoanalytic Theory." *Noûs* 14 (1980):307-385. (This is an enlarged version of Grünbaum 1979*b*.)

――― . "The Placebo Concept." *Behaviour Research and Therapy* 19 (1981): 157-167.

――― . *The Foundations of Psychoanalysis: A Philosophic Critique.* Berkeley: University of California Press, 1983.

Habermas, J. *Knowledge and Human Interests*. Boston: Beacon Press, 1971.

Hersen, M., and Barlow, D. H. *Single-Case Experimental Designs*. New York: Pergamon Press, 1976.

Hook, S., ed. *Psychoanalysis, Scientific Method and Philosophy*. New York: New York University Press, 1959.

Jones, E. *The Life and Work of Sigmund Freud*, vol. 2. New York: Basic Books, 1955.

――― . *The Life and Work of Sigmund Freud*, vol. 3. New York: Basic Books, 1957.

――― . *Editorial Preface to S. Freud, Collected Papers*, vol. 1. New York: Basic Books, 1959.

Kaplan, A. H. "From Discovery to Validation: A Basic Challenge to Psychoanalysis." *Journal of the American Psychoanalytic Association* 29 (1981):3-26.

Kaufmann, W. *Discovering the Mind*, vol. 3, *Freud Versus Adler and Jung*. New York: McGraw-Hill, 1980.

Kazdin, A. "Drawing Valid Inferences from Case Studies." *Journal of Consulting and Clinical Psychology* 49 (1981):183-192.

——— . "Single-Case Experimental Designs." In *Handbook of Research Methods in Clinical Psychology*, edited by P. C. Kendall and J. N. Butcher. New York: Wiley, forthcoming.

Kohut, H. "Introspection, Empathy, and Psychoanalysis." *Journal of the American Psychoanalytic Association* 7 (1959):459-483.

Kubie, L. S. *Practical and Theoretical Aspects of Psychoanalysis*. 2d ed. New York: International Universities Press, 1975.

Laplanche, J., and Pontalis, J. B. *The Language of Psychoanalysis*. New York: Norton, 1973.

Leo, J. "Cradle-to-Grave Intimacy." *Time* (September 7, 1981):69.

Levine, F. J. "On the Clinical Application of Heinz Kohut's Psychology of the Self: Comments on Some Recently Published Case Studies." *Journal of the Philadelphia Association for Psychoanalysis* 6 (1979):1-19.

Loftus, E. *Memory*. Reading, Mass.: Addison-Wesley, 1980.

Luborsky, L., and Spence, D. P. "Quantitative Research on Psychoanalytic Therapy." In *Handbook of Psychotherapy and Behavior Change*, edited by S. L. Garfield and A. E. Bergin. 2d ed. New York: Wiley, 1978.

MacKinnon, D. W., and Dukes, W. F. "Repression." In *Psychology in the Making*, edited by L. Postman. New York: Knopf, 1964.

Malan, D. H. *Toward the Validation of Dynamic Psychotherapy*. New York: Plenum, 1976.

Marmor, J. "Psychoanalytic Therapy as an Educational Process." In *Psychoanalytic Education*. Science and Psychoanalysis Series, edited by J. Masserman, vol. 5. New York: Grune and Stratton, 1962.

——— . "New Directions in Psychoanalytic Theory and Therapy." In *Modern Psychoanalysis*, edited by J. Marmor. New York: Basic Books, 1968.

——— . "Limitations of Free Association." *Archives of General Psychiatry* 22 (1970):161.

——— . *Psychiatry in Transition, Selected Papers of Judd Marmor*. New York: Brunner/Mazel, 1974.

Martin, M. *Social Science and Philosophical Analysis*. Washington, D.C.: University Press of America, 1978.

Meissner, W. W. *The Paranoid Process*. New York: Jason Aronson, 1978.

Meyers, S. J. "The Bipolar Self." *Journal of the American Psychoanalytic Association* 29 (1981):143-159.

Morse, S. J. "Failed Explanations and Criminal Responsibility: Experts and the Unconscious." *Virginia Law Review* 68 (1982):971-1084.

――――. *The Jurisprudence of Craziness*. New York: Oxford University Press, forthcoming.

Motley, M. T. "Verification of 'Freudian slips' and Semantic Prearticulatory Editing Via Laboratory-induced Spoonerisms." In *Errors in Linguistic Performance: Slips of the Tongue, Ear, Pen, and Hand*, edited by V. A. Fromkin, pp. 133-147. New York: Academic Press, 1980.

Munby, M., and Johnston, D. W. "Agoraphobia: The Long-Term Follow-up of Behavioural Treatment." *British Journal of Psychiatry* 137 (1980):418-427.

Ornstein, P. H., ed. *The Search for the Self: Selected Writings of Heinz Kohut: 1950-1978*. 2 vols. New York: International Universities Press, 1978.

Popper, K. R. *Conjectures and Refutations*. New York: Basic Books, 1962.

――――. "Replies to My Critics." In *The Philosophy of Karl Popper*, edited by P. A. Schilpp, Book 2. LaSalle, Ill.: Open Court, 1974.

Rachman, S. J., and Wilson, G. T. *The Effects of Psychological Therapy*. 2d enlarged ed. New York: Pergamon Press, 1980.

Rhoads, J. M., and Feather, B. W. "Application of Psychodynamics to Behavior Therapy." *American Journal of Psychiatry* 131 (1974):17-20.

Ricoeur, P. *Hermeneutics and the Human Sciences*. New York: Cambridge University Press, 1981.

Roazen, P. *Freud and His Followers*. New York: Knopf, 1975.

Robbins, M. "Current Controversy in Object Relations Theory as Outgrowth of a Schism Between Klein and Fairbairn." *International Journal of Psychoanalysis* 61 (1980):477-492.

Robinson, A. L. "Nuclear Evidence That Neutrinos Have Mass." *Science* 208 (1980):697.

Rosenthal, R. *Experimenter Effects in Behavioral Research*. Enlarged ed. New York: Irvington Publishers, 1976.

Rosenzweig, S. "An Experimental Study of Memory in Relation to the Theory of Repression." *British Journal of Psychology* 24 (1934):247-265.

————. "The Experimental Study of Psychoanalytic Concepts." *Character and Personality* 6 (1937):61-71.

Russell, B. *An Outline of Philosophy*. Cleveland, Ohio: Meridian Books, 1960.

Shapiro, A. K., and Morris, L. A. "The Placebo Effect in Medical and Psychological Therapies. In *Handbook of Psychotherapy and Behavior Change*. 2d ed., edited by S. L. Garfield and A. E. Bergin. New York: Wiley, 1978.

Slater, E., and Roth, M. *Clinical Psychiatry*. 3d ed. London: Baillière Tindall, 1977.

Stannard, D. E. *Shrinking History*. New York: Oxford University Press, 1980.

Sulloway, F. J. *Freud, Biologist of the Mind*. New York: Basic Books, 1979.

Sutherland, N. S. *Breakdown*. New York: Stein and Day, 1977.

Thomä, H. "Psychoanalyse und Suggestion." *Zeitschrift für Psychosomatische Medizin und Psychoanalyse* 23 (1977):35-56.

Timpanaro, S. *The Freudian Slip*. Translated by Kate Soper. Atlantic Highlands, N.J.: Humanities Press, 1976.

Von Eckardt, B. "On Evaluating the Scientific Status of Psychoanalysis." *Journal of Philosophy* 78 (1981):570-572.

Waelder, R. Review of *Psychoanalysis, Scientific Method and Philosophy*, edited by S. Hook. *Journal of the American Psychoanalytic Association* 10 (1962):617-637.

Watkins, J.W.N. "Corroboration and the Problem of Content-Comparison." In *Progress and Rationality in Science*. Boston Studies in the Philosophy of Science, edited by G. Radnitzky and G. Andersson, vol. 58. Boston and Dordrecht: D. Reidel, 1978.

Weitzman, B. "Behavior Therapy and Psychotherapy." *Psychological Review* 74 (1967):300-317.

Winokur, G. "Heredity in the Affective Disorders." In *Depression and Human Existence*, edited by E. J. Anthony and Teresa Benedek. Boston: Little, Brown, 1975.

Wolpe, J. "Behavior Therapy Versus Psychoanalysis." *American Psychologist* 36 (1981):159-164.

A Critical Examination of Motivational Explanation in Psychoanalysis

Morris N. Eagle

CLINICAL THEORY VERSUS METAPSYCHOLOGY: REASONS AND MOTIVES VERSUS CAUSES

Recently, psychoanalytic writers have discovered and appropriated the distinction between motive (or reason) and cause found in certain philosophical writings. In the psychoanalytic literature, this distinction has been made in the service of a parallel one drawn between the clinical theory and the metapsychology. Although the nature of and basis for this latter distinction is not always entirely clear, the general idea is that the clinical theory deals with such matters as intentions, wishes, reasons, and motives, and the metapsychology presumably deals with the mechanisms underlying those phenomena. The general view is that in the clinical theory Freud presumably dealt with the phenomena observed in the actual psychoanalytic situation and concepts closely tied to that situation, and in the metapsychology he attempted to explain these phenomena in what he considered to be the scientifically respectable terms of mechanisms, forces, and energies.[1]

The predominant position in recent discussions is to uphold the value of the clinical theory and to urge the scrapping of the metapsychology (e.g., see Klein 1970; Rycroft 1966; Gill 1976; Schafer 1976, 1978). The rationale for this position varies. Sometimes one reads that the metapsychology should be scrapped because it is unscientific and employs such pseudoscientific concepts as psychic energy and libidinal cathexis. At other times, the argument is that the metapsychology is to be abandoned because its natural science and causal mode of conceptualization and explanation is inappropriate to human action and to a person or agent who wishes, intends, strives, etc. On occasion, both criticisms of metapsychology are presented in a single work without any apparent recognition of some inconsistency (e.g., Schafer 1976).

The proposal to scrap the metapsychology because its concepts and explanations are pseudoscientific in no way entails a rejection of a natural-science mode of explanation for psychoanalysis, nor does it entail an exclusive emphasis on the clinical theory. On the contrary, the very basis for the proposal to scrap the metapsychology is that the concepts and explanations employed are scientifically unsound. This is the position inherent, for example, in Holt's (1967, 1976) criticisms of certain metapsychological concepts (e.g., psychic energy, drive) as unsound because they are inconsistent with current scientific knowledge. But the position that any version of metapsychology is unacceptable because "actions have no causes" (Schafer 1976), or because psychoanalytic explanation must deal only with reasons and motives, is, of course, quite a different matter. It explicitly rejects causal and natural-science modes of inquiry and explanation for human action and explicitly advocates limiting psychoanalytic accounts to what I shall call motivational explanations.

The basis for the distinction between explanation by way of reasons and motives, on the one hand, and causes, on the other, is not universally agreed upon, as is evident from the huge philosophical literature available on the subject. Some have argued for a thoroughgoing distinction between reason and cause explanations (e.g., Abelson 1977; Louch 1966); others have proposed reasons as a subspecies of cause (e.g., Davidson 1963; Goldman 1970; Moore 1978). In either view, however, *some* kind of distinction is made. What is of relevance in this article is the nature of the distinction made in the recent psychoanalytic (and the associated philosophical) literature calling for an autonomous and self-sufficient clinical theory for which motivational explanation will be appropriate and sufficient.

Let me try to make this distinction clear, for the purposes of the ensuing discussions. What I am calling *motivational explanation* is a variety of explanations in terms of the agent's own motives, reasons, intentions, purposes, and aims. I am aware that there are different shades of meanings among terms like *motives, reasons*, and *intentions*, but for the purposes of this article, I am using them interchangeably insofar as they share the common element central to motivational explanations—namely, accounting for an action by reference to the agent's purposes and aims. In addition, my interchangeable use of these terms accurately reflects the state of affairs in much of the recent psychoanalytic literature to which I refer. For example, while Schafer (1976) prefers to talk about reasons (because he believes that the term *motive* implies "a propulsive entity"), others talk about meanings or motives. But what all usages have in common is the emphasis on the agent's purposes or goals in carrying out the behavior. Such accounts emphasize in their explanation "making phenomena teleologically intelligible rather than predictable from knowledge of their efficient causes" (von Wright 1971: 8).

What is described as the causal or the natural-science mode of explanation—and they are often used interchangeably in the literature I am referring to—generally includes some or all of the following characteristics: explanation by reference to physical-chemical, including neurophysiological and biochemical, concepts, processes, and structures; explanation of an event from knowledge of antecedent conditions and relevant laws (Hempel's [1965] deductive-nomological explanation); "objective," external perspective, in which, to borrow Harré and Secord's (1972) description, the person is viewed "as an object responding to the push and pull of forces exerted by the environment" in contrast to "the person acting as agent directing his own behaviour."

It should be clear that I am not suggesting, by referring to "cause" and "causal explanation," that these concepts are simple and unproblematic. We all know that from Hume on, the concept of cause has had a long and complex history. Rather, I am adopting, for the purposes of the ensuing discussion, the definitions generally presented by certain recent philosophical and psychoanalytic writers who contrast motivational and causal explanation.

It will be clear from the following quoted passages that what most of these psychoanalytic and other writers mean by *causal* and *natural-science* mode of explanation is explanation in terms of "purposeless" physical conditions and processes and factors external to the person as agent, in contrast to explanation in terms of meaning, purpose, and intention. (It should be noted that in this view physiological and biochemical processes taking place within the organism are, of course, seen as factors external to the person.)

As noted earlier, some philosophers do not make the motive (or reason)-cause distinction as a distinction between causal and non-causal explanation, but prefer to describe reasons as a variety of cause (e.g., Davidson) or to refer to different kinds of causation (e.g,

Chisholm 1971). But—and this is the critical point—these writers make essentially the kind of distinction I am describing here, namely, explanation from the point of view of the agent's purposes and aims versus explanation from a perspective of impersonal conditions external to the agent. Thus, Davidson (1963) distinguishes between "agent causation" and "event causation," and Chisholm (1971) refers to Broad's (1952) distinction between "occurrent causation," defined as one state of affairs causing another, and "nonoccurrent causation," defined as a person causing a state of affairs.

Even if one prefers to reject altogether the concept of cause as no longer useful and wishes to replace it with the idea of functional relations among variables, the distinction I am describing would, nevertheless, continue to hold. Thus, while the relationship between antecedent (external) conditions and an action can be described in terms of functional relations among independently defined variables, it is not at all clear that the relationship between an agent (or rather, an agent's intention) and his action can be so described (see, e.g., Louch 1966). Whatever the terminology, the central point in the present discussion is the claim that for human action, the only proper mode of explanation is by reference to the agent's intentions, reasons, desires, and motives. This is the philosophical position taken by recent critics of psychoanalytic metapsychology.

Let me present a few passages from some recent psychoanalytic writings that reflect this distinction. Home (1966: 43) writes that "in discovering that the symptom had meaning and basing his treatment on this hypothesis, Freud took the psychoanalytic study of neurosis *out of the world of science* into the world of the humanities, because a meaning is not the product of causes but the creation of a subject." It should be clear that what Home means by a symptom having meaning is that it serves a purpose.

Quite similar to Home, Rycroft (1966:14) argues that "what Freud did...was not to explain the patient's choice causally but to understand it and give it meaning, and the procedure he engaged in was not the scientific one of elucidating causes but the semantic one of making sense of it." (It is clear that by "semantic" Rycroft means giving reasons and motives.)

Gill (1976:72) argues that "metapsychological points of view are posited in a natural-science framework, which is a reductionistic attempt to convert psychological discourse to a universe alien to it— the universe of space, force, and energy."

Finally, here are some passages from Schafer's recent work, which elaborates most fully the position examined in this article:

The terms of Freudian metapsychology are those of natural science.... It is inconsistent with this type of scientific language to speak of intentions, meanings, reasons, or subjective experience. [1976: 103]

In natural science that human being [described earlier as "sentient, self-determining, choice-making, responsible"] must be made into an object of observation, a mechanical or mindless object. [p. 112]

Schafer describes the content of the new action-language he proposes as

a universe of actions... which by definition are meaningful and goal-directed, as actions which have reasons rather than determinants [p. 142]. In this approach, we rely on reasons.... We do not rely on causes — causes that are the conditions regularly antecedent to the actions in question [p. 205]. Actions do not have causes. Although causes of actions, in the sense of their necessary and sufficient conditions, may seem to be ascertainable, this is simply not the case; for within the action system these causes must always be mediated by the person's interpretations, constructions, or understanding of them. [p. 369]

I will not burden the reader with many similar passages from the strictly philosophical literature. One can find discussion of the issue by, among others, Winch (1958); Peters (1950, 1958, 1965); Flew (1949); Mischel (1963); Toulmin (1948); Melden (1961); von Wright (1971); Cheshire (1975); Bernstein (1971); Goldman (1970); Landesman (1965); Davidson (1963); Louch (1966); Passmore (1966); C. Taylor (1964); R. Taylor (1966); Binkley, Bronaugh, and Marras (1971); Abelson (1977). A few illustrative passages from a recent book by Abelson (1977) should suffice:

[First], I shall argue that voluntary human actions of any kind... are not explainable by causes, not insofar as they logically could have causes though in fact they lack them, but in the stronger sense that either to affirm causes of action or to deny causes of action is semantically anomalous, amounting to what Ryle called a 'category mistake' [p. 28]. [Second], the concept of cause (in its natural scientific sense) cannot intelligibly be applied to the explanation of human action. [p. 30]

The broader philosophical distinction between motives (or reasons) and causes, of which the psychoanalytic distinction between the clinical theory and metapsychology is a specific concrete expression, and from which it wittingly or unwittingly draws its intellectual resources, has broadly and variously been characterized as Aristotelian versus Galilean (Lewin 1935), teleological versus causal, or finalistic versus mechanistic (von Wright 1971). Von Wright (1971) has recently discussed these distinctions in terms of the "two traditions," in epistemological and methodological thinking, of understanding and explanation, which, in turn, is broadly related to positivist and antipositivist philosophies of science. Understandably, the former tradition is associated with the natural sciences; the latter traditions grows out of the social sciences' concern with human behavior.

Frequently accompanying the apportioning of the human and inanimate domains to different explanatory systems is a methodological separation in which it is maintained that human phenomena are most appropriately investigated and known through methods of empathy, cognitive identification, intuition, etc., but the usual "objective" methods of the natural sciences are appropriate only to inanimate phenomena (e.g., see Home 1966).

The general idea of a separate explanatory mode and a separate method of investigation and knowing appropriate to man is, of course, not a new one and has found perhaps its fullest expression in the neo-Kantian distinction between historical or human sciences (Dilthey's *Geisteswissenchaften*, Rickert's *Kulturwissenchaften*, and Windelband's *Geschichte*) and natural sciences (*Naturwissenschaften*), and in related distinctions between understanding (*Verstehen*) and explanation (*Erklären*). (See, for example, Dilthey 1961; Hodges 1952; Collingwood, Taylor, and Schiller 1922; Collingwood 1946, for a discussion of the ideas of Dilthey, Rickert, and Windelband.) Indeed, the current distinction between the clinical theory and the metapsychology, and the accompanying apportioning of substantive and methodological domains, is, in certain regards, a most recent expression of this neo-Kantian program. As I have argued in a previous article (Eagle 1977), the call for a unique science of man, however frequently it has been sounded, has always had the quality of an unfulfilled promissory note, and there is no reason to believe that the present version will have a different fate. My own view is that this is so partly because of the failure of advocates of a separate-domain approach to address certain systematic issues, such as reliability and validity, and also because of the inherent limitations of motivational explanations. These are the issues I will discuss in the present article. I will also examine what I believe to be some of the tacit assumptions underlying the distinction between psychoanalytic clinical theory and metapsychology, and the rejection of the latter and espousal of the former. Finally, I will try to evaluate the claim that causal and/or natural-science modes of explanation are inappropriate to human action.

RELIABILITY AND VALIDITY OF MOTIVATIONAL
EXPLANATION IN PSYCHOANALYSIS

One glaring difficulty with the conception of systematic motivational explanation is that the problem of *criteria* for evaluating such explanations is not dealt with. With the exception of Sherwood (1969), in his book *The Logic of Explanation in Psychoanalysis*, I know of no psychoanalytic writer who has addressed systematically the problem of how one determines the adequacy or goodness of a motivational explanation. To a large extent, the fact that psychoanalysis does not simply limit itself to commonsense motivational explanations is what sharpens the problem of criteria for the reliability and validity of such explanations. In ordinary discourse, the agent's answer to the question, "Why did you do that?" is generally accepted as adequate. Thus, in ordinary discourse, the problems of criteria for reliability and validity generally do not arise with such sharpness, or they arise primarily in circumstances where the agent has reason to lie (e.g., he has committed a crime and is attempting to escape punishment), where the actions seem incomprehensible or gratuitous, or where there is a peculiar match between action and stated reason.[2]

The agent's reason is generally taken as *the* reason for the action. But in psychoanalytic explanations, the agent's stated reasons are not necessarily taken as *the* reasons. Rather, unconscious reasons and intentions are invoked and these are necessarily inferred. It is in the issue of how these inferences are to be made that the problems of criteria for reliability and validity arise.

How does one settle disagreements and disputes regarding different or even contradictory motive or reason explanations? How does one go about determining the validity of a motivational explanation? What are the criteria for deciding that a particular motivational explanation is valid or invalid? It seems to me that these simple and basic questions of reliability and validity, and the recognition of their importance, have more to do with science and scientific method than the characteristics often attributed to science by many critics.

One of the arguments used to demonstrate the presumed inappropriateness of the natural-science mode of explanation (and of metapsychology) to phenomena dealt with by psychoanalytic theory is that because the former uses impersonal forces and energies as its basic concepts, it is not suitable to explaining the actions and experiences of a person (e.g., Gill 1976; Schafer 1976). Aside from the question of whether the conclusion follows from the premise, it seems to me that such arguments confuse the content and terms of certain theories in the natural sciences with the *form* of scientific inquiry and testing. Surely, these critics must know of countless perfectly respectable, even elegant, scientific experiments and studies in the area of human perception, for example, which breathe not a word about physical forces and energies. They are considered to be scientific and to constitute a contribution to understanding and knowledge because they reflect systematic respect for such questions as "How do you know?" and "What is the evidence?" and for such considerations as experimental controls, prediction, and presentation of evidence.

To return to the original point — criteria for evaluating a motivational explanation — as noted, most psychoanalytic theorists tend not to concern themselves, in any systematic way, with this issue. Sherwood, who has given extensive thought to this issue, has proposed that one consider the "appropriateness" and "adequacy" as well as the "accuracy" of psychoanalytic accounts. He defines *appropriateness* as essentially concerned with whether the explanation is placed in the proper frame of reference, whether it addresses the specific questions raised, and whether it is formulated at the proper level of complexity. *Adequacy* includes self-consistency, coherence, and comprehensiveness. *Accuracy*, which constitutes a "truth claim," is concerned with whether the explanation yields an accurate "prediction of particular behaviour, past or present." I have tried to show, in a discussion of Sherwood's book (Eagle 1973a), that insofar as appropriateness and adequacy become relevant for evaluating a scientific explanation only after it is clear that the explanation is making a "truth claim," it is accuracy that is the bedrock criterion. But it is precisely on the issue of accuracy and the accompanying issues of prediction and generalization that Sherwood (and other psychoanalytic writers) is ambiguous and unconvincing. Sherwood (1969: 255) does not explain how the psychoanalytic narrative about a particular individual and the general theory are linked, except to say that the former "is independent of the general psychoanalytic theory of human behaviour, in the sense of not being dependent on the truth of it." He also does not make clear whether he believes that the narrative is intended to constitute the empirical base on which the theory is to rest. Finally, Sherwood offers no evidence of systematic efforts to determine the accuracy of even the individual psychoanalytic narrative.

Other psychoanalytic writers have proposed one or another variant of therapeutic effectiveness (e.g., reduction in symptoms) as a criterion for evaluating the validity of psychoanalytic accounts and interpretations. Aside from the fact that there are no systematic studies but only impressionistic accounts involving this criterion, there is an additional serious problem with it. As Sherwood points out, it may be that "truth is not even necessary for therapeutic efficacy" (p. 250). It is entirely possible that some clearly false statements are therapeutically effective. Further, this kind of criterion, however important it may be in a clinical situation, is useless outside that situation where one is interested in evaluating psychoanalytic explanation qua explanation.

Unless one intends to limit psychoanalysis to a therapeutic technique, the issue of evaluating psychoanalytic explanations outside the therapeutic context will be relevant. And even if psychoanalysis were limited to therapeutic technique and (as Schafer [1976, 1978] urges) dropped its claims and aspirations to a general psychological theory of human behavior, there would nevertheless remain *some theory* that guided therapeutic practice. One would, therefore, still confront the issue of criteria for evaluating the formulations comprising such a theory.

Problems similar to those outlined above plus additional ones arise in considering another suggested criterion: the recovery of early memories on the part of the patient. Without independent verification of the accuracy of the memories, which is almost never done, this criterion is useless. Furthermore, a false as well as a true statement can result in the report of early memories. Finally, the problem of suggestibility is ever present. Given the dynamics of the patient-therapist interaction, there is always the possibility, perhaps even likelihood, that patients will comply with the therapist's formulations by "recovering" appropriate memories.

Other criteria have also been proposed, such as how good a gestalt is formed by the explanation (Bernfield 1934; Schmidt 1955) and the empathic, intuitive understanding of the analyst (Home 1966; Baranger and Baranger 1966), but not one such proposal with which I am familiar has grappled seriously with the problem of intersubjective reliability—that is, with the question of what happens when one person's notion of a good gestalt and when one person's conception of empathic, intuitive understanding is radically different from another's.

Finally, Mischel (1963, 1966) has proposed that the agent's own acknowledgment, at least in the long run, is an essential criterion for establishing the validity of explanations in terms of the agent's motives and intentions, even if one is talking about unconscious motives and intentions. I have tried to show in an earlier paper (Eagle 1973) that the agent's acknowledgment cannot serve as a critical criterion. Suffice it to say here that some major problems with this criterion are the following:

(1) it assumes "privileged access" to one's motives, a situation certainly not applicable to unconscious motives; (2) acknowledgment may reflect persuasion and suggestion; (3) acknowledgment may never be forthcoming, as in the case of repressed material that remains repressed, or as in the very obvious case where the person to whom one is attributing unconscious (or, in this case, even conscious) motives is not available to either acknowledge or disavow; and (4) by Mischel's logic, the weakest status an interpretation could have is something like "awaiting acknowledgment" or "not yet confirmed," but never disconfirmed or falsified.

LIMITATIONS OF MOTIVATIONAL EXPLANATION

These problems of reliability and validity are in a sense "external," insofar as they apply equally to all explanatory accounts. In addition to these "external" problems, there are other "internal" ones, that is, problems that relate to the inherent limitations of motivational explanation. It is to this set of issues that I will now direct my discussion.

One of the more important observations about motivational explanations is contained in Black's (1967: 656) comment that "as soon as reasons for action have been provided, an enquiring mind will want to press on to questions about the provenance and etiology of such reasons." I take this comment to imply a number of things: for example, if one forgets for a moment the polemics regarding motive versus cause and looks at a human action only in terms of explaining it as fully as possible, it becomes clear that the fullest and most thorough explanation would include not only a formulation of the person's motives and reasons but a variety of other considerations. Even if one's initial orientation were to understand the motives or reasons for the action, one would want to know about such matters as the origin of these motives and reasons (e.g., Why is he so greedy? How did he come to be that way? What causes people to be greedy?), the external conditions under which the action occurred (e.g., He came upon the money and it was too much for him to resist), and perhaps even the person's neurophysiological condition.

In developing a theory of human behavior, would one ever want to restrict oneself to motive explanations on the polemical ground that causal explanations are not appropriate to human actions? Perhaps in the clinical work of psychoanalysis and other kinds of psychotherapy one might want generally to restrict oneself to the motivational language of wishes and intentions because of an assumed theory of what produces change in therapy and because of a concern with transforming what Schafer (1976) has described as "disclaimed actions" into "claimed actions." That is, because one believes that it is therapeutic for a person to claim and "own" his actions, motives, wishes, intentions, desires, etc., one might want to limit one's formulations and communications to motivational language.[3] But one must not confuse a strategic choice in therapy with a philosophical position regarding appropriate modes of explanation of human behavior. That, it seems to me, is what is being done by those who argue for an exclusively motivational mode of explanation in psychoanalysis. Because psychoanalytic *practice* may restrict itself to such language in no way argues for a similar restriction in a psychoanalytic *theory*, clinical or otherwise, of human behavior. Insisting on such a restriction implicitly defines clinical theory not as a theory about the clinical situation or a theory about psychopathology and its treatment, but as a theory limited to the terms and concepts employed in the clinical situation. Given the understandable and necessary limitations of the strictly clinical language, such insistence is like upholding the virtues of not knowing or understanding too much.

Insistence by certain psychoanalytic writers that one limit explanations of human behavior to the agent's intentions, wishes, wants, beliefs, and aims is not only related to therapeutic considerations but finds support in certain philosophical arguments regarding the relationship between motivational and nonmotivational explanations of human action. The autonomy of motivational explanation is defended on the basis of a number of considerations. Let us consider two basic related arguments. One has been called the irreducibility thesis; the other, the incompatibility thesis.

THE IRREDUCIBILITY AND THE INCOMPATIBILITY THESES

The irreducibility thesis states that action cannot be reduced to bodily movements, because the movements involved in different instances of an action may be indefinitely various. For example, there are an indefinite number of bodily movements that can be involved in carrying out different instances of signing-a-contract action (one can even use one's toes). Since, the argument goes, causal or natural-science explanations can explain only physical movements of the body, and since, as has been shown, human action cannot be reduced to such movements, it follows that action cannot be deterministically explained. At best, causal explanation will apply to one particular instance of an action, but not to action as such. This philosophical position, associated with, among others, Strawson (1963), is most clearly expressed, as far as the psychoanalytic literature is concerned, in the writings of Schafer (1976).

The related incompatibility thesis, stated clearly by C. Taylor (1964), for example, essentially argues that because they are logically incompatible, scientific nonteleological explanation and commonsense teleological explanation of human action cannot *both* be valid. Either one or the other is valid, and further, acceptance of the scientific explanation would radically alter our commonsense conception of action. When these arguments are combined with a claim that accounts of an action given in terms of the agent's reasons, aims, and purposes are adequate explanations, what follows is the presumed autonomy and sufficiency of motivational explanation.

First, I shall attempt a general reply to the incompatibility and irreducibility theses, and then shall offer an additional consideration of these arguments in the context of specific examples of behavior requiring explanation. My focus in the former task will be on the general issue of whether causal explanation is *relevant* to a theory of human behavior; or, to state it in a somewhat different manner, whether motivational explanation alone is sufficient for a full explanation of human action and for an adequate theory of human behavior.

Consider, first, the irreducibility thesis. As Bernstein (1971) tries to show, the philosophical position of what he calls the "new teleologists" can be seen, at least in part, as a historical reaction against a reductionism that tried to reduce action to physical, "colorless movements." They have succeeded in making us aware of categories relevant to intentionality and human action, and the likely nonreducibility of these categories to other simpler ones. But to proceed from the nonreducibility of, let us say, intentionality to the argument that only explanation by way of intentions and reasons is appropriate for human action, is an unwarranted extension. To put the matter simply, that intention is a nonreducible concept does not mean that only intentional concepts are relevant to explaining human action. Similarly, that human action cannot be reduced to physical movements of the body does not mean that action is not caused. For one thing, one can argue, as some do (e.g., Davidson 1963; Goldman 1970), that such things as reasons, wants, and beliefs function as causes of human action. As Goldman points out, those who argue that actions have no causes tend to have in mind a mechanical billiard-ball model of causality and, therefore, exclude the possibility that wants can function as causes of action. (But, as noted earlier, wants as causes are often taken to involve a special kind of causation, a causation very similar to, if not identical with, what is referred to in this article as motivational explanation.)

More pertinently, as will be shown, a full explanation of an action—and by full explanation I mean one that goes beyond the requirements of ordinary discourse—would include not merely an identification but an explanation of the wants, beliefs, aims, intentions, and reasons associated with the action. Any complete theory of human behavior would seek to account not only for overt actions but also for the intentions, etc., that people form. This would especially be true if wants, intentions, and so on are logically rather than contingently connected with actions and determine the definition of action. And it is, of course, evident that an adequate explanation of wants, beliefs, aims, etc.—an account of their "provenance and etiology"—cannot itself be limited to wants, beliefs, etc. An opening to explanation of action in terms of ordinary physical causation is provided by the fact that physical (including, of course, biological) causes play a part in determining the wants and beliefs we come to have as well as in shaping the knowledge we acquire regarding the kinds of actions (means) that will lead to particular ends.

Another argument against the "immunity" of action to causal explanation is similar to one presented by Goldman (1970). Since every specific action is implemented by a specific bodily movement and since bodily movements are caused, it follows that every specific instance of action is caused. Furthermore, since all the actions that could ever be carried out would be carried out in specific bodily movements, it follows that every action that could ever be carried out would have to be caused. What does it mean to say that "action as such" cannot be caused because no action can be reduced to a set of physical movements? To expect "action as such" to be caused is a "category mistake," in Ryle's (1949) sense, insofar as it is an abstraction, and abstract concepts are neither caused nor uncaused; the question simply does not apply. But what *is* caused is every instance of action, and in that sense, actions are caused.

Equally effective arguments can be marshaled against the incompatibility thesis. Let us assume that C. Taylor (1964) is correct in arguing that motivational (in his terms, teleological) and causal (nonteleological) explanations of human action are logically incompatible, or to take Strawson's (1963) version of this position, that the vocabularies for talking about human action and physical movements cannot effectively be correlated. As Taylor himself recognizes, the presumed incompatibility of teleological and nonteleological explanations does not guarantee the validity (or adequacy) of either one. But, Taylor argues, if our behavior could be accounted for by "mechanical theory," our present concept of action would be abandoned. This may or may not be true, but even if it is true, it is, again, no argument for the validity of teleological explanation (a point that Taylor would not dispute). For, as Bernstein (1971: 284) notes, in describing the response to this argument, "despite our strong convictions to the contrary, the most pervasive and basic types of assertions we make about our intentions, actions, reasons, motives are (or may be) *false* [emphasis in original]."

The same argument, it should be noticed, applies to the irreducibility thesis. That motivational accounts embedded in our ordinary discourse are irreducible to the terms of natural science has no bearing on their truth or correctness (Feyerabend 1962). Further, that intentionality and other related concepts play an indispensable role in what Sellars (1963) calls the "manifest image of man" does not mean that they will play a similar role in what he calls the "scientific image of man." It is likely, I believe, that while intentionality has primarily an explanatory role in the former "image," it will represent a phenomenon itself to be explained in the latter "image." That intentionality and the phenomena to which it is relevant will not be ignored or simply reduced away is now more likely because of the real contributions of the "new teleologists." This is all, however, that we can ask of a scientific treatment of man—i.e., that it not limit its explanatory concepts to intentionality.[4]

The incompatibility thesis is essentially a competitive model in which "horizontal" incompatibility is posited. That is, the argument claims that for a given action, a causal, nonteleological explanation and a motivational, teleological explanation cannot both be valid. One must, so to speak, choose one or the other. But, as I will try to show in the examples that follow, even if this "horizontal" incompatibility argument is correct, it is entirely possible that causal and motivational explanations are "vertically" compatible. That is, a full explanation of a given action may involve not only a motivational account of the agent's reasons and motives (and let us assume for the moment that such an account is logically incompatible with an account in terms of physical causes of movement) but also a nonmotivational explanation of the "provenance and etiology" of these reasons and motives. In this sense, even if causal and motivational explanations were competitively or "horizontally" incompatible, they could, nevertheless, be compatible in the sense of both contributing to a full and deep explanation of an action—an action in which motivational and causal accounts can be legitimately intermixed. That is, the validity of this approach is independent of the validity of the "horizontal" incompatibility thesis. It seems to me that those who have been intent on preserving the autonomy of teleological explanation have mistakenly equated the presumed irreducibility of teleological explanation to nonteleological explanation, and the presumed incompatibility between the two, with inapplicability and inappropriateness of the nonteleological.

It should be noted that an argument for the legitimacy of intermixing motivational and causal modes does not necessarily imply equal explanatory efficacy; for it is a feature of the motivational mode that wants, reasons, etc., serve an explanatory function on one level of discourse, but on a "deeper" level become themselves the phenomena to be explained. This is a serious limitation of motivational explanation, and I shall have occasion to return to this point.

SPECIFIC EXAMPLES OF LIMITATIONS OF MOTIVATIONAL EXPLANATIONS

I would now like to consider the issues just raised in the context of dealing with specific examples of behavior. Consider, first, the highly publicized and notorious actions of the criminal who called himself "Son of Sam." He provided a reason for his shooting rampage by telling us that he was ordered to carry out his shooting sprees. Sophisticated as we are, we might consider unconscious motives and reasons such as revenge for feeling jilted and abandoned. Let us even assume that we can cast Son of Sam's actions in the form of a practical syllogism—let us say, something like a desire to avenge and a belief that his shooting sprees would accomplish this end. That is, assume that we have found some reason in this bizarre unreason. But surely such an explanation would be an incomplete one. For would we not want to know how Son of Sam came to harbor such desires and aims, and how he came to believe that shooting randomly selected people would satisfy such aims? Or, if we focus on his explanation that he was ordered to shoot these people, would one not want to understand the etiology and the workings of a mind or cognitive structure in which delusions arise and are expressed in such actions? In short, *whatever his reasons*, one would want to know how Son of Sam came to want to plan and carry out such actions, and how there came to be such a strange match between certain aims and the action designed to carry out these aims.

People who believe that dogs and demons are giving them messages and orders have something wrong with their brains, even if we cannot, at present, be specific about the nature of the dysfunction. Or, if one prefers to remain entirely on a psychological level, people whose reality testing and behavior controls are as grossly disturbed as Son of Sam's have severe ego defects. Such a statement is a *structural* one—a metapsychological one, if you will—and says nothing about motives and reasons. Indeed, I do not see how it is possible to comprehend the oddness of the match between Son of Sam's reason and actions without such structural considerations. Many people have vengeful feelings toward women and society, but they generally do not go on shooting sprees, and that is generally so because most people have better reality testing and ego controls than Son of Sam had. We may hope—and this is an important feature of structural statements—to find increasing points of contact and correspondence between statements about reality testing and ego controls, on the one hand, and biochemical and neurophysiological statements, on the other.

It should be noted that the issue of whether or not Son of Sam's actions are reducible to physical movements, and whether or not reason and motive explanations for these actions are logically compatible with nonteleological causal explanations, has little, if any, bearing on the considerations raised here. For as noted earlier, even if motivational and nonteleological explanations are "horizontally" or competitively incompatible, a full understanding of Son of Sam's peculiar motives and aims, and his peculiar beliefs regarding the appropriate means to accomplish these aims, requires the "vertical" intermixing of motivational and nonmotivational explanations.

It seems difficult to understand why one would want to limit one's account to the incomplete form of motives and reasons and rule out any formulation regarding these kinds of structural considerations. I would also add that I find it difficult to understand why a "natural-science mode," which would attempt to operationalize and refine such concepts as reality testing, ego defects, and ego controls, and which would attempt to find physiological substrates or correlates for such constructs, is tantamount to rendering man a "mindless, mechanical object." After all, inanimate, mindless, and mechanical objects do not test reality and do not have ego controls and ego defects.

Let me provide a few examples that are closer to psychoanalytic formulations. One's reasons or motives for engaging in a variety of what can broadly be called oral behaviors, such as smoking, talking a lot, gum chewing, and teeth clenching, may vary with the specific action and behavior, but they may all be causally related to antecedent conditions of early oral deprivation. Whether the specific formulation is, in fact, correct is irrelevant to my argument. The point is that broad antecedent conditions may underlie specific reasons and motives, and that an elucidation of these conditions and their effects is necessary for an understanding of both the behavior and the reasons and motives for the behavior.

It may well be true that each of the oral behaviors is carried out because of certain specific wants and aims. But only a theoretical formulation explicating the process linking oral deprivation to wants and aims will permit an understanding of the origin and development of these wants and aims, and thereby provide a full explanation for the oral behaviors. Again, this is true independent of the validity of the irreducibility and incompatibility theses.

The second psychoanalytic example is taken from a recent book by Kohut (1977), who describes a case in which basic defects in the structure of the self are attributed, in large part, to the mother's flawed empathy and lack of responsiveness. He also discusses, in regard to this same case, issues of defensive and compensatory structures developed in response to these early traumata and early basic personality defects. Note that Kohut has no difficulty using and linking motivational and causal language. The early traumata and the basic defects they presumably lead to are cast in straightforward causal language, and the development of defensive and compensatory behaviors and structures can, at least in part, be cast in the language of motives.[5]

Let me now describe a *gedanken* experiment that illustrates clearly the incompleteness of motivational explanation in certain instances. Imagine that without one's awareness, an electrode were implanted in an area of the hypothalamus, which when stimulated, is known to be associated with aggression. Imagine that it is possible to stimulate this area by remote control (which, of course, is technically possible to do). Let us further imagine that the individual whose brain is so stimulated experiences anger during these periods of stimulation. My strong prediction is that the stimulated individual would generally find convincing reasons and motives for his experienced anger and whatever actions were associated with it. If he were driving, he might be full of unkind observations about the other "damn drivers." He might complain and explain his anger by referring to how awful the morning coffee tasted. He might not like the way this or that person spoke to him and account for his anger by mentioning this. I believe that something like what I'm describing is an everyday phenomenon. People experience different moods that are likely a function of such factors as hormonal shifts, fatigue, etc. (analogous to the brain stimulation in the hypothetical example), and, if they are somewhat inward looking, find themselves resisting the temptation to explain or find reason for their irritability and the actions linked to such irritability in, let us say, the behavior of their children or spouse.

An actual example, formally similar to the above *gedanken* experiment, is, in fact, available. Some years ago a number of pregnant women were given an androgen-related hormone, synthetic progestin, in order to prevent miscarriage (Money and Ehrhardt 1972). The behavioral and psychological characteristics of the fetally androgenized female offspring were investigated. The basic finding was that these girls tended to show a variety of common characteristics: tomboyism, lack of interest in feminine clothes and in playing with dolls, greater interests in career than in marriage and family, etc. Now, as far as we are concerned here, there is little doubt that each of the girls studied would have offered specific reasons and motives for being interested in athletics, for not playing with dolls, and for not giving marriage and family highest priority; but given the information available, is it not entirely appropriate to look to their intrauterine history in order to explain fully the behavior of these girls, *including* their reason-giving behavior?

In this example, an analysis and explanation, in terms of associated reason and motives, of each of the disparate behaviors studied would, by itself, yield little of interest. What brings order to the apparently disparate and unrelated behaviors, and what makes for an interesting contribution to knowledge and theory of human behavior, is the observation of what, from a certain perspective, constitutes a pattern or class of actions, a pattern or class of preferences, desires and beliefs (related to nonfeminine activity), and a systematic link between these patterns of action, desire, and belief and the earlier antecedent conditions of fetal androgen. Such an analysis, rather than simply matching behavior with reason or motive, reveals something systematic and of theoretical interest that we did not know before—namely, that fetal androgen predisposes girls to certain kinds of activities, desires, and beliefs. Further, such a finding then suggests the next important theoretical step of elucidating the *processes* that link fetal androgen to these activities, desires, and beliefs. It is these sorts of investigatory steps that form the basis for a systematic theory of human behavior.

In these examples, some interesting questions arise regarding the status of the motives and reasons given by the agent. How explanatory are the reasons given by the person undergoing hypothalamic stimulation for, let us say, yelling at someone? And how explanatory are the reasons given by the "fetal androgen girls" for, let us say, not wearing feminine clothes? One could say that the reasons given are rationalizations—that is, they are false—and that the "real" reasons for the behavior are hypothalamic stimulation, in the one case, and fetal androgen, in the other. Note that in this formulation the "real" reasons are nonmotivational, and that, in an important sense, in contrast to the psychoanalytic concept of rationalization, there are no (true) unconscious motives and motivational reasons for the actions in question. According to this formulation, the conscious motives and reasons given by the agent are false justifying and rationalizing constructions that mask not unconscious motives but nonmotivational physical events that are as inaccessible to the agent as unconscious motives.

Even if one accepts, however, the validity of the agent's reasons and motives, one would have to recognize that the factors involved in the "provenance and etiology" of these reasons and motives are unavailable to the agent. Thus, one could accept either anger at something X said or wanting to hurt X as valid reasons for yelling. And one could accept as valid reasons for not wearing feminine clothes, let us say, dislike of such clothes and women's-liberation ideology. But one would have to recognize that anger at what X said and wanting to hurt X, in the one case, and an ideological dislike of feminine clothes, in the other, are themselves linked to and in some way the product of hypothalamic stimulation and fetal androgen, respectively. Certainly, simply knowing the reasons given, even if one accepts them as valid, would not be especially enlightening. Rather, a deep understanding of these behaviors, *including an understanding of the reasons given*, would require that one go beyond the motivational, reason-giving mode of explanation. This would be true independent of the validity of the irreducibility and incompatibility theses, for it is meaningful to speak of causal links between the agents' reasons and such physical events as hypothalamic stimulation and fetal androgen whether or not the actions in question can be reduced to physical movements and whether or not the agents' reasons can be reduced to physiological events or are logically incompatible with such physiological events.

Recent highly informative experimental studies in social psychology give strong empirical support to this view and indicate that the limitations and unreliability of the agent's reasons as explanation for his behavior are not limited to esoteric instances of fetal androgen and hypothalamic stimulation. Rather, they are everyday occurrences. Nisbett and Wilson (1977), in an important and cogent article, review a large number of studies, all of which demonstrate that individuals very frequently cite as reasons for their behavior considerations that can be shown experimentally to have nothing to do with the stimuli that, in fact, did influence their behavior. Indeed, they almost never mention these actual stimuli to account for their behavior. Conversely, they often incorrectly attribute their behavior to stimuli that can be shown not to have influenced their behavior at all. As an example of the former use, although it can be shown that the probability of helpful intervention behavior by a bystander is a function of the number of people present, this factor is never mentioned among the individual's reasons for his behavior. Instead, the subject refers to such considerations as the "victim's" need and the likelihood of his own behavior being helpful. As another example, in one study on clothing preferences, a clear position-effect was observed which showed that individuals have a clear bias for the rightmost items. When, however, subjects were asked for the reasons for their preferences, position was never cited. More rational reasons, such as quality of the item, were given.

As an example of the reverse effect, in one study, subjects viewing a film under conditions of noise and distraction tended to report that their evaluation of the film was negatively influenced by these circumstances. Yet their ratings of the film were almost identical to those of a control group who viewed the film under standard conditions.

Nisbett and Wilson's explanation of these findings is consistent with a profound skepticism toward agents' reasons as adequate explanations of behavior. When, they argue, someone is asked to indicate why they responded as they did, they do so not by introspecting or by "consulting a memory of a mediating process, but by applying or generating causal theories" regarding how a particular response generally occurs, or *is supposed to* occur. These "causal theories" are derived from general models learned in a culture or subculture. For example, because people *believe* that the plight of the victim and the willingness of bystanders to help are good reasons for intervening, and because they believe that the number of others present is not a good reason, they give the former and not the latter (indeed, they reject the idea that the latter was at all a factor when it is suggested) as the reason for their behavior, even though the latter reason was the determining one. Similarly, because women believe that the knit, sheerness, and weave of nylon stockings are attractive characteristics, they offer these factors as reasons for their preference, even though it can be shown that position on the sales table is the determining factor. Finally, and conversely, because people believe that noise and distraction should affect one's reaction to a film, they offer this explanation in accounting for their rating of a film, when, in fact, it did not influence their rating at all.

It should be noted that in these examples, as in the previous ones, *the* best explanations for the behavior in question are not in terms of unconscious motives but in nonmotivational terms of external stimuli (e.g., position of merchandise on a table, number of people witnessing an assault), factors that are discounted by the individual but that are, nevertheless, effective and in terms of cognitive processes to which the individual has no access.[6]

Finally, it should be noted that these examples refute Schafer's (1976: 369) claim that "actions have no causes," because "these causes must always be mediated by the person's interpretations, constructions, or understanding of them." Since, in the examples, there is not necessarily an experienced event to be interpreted by the agent, one cannot say that the effects of hypothalamic stimulation and fetal androgen are mediated by the meaning these events have for the agent. Indeed, in both examples, the physiological factors strongly influence the meanings and interpretations the agent gives to events he confronts. This consideration highlights another weakness of Schafer's argument, one I have already discussed in an earlier context. It is undoubtedly true that the effects of many events we confront in the world are mediated through the meanings and interpretations we give to these events. But surely the story does not end there, for the kind of meaning one gives to an event, whether one interprets it this way or that way, has itself a "provenance and etiology." Hence, as in the earlier discussion of reasons and motives, one would have to say that the complete and adequate account of an action would not simply identify the relevant meanings and interpretations involved, but would probe the history and determination of these meanings and interpretations.

In the examples cited here, is it really true that causal explanation is irrelevant and that only motivational explanation is appropriate to human actions? In all these examples, causal explanations are relevant not only to fully understanding the actions in question but to fully understanding the motives and reasons given for the action. Further, insofar as it makes sense to speak only of the provenance or cause of motives and not of motives for causes, it is clear, contrary arguments notwithstanding, that motivational and causal languages simply do not belong to equally complete and equally efficacious explanatory systems, each with its own universe of relevant phenomena.

Finally, we have seen in these examples that motives and reasons have a dual status—in one context (everyday social interaction), they serve an explanatory function, and in another context, they are themselves the phenomena to be explained. This kind of consideration is undoubtedly what Black had in mind when making his comment about an enquiring mind wanting to know the provenance and etiology of motives.

METAPSYCHOLOGY RECONSIDERED

It seems to me that this dual-status notion is also something of what Freud had in mind when he felt it necessary to formulate a meta-psychological approach. That motives and reasons are themselves phenomena to be explained is what occasioned the need for an explanatory metapsychology—not simply the fact that Freud was influenced by a nineteenth-century conception of science. This conception of science probably influenced the particular content and terms of the meta-psychology—forces and energies, for example—but it did not, I believe, determine the need for the metapsychology itself. Freud looked at behavior, including the reasons people give for their behavior, and speculated about the kinds of processes and mental structures that would generate and make possible such behaviors. Compare this approach to contemporary ones—for example, Chomsky's deep structures, which can generate actual written and spoken sentences; or Harré's (1977) recent ethogenic approach, in which one tries to infer the so-called "template structures" underlying social interactions and the accounts of those interactions given by their participants—i.e, the explanations and justifications participants give for their actions. Note that in Harré's approach "accounts" parallel motive and reasons, and note further that these accounts, which in everyday social interaction serve to explain actions, constitute the data from which underlying structures are inferred. One can see that these contemporary approaches parallel Freud's attempt to infer the processes and structures (which constitute the metapsychology) underlying observable clinical phenomena (behavior and its accompanying reasons and motives).

The general distinction between appearance and underlying reality is at the heart of all theorizing. The particular distinction between reasons given by agents and underlying causes, or more broadly, between varying manifest behavior and more constant underlying realities, has always been of primary interest to theorists of human behavior. For Freud, the underlying realities involve psychic energies and structures and unconscious instinctual impulses and drives. For Marx, whatever reasons individuals may give for their behavior and their view of the world, the underlying determinants involve economic forces and class membership, which, because they shape the nature of our consciousness, necessarily determine the very reasons we give for our behavior. Pareto's (1966) concepts of "residues" and "derivatives" provide an example in sociological theory of an attempt to distinguish between the invariant springs and determinants of human conduct and the variable reasons people give to justify their behavior. For example, while Christian and pagan peoples may offer very different reasons and justifications for behavior, the very similar baptismallike rituals they practice suggest the operation of underlying inarticulate imperatives ("residues"). A very similar point of view, put somewhat differently, is expressed by Durkheim (1951) in his discussion of suicide, for example. Durkheim points out that the best predictors of suicide are such "impersonal" social factors as religious affiliation, family density, and strength and cohesiveness of the social group. Yet, if one looked only at individual accounts of reasons and motives for suicide, these predictive social factors would undoubtedly never appear as relevant: one would not expect an individual to cite these social factors as reasons. Rather, his reasons for suicide will, of course, involve the emotionally meaningful circumstances of his life. But any explanation of suicide that limits itself to individual reasons and does not include the antecedent conditions of religious affiliation, family density, and cohesiveness of group will necessarily be an inadequate explanation.

It has always been more possible for social thinkers to go beyond individual reasons and to look at general underlying determinants precisely because their perspective is social. That is, because they look for collective regularities that go beyond the individual, they are more likely to focus on determinants that are relevant to such regularities—economic forces, class consciousness, "residues," "collective sentiments," etc. By their very nature, these determinants are not accessible to the individual and will not be represented directly in his experiences and in his conscious reasons for behavior. (Of course, as Nisbett and Wilson have shown, even determinants that could be accessible—stimulus characteristics of the immediate situation—are often simply not cited among the reasons given for one's choices, judgments, preferences, etc.) Freud, too, attempted to find underlying regularities and reality behind appearances, not, however, in extraindividual collective determinants but in the intraindividual arena of unconscious psychic forces and in the quasi-biological arena of instinctual drives. But what he shared with Marx, Durkheim, and Pareto was a skepticism toward the reasons and accounts given by individual consciousness and a search for underlying determinants and regularities. And what he shares with contemporary theorists is the orientation that an adequate and theoretical explanation of what is manifest in reality must appeal to processes, structures, and entities that underlie the manifest.

Consider again Harré's ethogenic approach. Although he presents it as a counter to the "normal" science of experimental social psychology and bases his criticisms of the latter on grounds similar to those offered by critics of psychoanalytic metapsychology, Harré never suggests that one should limit one's explanation to the agent's account of his actions. Rather, he takes for granted that these accounts are themselves phenomena to be explained in terms of underlying generating structures. This insight is not achieved by the recent critics of metapsychology.

What also is not achieved by these recent critics is the insight that even explanations on a purely psychological level are not necessarily limited to motives and meanings. For example, certain psychological explanations, those concerned with cognitive models, for example, focus on the logical characteristics of cognitive structures necessary to generate such-and-such behaviors, much as one can describe the logical characteristics of computer programs necessary to generate particular outcomes. Note that in such descriptions nothing need be said of hardware, in the case of computers, or neurophysiology, in the case of human and animal behavior. Hence, such explanations are nonreductionist. Note also, however, that such explanations are not characterized by reference to motives and reasons.

One could argue that I am misrepresenting the position of the critics of metapsychology insofar as they, too, could recognize that agents' accounts are themselves phenomena to be explained, however, not by reference to underlying causal mechanisms or structures but by uncovering unconscious motives and reasons and thus preserving a self-sufficient motivational mode of explanation. In other words, they would argue that when *his* reasons are incomplete, inadequate, or dissimulating, one finds *the* reasons for behavior by identifying the operative unconscious motives.

UNCONSCIOUS MOTIVATION AS EXPLANATION

Aside from the problems of reliability and validity of motivational attributions discussed earlier, there are additional difficulties with the notion that unconscious motives can provide a universal underlying explanation of behavior. First, as indicated in our earlier examples and discussion, certain behaviors are best explained in terms of underlying conditions (e.g., neurophysiological, hormonal, situational, social factors) rather than in terms of reasons and motives. Secondly, certain behaviors are best conceptualized as "intrinsically motivated," "conflict-free," and relatively autonomous and independent of unconscious motives (Hartmann 1958). Thirdly, one must raise the question of the kind of explanation given when one explains behavior in terms atural-science mode (and its concrete metapsychological expression) and an insistence on the autonomy and sufficiency of the motivational mode (and its concrete expression in the clinical theory) is the general philosophical assumption that psychoanalytic, as well as other theories of human behavior, if they are to preserve the personhood and agential nature of human behavior, must limit their explanatory terms to the *agent's point of view*, motives, reasons, and aims (see, for example, Home [1966] and Schafer [1976] for explicit presentations of this view). According to this view, to do otherwise, to employ explanation characteristics of the natural sciences is to render man a "mindless and mechanical object" (Schafer 1976).[9]

The grounds for the insistence on preserving the agent's point of view in explanation often intermix moral and pragmatic arguments. The ethical ground, derived from the Kantian formula that no man must ever become solely a means to an end, is based on the belief that explanations other than those formulated from the agent's point of view render man an object and thus are morally unjustified. The other ground is that because these other modes of explanation are inappropriate to human action, they fail as explanations. According to the former position, however powerful the natural-science mode of explanation might be, its application to human behavior is unethical because it treats man as object and thus violates a moral imperative. The latter position simply argues that the natural-science mode of explanation, when applied to human behavior, is not good explanation. I do not want in this article to evaluate the ethical argument, but I do believe that it is an invalid one. The fact is that nonagentic factors and happenings *do* influence our behavior, and it is neither particularly moral to ignore them nor particularly immoral to recognize them in one's plan, and it is complex and theory. But the issue cannot be fully discussed now; it is complex and merits full discussion. I do merely want to point out in passing that the ethical and pragmatic arguments are often intermixed, and this tends to confuse matters.

The question I have focused on here is whether explanation in terms of unconscious motives is explanation from the agent's point of view. What is central, of course, to unconscious motives and wishes is that they are neither experienced nor acknowledged. In fact, they are most frequently disavowed by the agent to whom they are attributed and therefore, would seem to be an instance where motivational explanations are not from the agent's point of view.

Frequently, when unconscious purposes and aims are inferred/ attributed to the agent by an outside observer to explain something a symptom or a slip of the tongue, the symptoms are experience

---

of unconscious motives. Is such an account always *motivational* in the ordinary sense of motivational explanation (and in the sense in which I am using the idea in this article), where one explains a behavior in terms of agents' desires, aims, and beliefs?[7] That is, do such accounts fit the model of a practical syllogism in which the major premise is that agent A desires Y, the minor premise is that A believes that doing action X will achieve Y, and the conclusion is doing action X?

In order to deal with these issues, I want to consider briefly Freud's principle of psychic determinism, which has been viewed by some as one of the most important foundations and principles of psychoanalytic theory. As Schafer (1976) points out, there is some ambiguity regarding what precisely is meant by psychic determinism. By some, the concept has been interpreted as essentially expanding the domain of scientific determinism of psychic life, and some of Freud's writings support this interpretation. But by that interpretation, the principle of psychic determinism is hardly the original contribution it is often made out to be. For surely, every scientist or scientifically inclined thinker of the late nineteenth and early twentieth century would have implicitly or explicitly taken that position. Other of Freud's writings suggest, however, that what he meant by psychic determinism was the principle that all psychic events—however seemingly trivial, irrational, or "accidental" (such as slips of the tongue or bizarre dream images)—are motivated. That is, psychic determinism is actually motivational determinism (Rubinstein 1967). Here the concept of unconscious motivation is critical, for in order to show that there are no exceptions to the doctrine of psychic determinism, Freud appealed to unconscious motives and meanings. Thus, he tried typically to show, for example, that a seemingly accidental slip of the tongue or non-understandable bizarre dream content could be shown to have an unconscious meaning and motive.

Schafer and others who uphold the primacy of the clinical theory, and who believe in the possibility of a comprehensive psychoanalytic theory that limits itself to motivational accounts, base their belief, to an important degree, on some version of this latter conception of motivational determinism—that is, on the premise that every action, by definition, is intentional, goal directed, and done for a reason.

To say, as Schafer does, that every action has a reason is, by one interpretation, a trivial statement, for it can be understood as a reiteration of general determinism. What Schafer really wants to emphasize is that the acting *agent* has a reason (or a purpose) for every action he carries out—and that, of course, is what makes clear that Schafer's principle of every action having a reason is a version of Freud's motivational determinism. Further, what Schafer does, as the earlier quoted passage shows, is to widen, by definition, the domain of motivational determinism by radically extending what counts as action ("all human activity with a point").

But does explanation in terms of unconscious motives (or reasons) necessarily constitute motivational explanation in any ordinary sense of the term, in which one explains an action by reference to agents' reasons (as well as beliefs and desires)? Consider the classic example in psychoanalytic theory of explanation in terms of unconscious motivation—namely, the account of dreaming and dreams. Freud claimed that the motive force for dreams is wish fulfillment, and he clearly suggested that without the wish there is no dream. Recent research on dreams has revealed enormous information regarding the phenomenon of dreaming. We now know, for example, that we dream every ninety minutes, that all mammals so far studied do dream, and that dreaming is part of a complex neurophysiological system not yet fully understood. In order to stick to the wish-fulfillment theory of dreams, one would have to propose that the strength of infantile wishes somehow surges every ninety minutes and that animals have unacceptable wishes that await the weakening of the censor to appear in dreams.

Freud's problematic use of motivational explanation is particularly reflected in the idea that one dreams in order to preserve sleep. As Moore (1978) convincingly shows, Freud implicitly equates motivational with functional explanation. Thus, it may well be that dreaming protects sleep, but it does not follow from that fact (assuming it is a fact) that the sleeping agent wishes to preserve sleep and dreams in order to achieve that wish (just as it does not follow from the fact that the heart circulates blood that one wishes it to do so, or that its operation depends upon one's wishes).[8]

What about the *content* of dreams? Surely, it will be argued, the content of dreams reflects unconscious wishes and motives, and thus can be said to be motivated. Here we have another problematic use of *motivational*, not only by Freud but also by many contemporary psychoanalytic theorists. Here the implicit equation is between *personally meaningful* and *motivated*. The assumption is that because dreams are personally meaningful and appear to reflect our innermost preoccupations, concerns, and desires, they are motivated. But, of course, the fact that dream contents are made up of our most pressing preoccupations and desires (and let us assume that they are) does not mean that we *wanted* to dream these contents or that these contents were dreamt in order to fulfill certain desires and wishes. It could mean simply that

---

pressing preoccupations and desires continue to infl[ ] perhaps even especially influence thought) in the [ ] point can be brought out with the use of an analogy: ev[ ] we see in Rorschach inkblot cards may reflect our pers[ ] desires, etc., this does not mean that we *wanted* to see the[ ] that they were intended to fulfill certain aims. Indeed, th[ ] which pressing preoccupations influence dream content [ ] content in general) would seem to be best described in a s[ ] ward causal rather than a motivational account. Dreams ar[ ] carrying out of intentions and aims; rather, they are happeni[ ] *reflect* intentions and aims (see Shope 1967, 1970, 1973).

That dreams reflect personal aims and intentions seems to be a[ ] support for the view that they are best understood as motivated [ ] acts carried out by the agent. In support of this position, Sch[ ] (1976:234) cites Freud's (1925) comment that we are responsible for [ ] dreams and takes Freud to mean that we are responsible because "th[ ] dreamer dreamt the dream, i.e., . . . it was his or her action." Whateve[ ] Freud intended, however, there are at least two ways to understand [ ] this way of referring to responsibility. One way, exemplified by Schafer, is to take the position that the agent is responsible for his dreams in the same way that he is responsible for his other actions, including actions with unconscious reasons. Another (and in my view, more meaningful) way is to recognize that although dreams are involuntary happenings, we are nevertheless, in a certain sense, "responsible" for dream contents insofar as they reflect what we are concerned with, preoccupied with, desire, and wish. That is, they reveal the kind of people we are. If being hungry "produced" dreams with food content, one could, in a certain sense, say that we are "responsible" for these contents insofar as they reflect our hunger and preoccupation with food. But one need hardly consider the dream an act in order to assign this kind of "responsibility" or in order to accept the proposition that "the dreamer dreamt the dream."

UNCONSCIOUS MOTIVATION AND THE AGENT'S POINT OF VIEW

What is critical in a motivational account is not simply whether the behavior was purposive (heartbeat and reflexes are purposive) or ordered in a personally meaningful way, but whether the behavior was *intended to achieve a goal or aim set by the agent*. This latter test is particularly important, because often underlying a rejection of the

the agent as purposeless (certainly not his purposes or aims)—as caused happenings rather than intended actions (see Eagle [1977] for a further discussion of this issue). In a certain sense, the agent's point of view in this case is to experience and explain his behavior as an unintended happening, and it is the outside observer's point of view to explain the behavior in terms of purposes and aims.

One can argue that unconscious reasons and motives are still, to use Mischel's (1966) phrase, reasons and motives "in a widened sense"— that is, they remain explanations from the agent's point of view insofar as the agent would acknowledge them if he were fully self-aware, unhindered by repression and other defenses. The basic argument, then, is that explanations in the clinical theory are given in terms of the purposes and aims held by the agent whether or not he is aware of them. What does it mean, however, in the circumstance of disavowal and denial to say that the attributed purposes and aims are, nevertheless, *his* purposes and aims? It could mean that the agent would acknowledge these purposes and aims under such-and-such specifiable conditions, e.g., if repression were lifted. But what if repression were not lifted? Will the attributed purpose and aims continue to be from the agent's point of view?

One could say further that, even if the attributed purposes and aims are not *his*, simply speaking in terms of purposes and aims is speaking in terms of the agent's point of view, because these are the kinds of terms that are only applicable to agents. That is, one could say: "Even if I'm wrong about what specific aims I attribute to X, my account of X's behavior is cast in terms of *his* aims (rather than in terms of external stimulus conditions or neurophysiological factors, for example) and thus is from his point of view."

Characteristic of formulations in psychoanalytic theory dealing with unconscious motives is discussion of aims, wishes, and purposes. Indeed, it is this characteristic that recent critics of metapsychology consider the heart of psychoanalysis and the core of its clinical theory. But, as I have tried to show earlier, simply discussing aims, wishes, and purposes being reflected in behavior does not necessarily mean that one is explaining that behavior from the point of view of what the agent is trying and aiming to do. Thus, also as I have tried to show, an outside observer may explain my dreams causally in terms of my preoccupations and wishes that cause my dream content, rather than in terms of what I am trying to accomplish. (It is a mistake to assume that nonmotivational must preclude the personally meaningful.)

A closer look at how the language of unconscious motives is used in Freudian theory indicates that in the operation of unconscious motives in dreams, parapraxes, etc., there is discussion of impersonal entities (such as wishes) pressing for discharge rather than of persons trying to achieve certain aims. And the formulation that unconscious wishes press for discharge is made not primarily on the inductive basis that this has been observed to be true in all instances of behavior studied, but on the basis of a theoretical-conjectural model regarding the operation of the presumably universal sexual and aggressive instincts. In other words, the very concept of unconscious motives and the principle of universal motivational determinism are linked to a theory of instincts. Thus, when one is certain that one will find unconscious wishes operative in dreams, parapraxes, symptoms, indeed, in all behavior, one is not explaining behavior from the agent's point of view or from the point of view of what the agent is trying to achieve, but rather from the point of view of a theory regarding the agent's biological nature. In this sense, aspects of the Freudian theory of unconscious motivation and of universal psychic (motivational) determinism are misnomers, for we are not really being told that all behavior is motivated (unless "motive" is used in the special sense mentioned by Shope [1973]), but only that all behavior presumably reflects the operation of specieswide instincts. Upon analysis, then, it appears that Freud's psychic determinism really constitutes a claim that all behavior—including behavior such as dreams, parapraxes, and certain symptoms, which were thought to be meaningless—reflects the operation of instinctual wishes constantly pressing for discharge.

To put the above point in a somewhat different manner, Freud may have shown that dreams, parapraxes, and symptoms are ordered and goal directed, but he did not show that these behaviors are actions; for to show that they are actions, he would have had also to show that these behaviors are envisaged by the agent as a means to his goals. As Peters (1965) points out, the very concept of 'wish' implies that a practical or realistic means to the wished-for goal has not really been considered. And the concept of 'unconscious wish' employed by Freud, given its links to instinctual drives and its operation according to primary-process thinking, implies even less the idea of action carried out to achieve particular ends (see Shope 1967, 1970, 1973). The way Freud uses 'unconscious wish,' it is more a statement of our biopsychological nature than a description of motives and reasons for action.[10] By declaring all "behavior with a point" to be action, Schafer has implicitly reduced the criterion of action solely to goal directedness and has ignored the issue of whether the behavior is envisaged by the agent as a means to the goal. By doing so, he essentially obliterates the distinction between secondary and primary process, between carrying out something in reality and fantasy, between plan and wish.

Those like Schafer, who favor Freud's clinical theory and reject his metapsychology, could say that they reject Freudian instinct theory and that when they talk about unconscious wishes, motives, and reasons, they are talking only about a person's disclaimed and disowned desires, aims, wishes and, reasons. But the kinds of wishes, aims, etc., that analysts, including Schafer, focus on as important in their clinical work are not simply determined by the data patients present, but are determined by a psychoanalytic theory about the kinds of wishes and aims people tend to have. More specifically, like other analysts, Schafer maintains that the sexual and aggressive wishes and aims are particularly important in clinical work. Are they judged to be important simply because patients frequently present such wishes and aims, or, at least in part, because of Freudian instinct theory and its postulate regarding the ubiquitousness of sexual and aggressive wishes and aims? Given the opaqueness of behavior with regard to underlying motives, wishes, and aims, particularly unconsciously motivated behavior such as dreams, parapraxes, and symptoms, it would appear that only a theory concerning the aims and wishes all people presumably have would account for the emphasis given to one set of themes rather than another. Surely, for example, the frequency with which unconscious sexual aims are presumed to constitute the latent thoughts underlying manifest dream content is not accounted for by the obvious appearance of such aims in dreams, but rather by a theory of the kinds of aims that are presumably ubiquitous (see Moore 1978, for a further discussion of this issue). In short, a "reject everything but the clinical theory" approach ironically removes some of the very foundation on which clinical work is based.

On the basis of this discussion, we must reject the argument that because unconscious motives are still motives and reasons, even if "in a widened sense" (Mischel 1963, 1966), they operate in the same manner as conscious reasons and motives and meet the requirements that explanations of human behavior be given from the agent's point of view and reflect the agential nature of human behavior.

Indeed, as I have tried to show, some characteristics of unconscious motives—their peremptory and driven quality, for example—described in psychoanalytic theory resemble propelled events and a billiard-ball model of caused happenings more than they resemble actions planned with a particular purpose or aim in mind. Indeed, it is these characteristics that are evoked when patients describe ego-alien

symptoms and actions (e.g., a hand-washing compulsion) as propelled happenings not subject to plan, choice, or desire. As Flew (1956)
points out, the concept of unconscious motives combines characteristics that normally do not go together: intentionality and lack of volition. That is, in psychoanalytic theory, a hallmark of unconsciously
determined behavior is that it is both intentional or at least purposive,
on the one hand, and involuntary, on the other. Normally, we do not
expect these qualities to appear together in human action.

   This paradoxical feature of unconsciously motivated behavior
(including symptomatic behavior) suggests that explanation of behavior in terms of unconscious motives is not explanation from the agent's
point of view in any simple way, if, indeed, it is at all. Thus, many of the
psychoanalytic formulations of presumably typical unconsciously
motivated behavior—dreams, parapraxes, and symptomatic behavior,
for example—are not of a motivational character at all, in the sense of
specifying the agent's desires and beliefs regarding how the behavior
in question fulfills those desires. (That is, they do not constitute a
practical syllogism.) Simply referring to these sorts of behaviors as
disclaimed or disowned actions, as Schafer (1976, 1978) does, is an
arbitrary and purely verbal "solution" of this paradox. It does not
address the critical issue of the differences between these so-called
disclaimed actions and what we normally mean by actions, and
whether these differences disqualify the former from being viewed as
actions in any normal sense of the term.

THE DUALITY OF UNCONSCIOUS MOTIVATION

The above ambiguity, namely, that formulations of unconsciously
motivated behavior appear to be from the agent's point of view and yet
are not so in any simple way (or, to put it another way, the ambiguity of
unconsciously motivated behavior with regard to its proper membership in the realm of the personal) is reflected in the dual nature of
psychoanalytic theory—in Freud's concern with, if you will, meaning
and mechanics, clinical theory and metapsychology. (As far as I am
able to understand him, Ricoeur [1970], of all recent philosophically
oriented commentators on psychoanalytic theory, is most acutely and
abidingly aware of this duality; see also Shope [1973].)

   Attempts to resolve this ambiguity and tension by eliminating or
declaring the illegitimacy of one or the other end of the polarity—
either the "ordinary discourse" clinical theory or the metapsychol-

ogy—ignores a central feature of psychoanalytic theory, namely, its insight into the duality of human behavior. Whether or not he succeeded, whether or not the specific concepts were heuristic and scientifically sound, and whether or not he was reflectively aware of all the ramifications of what he was attempting to do, by employing both a language that represents essentially a refined common sense (the so-called clinical theory) and a metapsychological language of impersonal and imperceptible concepts, Freud was responding to the duality of human behavior and was implicitly attempting to integrate, to use Sellars's (1963) terms once again, the "manifest image" and the "scientific image" of man. Or, to use a formulation recently used by Rubinstein (1976), Freud recognized and struggled with the fact that we are both, according to the perspective one takes, persons and organisms.

The history of theories of human behavior are replete with attempts to exclude one or the other of these perspectives, and I must confess that in a broad historical context, I view much of the current formulations of the "new teleologists" and much of the insistence on the exclusive legitimacy of the clinical theory as the most recent expression of the rejection of the organismic. The real challenge, however, has always been over how to integrate these two perspectives into a unified image of man; or, stated more modestly, over how to enrich one perspective by linking it to the other. As Sellars (1963:40) put it in broad form:

Thus, the conceptual framework of persons is not something that needs to be *reconciled with* the scientific image, but rather something to be *joined* to it. Thus, to complete the scientific image we need to enrich it *not* with more ways of saying what is the case, but with the language of community and individual intentions, so that by construing the actions we intend to do and the circumstances in which we intend to do them in scientific terms, we *directly* relate the world as conceived by scientific inquiry to our purposes and make it *our* world and no longer an alien appendage to the world in which we do our living. We can, of course as matters now stand, realize this direct incorporation of the scientific image into our way of life only in imagination. But to do so, if only in imagination, is to transcend the dualism of the manifest and scientific images of man-of-the-world.

Returning to the specific issue of causal and motivational modes of explanation, the point is that psychoanalytic formulations of unconscious motives often partake of and have features of both modes. If the program of those who want to limit psychoanalysis to what I am calling *motivational explanations* is to exclude causal explanation and include only terms that deal with the agent's reasons, motives, and purposes, they will have to examine closely the conceptual challenges presented by the psychoanalytic notion of unconscious motives. They cannot assume that unconscious reasons and motives are identical to conscious ones, save for the simple difference that one is unaware of them in the former case and aware of them in the latter. As Rubinstein (1976:256) puts it, "With regard to unconscious mental events, the expanded clinical theory, in however general terms it may be phrased, makes use of what we traditionally refer to as metapsychology." He also notes, as I have been arguing above, that discussion of unconscious mental events "straddles two worlds—our everyday human world and the world of natural science" (p. 256). It is ironic, then, that the critics of metapsychology, if they are to be consistent in their rejection of metapsychology, may find that they will have to do without a concept—i.e., unconscious mental events—that is central to clinical psychoanalysis. They will then have to remain entirely with a commonsense psychology of reasons and motives. That is, by removing the sustenance that would come from a body of thought whose perspective is the organismic, they will have resolved the tension and ambiguity in psychoanalytic theory by impoverishing rather than enriching it.

Even if one is concerned only with adequately describing certain clinical phenomena, one must retain a dual perspective. One can observe, for example, certain psychopathological symptoms in which it seems quite clear that the person is subjugated by the symptoms and where consideration of reasons and motives seems at first flush irrelevant. Yet, the appearances and disappearances, the ebb and flow of the intensity of the symptoms, seem so clearly related to particular purposes and aims that it is difficult to resist the conclusion that the symptoms represent, in some respects, purposive quasi action. It is this paradoxical duality that is captured by the concept of unconscious motives and reasons, and is not characteristic of conscious motives and reasons. In any case, advocates of the "clinical theory only" approach cannot assume that explanation by way of unconscious wishes, motives, and reasons in psychoanalytic theory is purely motivational from the agent's point of view in the same sense that explanation by way of conscious motives and reasons is purely motivational.

AGENT AS UNITARY ENTITY

I want to raise one final difficulty in considering explanation in terms of unconscious motives as explanation from the agent's point of view, and here I want to focus on the concept of agent rather than on the issue of motives versus cause. Consider the situation I described earlier: one explains an action by attributing an unconscious motive to an individual, who disavows the attribution; one insists, however, that because it is *his* motive, whether or not he avows it, one's explanation is from the agent's point of view. A strange but, it seems to me, legitimate question to ask in this case is: which part of the agent? That is, what I am suggesting is that for any complex, *or* "component," theory of personality that recognizes conflicting motives—avowed and disavowed—or that recognizes that the heart has reasons the mind knows not of, it is difficult to speak accurately of any single agent from whose point of view one is formulating motives or reasons. This, I believe, is implicitly recognized in Freud's tripartite structural model of personality and in his specific suggestion that repression necessarily involved some splitting of the ego. The simple notion of personhood, or more accurately, of a unitary person or agent is meaningful and possibly unproblematic in most contexts (as seen for example, in the statement, He went to the movies); but if one takes the idea of unconscious motives seriously, I don't believe it is at all a simple matter in the context of formulating motives and reasons for actions, or in the context of speaking of unconscious motives, wishes, and desires. This is a complex issue, and I intend only to bring it up in passing here (for a recent discussion critical of approaches that partition the self, see Thalberg [1977]). I suggest, however, that the concept of agent and person may not be entirely unproblematic and "primitive" even if one takes the purely personal perspective, particularly if that perspective is open to influence by such considerations as the meaning of unconscious conflict, which is among the implications of recent split-brain research (for a discussion of the philosophical implications of this research, see Galin [1974] and Nagel [1971]). This issue however, is complex and should be dealt with in an entirely separate discussion.

CONCLUSION

I want to close this article by returning to and reiterating a central theme. I believe that by limiting itself to a motivational mode of explanation and by disclaiming any links to the natural-science mode, psychoanalysis must renounce any aspirations to a general theory of human behavior. Human behavior simply cannot be adequately explained by such a single mode of explanation, particularly a mode of explanation characterized by inherent problems of reliability and validity, and one that, however useful and necessary in the context of ongoing social interaction (and psychotherapy), is limited in a broader explanatory context. Motivational explanations arise out of, to use Wittgenstein's phrase, our "forms of life," and their main function belongs in that arena. As explanation, they are noncumulative. One does not discover new motives as one discovers a new star or a new physiological process or new facts about perception or memory. One simply "matches," so to speak, already known motives to particular actions.

As noted earlier, motivational accounts represent both explanation for an action and data and phenomena themselves to be explained. It may certainly help our understanding of an action to know the agent's desired aim and his beliefs regarding the kind of action that will achieve these aims. But once we are able to identify these reasons and aims, then begins the theoretical work of addressing such issues as how we come to have the desires we have, how we come to acquire beliefs regarding means/ends relationships, and the nature of the processes not only underlying desires and beliefs but those underlying the *links* between desire and belief, on the one hand, and action, on the other. This is, I believe, the main import of Black's comments regarding "provenance and etiology" of motives, comments that have served as an organizing theme for this article.

One may now get a glimpse of why motivational explanations have such limited theoretical status. By themselves, they tell us nothing about the "provenance and etiology" of motives, reasons, and desires, and they tell us nothing about the *processes* underlying reasons, actions, or the link between reasons and actions. They do not allow us to build a theory that, going beyond the "manifest image" of man, will enable us to understand why and how people do what they do, why and how they come to have the motives, reasons, and desires they do, and the complex relationship between desires and actions.

The noncumulative and theoretical properties of motivational explanations are also important to consider in the context of psychotherapy. One must remember that psychoanalysis is a form of treatment as well as a theory of behavior. It is one thing to argue that psychoanalysis properly belongs to the humanities or is a hermeneutic discipline. But I know of no other hermeneutic discipline or discipline within the humanities that, in one of its guises, claims special province in treating disturbed and troubled people. Given this fact, there is simply no way that psychoanalysis can shrug off problems of accountability—which, after all, is the pragmatic side of reliability and validity—and there is no way, I believe, that psychoanalysis can legitimately and comfortably content itself with the status of a simply hermeneutic endeavor. For, implicitly or explicitly, psychoanalysis claims to be therapeutically effective, and the evaluation of such claims already carries one beyond the motivational mode of inquiry and explanation favored by those conceiving of psychoanalysis as a hermeneutic discipline or as belonging to the humanities. As Grünbaum (1977) points out, the claim to therapeutic efficacy is a causal one, and the evaluation of such claims immediately takes one beyond the modes and methods of the humanities. In this sense, it is analogous to the situation existing outside the therapeutic context: the very acts of probing the "provenance and etiology" of motives and of evaluating the reliability and validity of motive attribution carry one beyond the mode of motivational explanation itself. Only if we fail to carry out these acts of probing and evaluating—an indefensible position, in my view—and, as I have tried to show, only if we restrict ourselves to a commonsense psychology, can we remain within the mode of motivational explanation.

NOTES

1. Freud (1957: 181) wrote that "when we have succeeded in describing a physical process in its dynamic, topographical, and economic aspects, we should speak of it as a *metapsychological* presentation." Interpreted closely, this would mean that a metapsychological presentation would describe a process from the point of view of conflict among forces and structures (i.e., among id impulses, ego reality-testing and ego defense, and superego valuations), distribution of so-called psychic energy, and its place in the unconscious/preconscious/conscious dimension. Stated more broadly, "metapsychology has generally referred to those parts of psychoanalytic theory that are not immediately referrable to the evidence of conscious behaviour, but that employs instead mediating concepts such as 'structure,' 'drive,' 'libido,' and so forth" (Kovel 1978: 25). The parallel between these "mediating concepts" and the imperceptible explanatory entities postulated in the natural sciences should be evident.
2. It can be noted that psychoanalysis is especially concerned with precisely circumstances of this sort. However, the "lying," the incomprehensibility, and the odd relation between stated reason and action occur primarily in relation to oneself rather than to others.
3. The claim that only motivational accounts are therapeutic is a debatable one. I believe there are occasions when causal explanations are therapeutic. It has been argued (by Fingarette [1963], for example) that the provision of a coherent meaning scheme is what is therapeutic about psychoanalytic interpretations. If this is so, the meaning scheme provided by causal explanations can be as therapeutic as that provided by motivational accounts. Indeed, it may well be that the causal type of explanation provided to the patient in behavior therapy is one of the unwitting factors in positive therapeutic effects in this area.
4. I am indebted to Michael Moore for a clarifying discussion of this issue.

5. It is my strong impression that even entirely clinical psychoanalytic explanations of narcissistic personality disorders, schizoid and borderline conditions, and psychosis, influenced by recent developments in ego psychology and object-relations theory, have come to be characterized more and more by a mixture of motivational and causal languages. Generally, these explanations are causal in outlook in accounting for early defects in ego structure or, in the example given, in the structure of the self (defects that are generally attributed to early trauma and/or genetic predispositions), and motivational in accounting for subsequent defensive and compensatory reactions to these early defects.

6. The Nisbett and Wilson (1977) article and the hypothalamic-stimulation and the fetal-androgen examples raise the question of whether one can speak meaningfully of unmotivated action and behavior. In discussing the various functions of "motive terms," Wittgenstein (1967) claimed that motives are often a way of justifying an action and are generated only after one is asked or after one asks oneself to explain an action. If I am interpreting Wittgenstein correctly, he is suggesting that it is quite possible for there to be no motives for certain actions we carry out, and that our strong propensity to find and provide motives for our own and other people's actions springs from our need to justify and rationalize—in the nonpsychoanalytic sense—human actions. The issue of unmotivated behavior also arises in regard to "intrinsically motivated" behavior. As has been pointed out (Hunt 1965), there are a class of behaviors that are carried out not for the purpose of achieving a goal external to the behavior but, so to speak, for their own sake. In these behaviors, the doing, the carrying out of the action, is its own reward and its own motivator. Or, as formulated by Piaget, exercising a capacity is its own reward. Much of play can be characterized in this way. These "intrinsically motivated" behaviors do not easily fit the model of the practical syllogism in which an action A is carried out because of a desire to accomplish goal X and a belief that doing A will accomplish goal X. There is no goal to be accomplished unless one wants to posit some state, such as "pleasure," as a generalized goal for an indefinitely large class of behaviors. Such accounts would hardly constitute sharp and enlightening explanations for specific behaviors. It should also be noted that these behaviors are directed by goals intrinsic to the activity (or, if put another way, these behaviors are rule following). For example, in tennis one hits the ball *in order to* get it across the net and to score points. But the playing of tennis is not necessarily done for the purpose of accomplishing a goal external to the playing of tennis itself. One must not confuse goal directed from an internal or intrinsic perspective with goal directed from the perspective of an external goal. Within psychoanalytic theory, the same issue is dealt with by Hartmann's (1958) formulations to the effect that some behaviors can be relatively "conflict free" and "autonomous" of instinctual drive. This comes very close to saying that certain behaviors are engaged in for their own sake (and not because they gratify or discharge a drive), and, whether acknowledged or not, this notion certainly modifies and perhaps contradicts the Freudian principle that all behavior, either directly or indirectly, serves to gratify instinctual drives. In the present context, the possibility of unmotivated behavior, whether construed as "autonomous" or "intrinsically motivated," further suggests the difficulties with a position that argues for the tenability of a self-sufficient and thoroughgoing motivational account of behavior.

7. Shope (1973) makes a convincing case that Freud used *motive* in a somewhat different and now archaic sense.

8. For a discussion of functional explanation, see Hempel (1965).

9. So there is no misunderstanding, I repeat here a point made earlier. In the context of psychoanalytic psychotherapy, to the extent that one construes one's task to be an extension of the domain of the personal, an obviously strong case can be made for the near exclusive use of a motivational mode. Indeed, Schafer (1976, 1978) makes quite clear that he conceives of his action language as constituting such an extension — from unclaimed to claimed, from disowned to owned actions, from "I can't" to "I won't." If Schafer limited his program to a therapeutic strategy, there might be little quarrel with his treatment of action (or, at least, there would be a different kind of quarrel). But he goes far beyond such limits to a discussion of such broader issues as the nature of action and the proper mode of explanation for action.

10. It can be argued that unconscious motives and wishes, at least in part, operate in the same manner as hypothalamic stimulation and fetal androgen in the earlier examples, namely, by influencing the conscious wants one experiences (see Goldman 1970). It seems to me that this is inherent in Freud's conception of instincts, for however one conceptualizes Freudian instincts, it is likely that they operate via such processes as hypothalamic stimulation and hormonal production.

BIBLIOGRAPHY

Abelson, R. *Persons: A Study in Philosophical Psychology.* London, N.Y.: Macmillan, 1977.

Baranger, M., and Baranger, W. "Insight in the Analytic Situation." In *Psychoanalysis in the Americas*, edited by R. E. Littman. New York: International Universities Press, 1966.

Bernfield, S. "Die Gestalt Theorie." *Imago*, no. 20 (1934).

Bernstein, R. J. *Praxis and Action.* Philadelphia: University of Pennsylvania Press, 1971.

Binkley, R., Bronaugh, R., and Marras, A. *Agent, Action and Reason.* Toronto: University of Toronto Press, 1971.

Black, M. Review of A. R. Louch's *Explanation of Human Action. American Journal of Psychology* 80 (1967):655-656.

Broad, C. D. "Determinism, Indeterminism, and Libertarianism." In *Ethics and the History of Philosophy.* London: Routledge and Kegan Paul, 1952.

Cheshire, N. M. *The Nature of Psychodynamic Interpretation.* New York: Wiley, 1975.

Chisholm, R. "On the Logic of Intentional Action." In *Agent, Action and Reason*, edited by R. Binkley, R. Bronaugh, A. Marras. Toronto: University of Toronto Press, 1971.

Collingwood, R. G. *The Idea of History.* Oxford: Oxford University Press, 1946.

Collingwood, R. G., Taylor, A. E., and Schiller, F.C.S. "Are History and Science Different Kinds of Knowledge?" *Mind* 31 (1922):443-466.

;on, D. "Actions, Reasons and Causes." *Journal of Psychology* 23
):685-700.

W. *Meaning in History,* edited by H. P. Rickman. London: Allen and
n.

m, E. *Suicide: A Study in Sociology,* translated by J. A. Spaulding and G.
on. Glencoe, Ill.: Free Press, 1951.

. "Sherwood on the Logic of Explanation in Psychoanalysis." In
nalysis and Contemporary Science, edited by B. B. Rubinstein. New
acmillan, 1973a.

alidation of Motivational Formulations: Acknowledgement as a
." In *Psychoanalysis and Contemporary Science,* edited by B. B. Rubin-
v York: Macmillan, 1973b.

ne Conceptual Issues in Psychotherapy. In *Science and Psychother-*
, edited by R. Stern, L. S. Horowitz, and J. Lynes. New York:
Haven, 1977.

Feyerabend, P. "Explanation, Reduction, and Empiricism." In *Minnesota Stu-*
dies in the Philosophy of Science, edited by H. Feigl and G. Maxwell. Minneapolis: University of Minnesota Press, 1962

Fingarette, H. *The Self in Transformation.* New York: Basic Books, 1963.

Flew, A. "Psychoanalytic Explanation." *Analysis* 10, 1 (1949). (Also in Mac-
Donald, M., ed. *Philosophy and Analysis.* Oxford: Basil Blackwell, 1954.)

——— . "Motives and the Unconscious." In *The Foundation of Science and the*
Concepts of Psychology and Psychoanalysis. Minnesota Studies in the Philosophy of Science 1, edited by H. Feigl and M. Scriven. Minneapolis: University
of Minnesota Press, 1956.

Freud, S. *The Unconscious.* Standard Edition, vol. 14, London: Hogarth Press,
1957a. (originally published in 1915)

——— . "Some Additional Notes on Dream Interpretation as a Whole." Standard Edition, vol. 19. London: Hogarth Press, 1957b. (originally published in
1925)

Galin, D. "Implications for Psychiatry of Left and Right Cerebral Specializa-
tion. A Neurophysiological Context for UCS Processes." *Archives of General*
Psychiatry 31 (1974):572-583.

Gill, M. "Metapsychology Is Not Psychology." In *Psychology versus Meta-*
psychology: Essays in Memory of George S. Klein, edited by M. M. Gill and P. S.
Holzman. New York: International Universities Press, 1976.

Goldman, A. I. *A Theory of Human Action.* Englewoods Cliffs, N.J.: Prentice-
Hall, 1970.

Grünbaum, A. "How Scientific is Psychoanalysis?" In *Science and Psychother-*
apy, vol. 1, edited by R. Stern, L. J. Horowitz, and J. Lynes. New York: Haven,
1977.

Harré, R. "The Ethnogenic Approach: Theory and Practice." In *Advances in*
Experimental Social Psychology, edited by L. Berkowitz. New York: Academic
Press, 1977.

Harré, R., and Secord, P. F. *The Explanation of Social Behavior.* Oxford: Basil
Blackwell, 1972.

Hartmann, H. *Ego Psychology and the Problem of Adaptation*. New York: International Universities Press, 1958.

Hempel, C. G. *Aspects of Scientific Explanation and Other Essays in the Philosophy of Science*. New York: Free Press, 1965.

Hodges, H. A. *The Philosophy of Wilhelm Dilthey*. London: Routledge and Kegan Paul, 1952.

Holt, R. R. "Beyond Vitalism and Mechanism: Freud's Concept of Psychic Energy." In *Science and Psychoanalysis*, vol. 2, pp. 1-41. New York: Grune and Stratton, 1967.

————. "Drive or Wish? A Reconsideration of the Psychoanalytic Theory of Motivation." In *Psychology versus Metapsychology: Psychoanalytic Essays in Memory of George S. Klein*, edited by M. M. Gill and P. S. Holzman. New York: International Universities Press, 1976.

Home, H. G. "The Concept of Mind." *International Journal of Psychoanalysis* 47 (1966):42-49.

Hunt, J. "Intrinsic Motivation and Its Role in Psychological Development." *Nebraska Symposium on Motivation*, vol. 13, edited by D. Levine. Lincoln: University of Nebraska Press, 1965.

Klein, G. S. "Two Theories or One?" *Menninger Clinic Bulletin* 37 (1970):102-132.

Kohut, H. *The Restoration of the Self*. New York: International Universities Press, 1977.

Kovel, J. "Things and Words." *Psychoanalysis and Contemporary Thought* 1 (1978):21-88.

Landesman, C. "The New Dualism in the Philosophy of Mind." *Review of Metaphysics* 19 (1965):329-345.

Lewin, K. "Aristotelian and Galilean Modes of Thought." In *A Dynamic Theory of Personality: Selected Papers*, translated by D. K. Adams and K. E. Zener. New York: McGraw-Hill, 1935.

Louch, A. R. *Explanation and Human Action*. Oxford: Basil Blackwell, 1966.

Melden, A. I. *Free Action*. New York: Academic Press, 1961.

Mischel, T. "Psychology and Explanations of Human Behaviour." *Philosophical and Phenomenological Research* 23, 4 (1963).

————. "Pragmatic Aspects of Explanation." *Philosophy of Science* 33 (1966): 40-60.

Money, J., and Ehrhardt, A. *Man and Woman, Boy and Girl*. Baltimore, Md.: Johns Hopkins University Press, 1972.

Moore, M. "The Nature of Psychoanalytic Explanation." *Psychoanalysis and Contemporary Thought* 3 (1980):459-543.

Nagel, T. "Brain Bisection and the Unity of Consciousness." *Synthese* 22 (1971):396-413.

Nisbett, R. E., and Wilson, T. D. "Telling More Than We Can Know: Verbal Reports on Mental Processes." *Psychological Review* 84 (1977):231-259.

Passmore, J. *A Hundred Years of Philosophy*. Rev. ed. New York: Basic Books, 1966.

Pareto, V. *Sociological Writings*. Selected and introduced by S. E. Finer. Translated by D. Mirfin. New York: Praeger, 1966.

Peters, R. S. "Cause, Cure and Motive." *Analysis* 10, 5 (1950). (Also in Macdonald, M., *Philosophy and Analysis*. Oxford: Basil Blackwell, 1954.)

———— . *The Concept of Motivation*. London: Routledge and Kegan Paul. New
York: Humanities Press, 1958.

———— . "Emotions, Passivity and the Place of Freud's Theory in Psychology."
In *Scientific Psychology*, edited by B. B. Wolman and E. Nagel. New York: Basic
Books, 1965.

Ricoeur, P. *Freud and Philosophy: An Essay on Interpretation*. Translated by Denis
Savage. New Haven, Conn.: Yale University Press, 1970.

Rubinstein, B. B. "Explanation and Mere Description: A Metascientific Exami-
nation of Certain Aspects of the Psychoanalytic Theory of Motivation." In
Motives and Thought: Essays in Honor of David Rapaport, edited by R. R. Holt.
Psychological Issues Monograph no. 18/19, vol. 5. New York: International
Universities Press, 1967.

———— . "On the Possibility of a Strictly Clinical Psychoanalytic Theory: An
Essay in the Philosophy of Psychoanalysis." In *Psychology versus Meta-
psychology: Essays in Memory of G. S. Klein*, edited by M. M. Gill and P. S.
Holzman. New York: International Universities Press, 1976.

Rycroft, C. "Causes and Meanings." In *Psychoanalysis Observed*, edited by C.
Rycroft. London: Constable, 1966.

Ryle, G. *The Concept of Mind*. New York: Barnes and Noble, 1949.

Schafer, R. *A New Language for Psychoanalysis*. New Haven, Conn.: Yale University Press, 1976.

———— . *Language and Insight: The Sigmund Freud Memorial Lectures 1975-76*.
University College London. New Haven, Conn.: Yale University Press, 1978.

Schmid, F. "The Problem of Scientific Validation in Psychoanalytic Interpretation." *International Journal of Psychoanalysis* 36 (1955):105-113.

Sellars, W. *Science, Perception and Reality*. London: Routledge and Kegan Paul,
1963.

Sherwood, M. *The Logic of Explanation in Psychoanalysis*. New York: Academic
Press, 1969.

Shope, R. "The Psychoanalytic Theories of Wish-Fulfillment and Meaning."
Inquiry 10 (1967):421-438.

———— . "Freud on Conscious and Unconscious Intentions." *Inquiry* 13
(1970):149-159.

———— . "Freud's Concept of Meaning." In *Psychoanalysis and Contemporary
Science*, vol. 2, edited by B. B. Rubinstein. New York: Macmillan, 1973.

Strawson, P. F. "Determinism." In *Freedom and the Will*, edited by D. F. Pears.
New York: St. Martin's Press, 1963.

Taylor, C. *The Explanation of Behavior*. London: Routledge and Kegan Paul; New
York: Humanities Press, 1964.

Taylor, R. *Action and Purpose*. Englewood Cliffs, N. J.: Prentice-Hall, 1966.

Thalberg, I. "Freud's Antinomies of the Self." In *Philosophers on Freud*, edited
by R. Wollheim. New York: Jason Aronson, 1977.

Toulmin, S. "The Logical Status of Psychoanalysis." *Analysis* 9, 2 (1948). (Also in Macdonald, M., ed. *Philosophy and Analysis*. Oxford: Basil Blackwell, 1954.)

Von Wright, G. H. *Explanation and Understanding*. Ithaca, N. Y.: Cornell University Press, 1971.

Winch, P. *The Idea of a Social Science*. London: Routledge and Kegan Paul, 1958.

Wittgenstein, L. *Lectures and Conversations in Aesthetics, Psychology and Religious Belief*. Berkeley and Los Angeles: University of California Press, 1967.

CONTRIBUTORS

Morris Eagle is Professor of Psychology and Chairman of the Department of Psychology at York University (Ontario). He has done clinical work at the Clarke Institute of Psychiatry and in private practice. He has published extensively on the conceptual problems of psychotherapy and on the logic of motivational explanation.

Adolf Grünbaum is Andrew Mellon Professor of Philosophy, Research Professor of Psychiatry and Chairman of the Center for Philosophy of Science at the University of Pittsburgh. He is author of *Philosophical Problems of Space and Time* and other works. He is president of the American Philosophical Association (Eastern Division) and past president of the Philosophy of Science Association.

Larry Laudan is Professor of History and Philosophy of Science at the University of Pittsburgh and Visiting Research Professor in the Science Studies Center at Virginia Polytechnic Institute. He is author of *Progress and Its Problems* and *Science and Hypothesis*.

Joseph Margolis is Professor of Philosophy at Temple University. His recent books include *Persons and Minds*, *Art and Philosophy*, and *Philosophy of Psychology*.

Michael Moore is Robert Kingsley Professor of Law at the University of Southern California Law Center. He has written extensively on legal conceptions of mental illness and on the legal ramifications of unconscious motivation.

Kenneth Schaffner is Professor of History and Philosophy of Science and Director of the Program on the Social and Conceptual Foundations of the Bio-Medical Sciences at the University of Pittsburgh. He is author of *19th-Century Ether Theories* and former general editor of *Philosophy of Science*.

Index

Abel, R., 300

Abelson, R., 312, 315

Action: agent's inadequate account of, 327-330, 334; based on purpose, 312, 313, 314, 321; basic, 50-51, 133, 134-135, 136; belief/desire sets in, 40, 41, 51-52, 53-54; and bodily movement, 134-135, 136, 139; causally explained, 125-141, 315; complex, 50, 51; dreaming as, 50, 53; and effect, 131; and events, 34-35, 52, 130, 134; free, 131-133, 134, 135, 136, 137, 138, 139; function of, 40-41, 136; generated, 134; has no cause, 315, 322-323, 331; individuating, 132-133; intentionality of, 18, 19, 24-25, 28, 71 n. 51, 131-132, 134, 137, 139, 321, 322, 323, 324; and motive, 34-35, 40,41 46, 49-50, 52, 317, 320; physically explained, 134-137; planned, 340, 341; primitive, 134, 135; rational, 40; rationalization of, 11-12, 13-14; responsibility for, 337; theory of, 50-53. *See also* Behavior

Adler, Alfred, 149, 150, 160, 161, 162, 297; psychology of, 152, 153, 154

Agency/agent, 312, 313-314, 319-320; animal, 128; causal/causation, 127-128, 314; effect and, 126, 128; human, 125, 127, 128, 129, 130, 131-132, 133, 139; inadequate account of actions by, 327-330, 334; inanimate, 128-129; model of, 127, 128, 130; point of view of, 337-342, 344-345

Ambivalence, 171-172, 300

Amentia, 55-56

Analyst: as catalyst, 215, 266, 268, 273; influences patient (*see* Suggestion; Transference); interferes in free association, 240-244, 245, 261, 262, 265-267, 296, 301; interpretation by, 21, 174, 175-176, 183-185, 191-192, 240, 265-266, 267, 270, 272, 292-293, 294-297; reconstruction by, 293-294; role of, 146, 187, 292-294; on unconscious motives, 27. *See also* Psychoanalysis

Anderson, J., 86, 87

Anxiety, 157, 207; causes memory lapse, 223-224, 229-230; causes parapraxes, 223-224; dreams, 262, 264; repressed, 223-224; sexual, 236

Anxiety neurosis, 292; acquired, 165, 166, 167; v. depression, 168-169; Freud on, 164-168, 169, 209-211, 212; as hereditary, 165, 166; v. neurasthe-

Designer: UC Press Staff
Compositor: Trigraph Inc.
Printer: Thomson-Shore
Binder: Thomson-Shore
Text: Palatino
Display: Palatino